FUNCTIONAL CHEMISTRY OF THE BRAIN

Monographs in Modern Neurobiology
edited by Walter B. Essman

PSYCHOPHARMACOLOGY
An Introduction to Experimental and Clinical Principles
Luigi Valzelli

NEUROCHEMISTRY OF CEREBRAL ELECTROSHOCK
Walter B. Essman

CURRENT BIOCHEMICAL APPROACHES TO LEARNING AND MEMORY
Edited by Walter B. Essman and Shinshu Nakajima

FUNCTIONAL CHEMISTRY OF THE BRAIN
Adrian Dunn and Stephen C. Bondy

FUNCTIONAL CHEMISTRY OF THE BRAIN

Adrian J. Dunn

Department of Neuroscience
University of Florida College of Medicine
Gainesville, Florida

and

Stephen C. Bondy

Department of Neurology
University of Colorado Medical Center
Denver, Colorado

S P Books, Division of
SPECTRUM PUBLICATIONS, INC.
Flushing, New York

Distributed by Halsted Press
A Division of John Wiley & Sons
New York   Toronto   London   Sydney

Copyright © 1974 by Spectrum Publications, Inc.

All rights reserved. No part of this book may be reproduced in any form, by photostat, microform, retrieval system, or any other means without prior written permission of the copyright holder or his licensee,

SPECTRUM PUBLICATIONS, INC.
86-19 Sancho Street, Holliswood, N.Y. 11423

Distributed solely by the Halsted Press division of John Wiley & Sons, Inc., New York

Library of Congress Cataloging in Publication Data

Dunn, Adrian.
   Functional chemistry of the brain.

   (Monographs in modern neurobiology)
   Includes bibliographies.
   1. Brain chemistry. I. Bondy, Stephen C., joint author. II. Title. [DNLM: 1. Brain – Physiology. 2. Brain chemistry. WL300 D923f]
QP376.D86   612'.822   74-16049
ISBN 0-470-22695-1

To Glenda
and Joan
and Julian
and Sharon

Preface

The essence of neurobiology is the integration of a spectrum of information from many different disciplines. It is not adequate to have the specialized viewpoint of a physiologist, biochemist, anatomist, neurologist or psychologist; a more holistic approach is needed in order to conduct meaningful research. In general, the brain should ultimately be studied in relation to its output in the form of behavior.

This book attempts to review concisely the present status of brain biochemistry. It is intended to be comprehensive, but not excessively detailed. While the book is primarily intended for students of biochemistry unfamiliar with the brain and students of the brain unfamiliar with its biochemistry, we believe that it will be of use to neuroscientists of all disciplines. Cerebral chemistry is the main concern of this book, but it is basically a tool with which to approach the understanding of brain function. Thus, we have attempted to show the significance of the chemstry to the brain as a whole. Chapters are arranged to relate the chemistry to structural and functional features, rather than to deal with chemical classes. Nevertheless, advocates of the classical approach will find all classes represented.

During ontogenesis the germ cells of cerebral tissue become differentiated, developing distinctive morphology and anatomical relationships. This process is parallelled by considerable chemical specialization involving the appearance of many different substances. Features that are specific to nerve tissue are the most likely to be directly and intimately concerned in nerve function. For this reason we have tended to stress those chemicals that are found solely in mature nervous tissue or are present there in unusual concentrations. We have also been concerned, especially in later chapters, with biochemical reactions that seem to respond to nervous system function.

A special note on the use of references. In a book of this scope it would obviously be very difficult to supply exhaustive references. We have tried instead to cite references sparingly, but such that any source can be retrieved. We have tried where possible to reference the most recent and comprehensive reviews from which the source references may be obtained. Where reviews do not exist, we have normally chosen to cite the most recent of a series of papers, from which earlier references may be obtained. In addition to the specific references cited at the end of each chapter, we strongly recommend as general neurochemistry references:

Handbook of Neurochemistry in eight volumes (edited by A. Lajtha), Plenum Press, New York, 1969-1972.

Biochemistry and the Central Nervous System, 4th edition. H. McIlwain and H. S. Bachelard, Churchill-Livingstone, London, 1971. (Obtainable in the U.S.A. from Williams and Wilkins, Baltimore.)

Basic Neurochemistry (edited by R. W. Albers, G. J. Siegel, R. Katzman and B. W. Agranoff), Little, Brown and Company, Boston, 1972.

Adrian J. Dunn
Gainesville, Florida

and

Stephen C. Bondy
Denver, Colorado
November 1974

Acknowledgements

We wish to express our sincere gratitude to the large number of people who contributed in one way or another to this book. In particular we thank Dr. Rainer Foelix for the electronmicrographs; Mrs. Ann Jennings for drawing most of the figures; Professors James H. Austin, J. Logan Irvin, Frederick A. King and John E. Wilson who encouraged us; the army of colleagues who read, criticized and added to the text; and our publisher, Spectrum Publications. We are also exceedingly grateful for the many friends who tolerated us during the year or so of writing and who still regard us as friends.

CONTENTS

Preface — vii

I. Anatomical Features of the Brain — 1

   A. The Privileged Relationship of the Brain to the Body — 2
      i) The Blood Supply
      ii) The Cerebrospinal Fluid
   B. Cells of the Brain — 5
      i) Neurons
      ii) Neuroglia
         Summary of glial function
      iii) Separation of Cell Types
   C. Chemical Analysis of Cerebral Anatomy — 17
   References — 21

II. The Basic Biochemistry of the Brain — 23

   A. The Generation and Use of Energy — 23
   B. The Nutritional Requirement — 30
   C. Chemicals of Special Significance for the Brain — 32
      i) Amino Acids
         Glutamate
         Glutamine
         Aspartate
         N-acetylaspartate
         Gamma-aminobutyrate
         Taurine and cystathionine
         N-acetylhistidine
         Urea
      ii) Peptides
         Glutathione
         Other peptides
      iii) Nucleotides
         Cyclic nucleotides
   D. Metabolic Compartmentation — 47
   References — 49

III. Genetic Expression in the Brain — 51

   A. Genome to Protein — 51
      i) Nuclei
      ii) Deoxyribonucleic Acid, DNA

      iii) Chromosomal Proteins
      iv) Ribonucleic Acid, RNA
      v) Mitochondria
      vi) Ribosomes
      vii) Protein Synthesis
      viii) Brain Proteins
      ix) Protein Catabolism

  B. Regulation   62
      i) Degeneration and Regeneration of Neurons, and Chromatolysis
      ii) Enzyme Induction

  C. Genetic Approaches to Brain Function   65

References   67

IV. Neuronal Processes   71

  A. Axons and Dendrites   71
  B. Neuronal Conduction   73
      i) Mechanism
      ii) Models
      iii) The Sodium Pump
  C. The Structure of Membranes   78
  D. Membrane Molecules   81
      i) Fatty Acids
      ii) Phospholipids
      iii) Sphingolipids
      iv) Gangliosides
      v) Cholesterol
      vi) Glycoproteins
  E. The Myelin Sheath   97
  F. Axoplasmic Transport   102
      i) Molecules Transported
        Neurotransmitters
        Proteins
        Glycoproteins, glycolipids and phospholipids
        RNA
      ii) Mechanism
      iii) Transneuronal and Retrograde Transport

References   110

V. The Synapse   113

  A. Chemical Neurotransmission   113
  B. Synaptosomes   121

C. Neurotransmitters	123
Criteria for the establishment of a chemical substance as neurotransmitter at a particular junction	
i) Acetylcholine	
Acetylcholine receptors	
Membrane effects	
Assay of acetylcholine	
ii) Catecholamines	
Synthesis	
Storage and release	
Receptors	
Catabolism	
Assay of catecholamines	
iii) Serotonin	
Assay of serotonin	
iv) Glutamate	
v) Gamma-aminobutyrate (GABA)	
vi) Glycine	
vii) Histamine	
viii) Other Neurotransmitters	
ix) Turnover of Neurotransmitters	
D. Synaptic Components Other than Neurotransmitters	147
i) Gangliosides	
ii) Proteins	
iii) Glycoproteins	
E. Synaptic Modification	150
References	151
VI. Cell-Cell Interaction	155
A. The Development of Nerve Connections—Neurotropism	156
B. Effects of Nerve on Innervated Tissues—Neurotrophism	158
i) Effects of Nerve on Muscle	
C. Effects Between Neurons and Cells That They Do Not Innervate	164
i) Neuronal-Glial Interaction	
ii) Neurosecretion	
D. Prostaglandins	172
References	174
VII. The Biochemistry of Neural Stimulation	177
A. Electrical Stimulation of Nervous Tissue	177
i) Energy Metabolites and Convulsions	
ii) Neurotransmitters	
iii) RNA	

   iv) Protein
   v) Cyclic Nucleotides
   vi) Inositol Phosphatides
 B. Sensory Deprivation and Stimulation   190
   i) Short-term Studies
   ii) Long-term Studies
References   193

VIII. The Biochemical Basis of Behavior   197

 A. Experimental Approaches   200
 B. Learning and Memory   201
   i) Agents That Affect Learning
   ii) Biochemical Correlates of Learning
    RNA
    Protein
    Glycoproteins, glycolipids and phosphoproteins
    Neurotransmitters
   iii) Memory Transfer
 C. Environmental Enrichment   218
 D. Affective Disorders and Schizophrenia   219
 E. Sleep   221
 References   224

IX. Development of the Brain   229

   Early development
   The middle stage of development
   Later development
 A. Genetic Factors   231
 B. Humoral Factors   233
 C. Impulse-related Factors   236
 References   237

Appendix   239

 Glossary   241
 Abbreviations   249
 Actions of Commonly Used Drugs   253

Index   263

FUNCTIONAL CHEMISTRY OF THE BRAIN

I. Anatomical Features of the Brain

Recently, the traditional view of the relationship between the brain and the body has been revised. Originally, the brain was considered to control the functions of the body, with little humoral feedback. The brain took from the blood those substances it needed and ignored those it did not, maintaining itself in a homeostatic state insensitive to fluctuation in plasma composition. It has now become apparent that the brain does indeed respond metabolically to activities of the body and to substances in the blood. The relationship between the brain and the body is the product of numerous complex interactions that can no longer be regarded as one-sided. Nevertheless, the view of the brain as a nurtured organ with sophisticated protective mechanisms is still valid.

The structure of the brain and the way in which the brain operates reflect the properties of its underlying chemical constituents. Thus information concerning molecular events within the brain can be important for understanding its complex mechanisms. In this first chapter we shall briefly outline the major structural features of the brain, as well as the cells of which it is composed, and indicate the ways in which its chemistry can be studied. This will form the groundwork for the subsequent chapters, in which the chemistry will be examined in relation to particular structural and functional features of the brain and the nervous system.

A. THE PRIVILEGED RELATIONSHIP OF THE BRAIN TO THE BODY

The brain is the most protected organ in the body and is heavily shielded from physical or chemical stress. The anterior position and fragile nature of brain substance make it peculiarly vulnerable to physical damage. Especially important is its very limited capacity for regeneration following damage. Also, cerebral function depends on the maintenance of the fine structure of the brain and the precision of its connections. Thus the brain is almost totally surrounded by a bony exoskeleton — the skull. A disadvantage of this exoskeleton is that it is more difficult to accommodate tissue growth within a rigid structure than on the surface of an interior supporting structure. During embryogenesis, the brain grows early in relation to the rest of the body. Even at eighteen months of age, the head circumference of the human infant has already reached about 87 percent of its final adult size. This disproportionately early growth is necessary because later on, after the fontanelles close and partial fusion of the cranial sutures occurs, no major expansion will be possible.

The brain is further protected by being suspended in a liquid medium — the cerebrospinal fluid. As a floating organ it is able to move within the skull to a limited degree and therefore can recoil following a blow to the head.

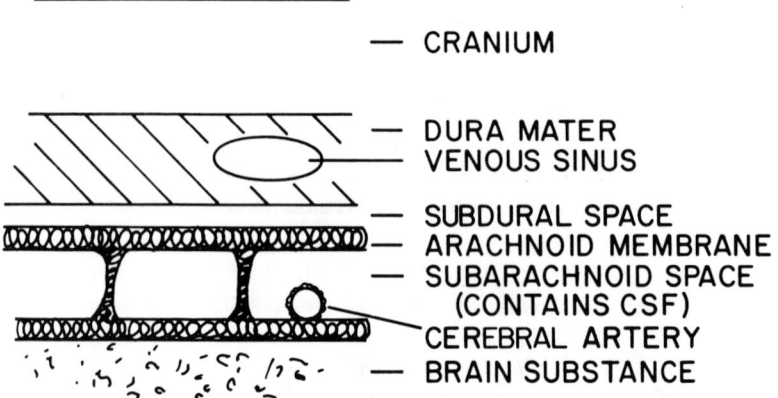

Figure 1.1 Diagrammatic cross-section of the surface of the brain showing the arrangement of covering membranes and vessels.

Within the skull, three membranes enclose the brain: the outer dura mater, the arachnoid and the inner pia mater (Figure 1.1). Major blood vessels supplying the brain course between the dura and the arachnoid in the arachnoid space.

i) The blood supply

The cerebral vascular system exhibits several distinctive features that relate to the requirement of the brain for a continuous high nutrient supply and to the need to maintain a constant chemical environment. Short periods of glucose deprivation or anoxia that can easily be survived by other tissues cause profound effects on the brain and can rapidly and irreversibly damage it. Cerebral tissue contains very low reserves of dissolved oxygen which fall to an insufficient level less than a second after occlusion of a vessel.[13] Since the capacity for anaerobic metabolism is limited, cutting off the blood supply to the human brain causes loss of consciousness in six seconds.

The blood enters the brain by way of a ring of blood vessels at its base — the circle of Willis. The arrangement is such that following the occlusion of a major cerebral artery, anastomotic connections can be made permitting regional cerebral circulation to be maintained relatively unimpaired. Because the diameter of cerebral arterioles may vary, the rate of blood flow through brain tissue can be modified. This regulation is largely effected by the local concentration of vasodilatory chemicals such as CO_2 (see p. 24). There is, however, some control of cerebral blood flow by autonomic nerves (sympathetic and parasympathetic) within the walls of blood vessels. The supply of blood to the brain is less susceptible to general physiological state than that of muscle or visceral organs. In contrast to most other tissues, the brain's energy requirement remains at a constant high level, largely irrespective of the degree of functional activity.

Dyes such as trypan blue injected into the bloodstream permeate all regions of the body except the central nervous system.[1] This observation suggested the existence of a permeability barrier between the blood and the brain. When the trypan blue was injected into the cerebrospinal fluid, it had complete access to the brain; this suggested that the barrier existed specifically between the blood and the brain and was not a property of brain tissue itself. Later, studies of the incorporation of intravenously injected radioactive glutamic acid or radioactive phosphate showed that much less radioactivity was incorporated into the proteins and nucleic acids of the brain than into such macromolecules in other tissues. These results appeared to confirm the concept of the brain as a chemically stable organ, a concept formed by early researchers who found that the bulk of cerebral lipids were renewed rather infrequently. However, consideration of the trypan blue results suggested that an important factor may have been the limited access of the radioactive precursors to the brain. When the precursors were injected intracerebrally, very much higher rates of incorporation were observed. These results suggested the existence of a functional *blood-brain barrier*.[1] The barrier is now known to be highly selective: while some substances may pass freely between the blood and the brain, the passage of many others is severely hindered. The selective nature of the barrier suggests that the capillaries of the mature brain may have a restricted permeability. Brain capillaries are never in direct contact with neurons, but are largely surrounded by astroglial processes which intervene as a buffer. Thus the blood-brain barrier may reflect the sum of the permeability properties of the capillaries, the astroglia and the neurons.

The blood-brain barrier is absent from very young animals and appears relatively late in the developing nervous system. It provides another mechanism for the protection of the brain, in this case from fluctuations in the composition of the plasma and from toxic substances that it may contain. The barrier isolates not only the brain from the bloodstream, but also the body from the brain. During maturation it prevents contact between the proteins of brain tissue and the antibody-forming system. This means that if cerebral proteins leak into the plasma they may not be recognized by the immune system as "self." Proteins regarded as "foreign" could induce the formation of antibodies to themselves. The potential of some cerebral proteins and perhaps lipids to be antigenic in this manner may account for the underlying mechanism of certain autoimmune diseases such as allergic encephalomyelitis (p. 100).

ii) The Cerebrospinal Fluid (CSF)[2]

As mentioned above, trypan blue and other such dyes injected into the CSF have complete access to the brain, so that the CSF may be regarded as being on the brain side of the blood-brain barrier. CSF has a composition distinct from that of lymph or plasma, although it is produced from plasma in the highly vascular choroid plexus which lines the ventricles.[3] Serum contains 60 mg protein per ml, while CSF contains only 0.35 mg protein per ml. Serum proteins are absent from the CSF and its ionic composition is similar to that of plasma but contains less K^+ and Ca^{2+}. However, it should not be assumed that the cells of the choroid plexus merely filter out the protein from the blood, since certain ions such as sulfate, iodide and thiocyanate readily penetrate the brain tissue from the blood but do not appear in CSF. The production of CSF involves the active transport of Na^+ from the cells of the choroid plexus into the ventricular space. Inhibitors of

Na^+ transport (such as ouabain) or of carbonic anhydrase (such as acetazolamide) severely decrease the production of CSF. The effects of the two inhibitors are non-additive, indicating that they affect the same process. The HCO_3^- diffuses out to balance the charge on the Na^+ and is then split into CO_2 and water by carbonic anhydrase. Thus a gradient of HCO_3^- is formed across the membrane. Osmotic pressure then causes the passive diffusion of water into the CSF. The continuous production of CSF is paralleled by an equivalent drainage which takes place at the arachnoid villi on the surface of the brain.[2] The rapid circulation of CSF (it has a half-life of three hours in man) suggests that its role is not merely one of physically cushioning the brain, but that it also functions in maintaining the stable chemical environment required by the brain. In addition to preventing many substances from passing from the blood to the CSF, the choroid plexus actively transports many chemicals from the CSF to the blood. This makes possible the rapid elimination from the CSF of toxic chemicals such as thiocyanate.[3]

The blood-brain barrier may break down in pathological conditions such as multiple sclerosis, neurosyphilis or necrosis following a cerebral infarction. In such cases plasma proteins (such as γ-globulin) or enzymes normally contained within nerve tissues (such as lactic dehydrogenase) may be present in the CSF. The protein and enzyme composition of CSF is often used as a diagnostic test for several cerebral disorders.[4]

The privileged status of cerebral tissue is also reflected in a variety of other ways. The supply of nutrients to the brain is given high priority: in undernourished young animals brain development is less impaired than bodily growth; under starvation conditions, large weight losses occur from muscle tissue and visceral organs, but the weight of the brain and its protein content fall by only about 2 percent.[5] This implies that the mechanisms for the supply of materials to the brain are favored. A good example of such a mechanism is the cerebral uptake of glucose. All tissues actively take up glucose from the bloodstream. In several tissues such as muscle, insulin can increase this uptake. However, insulin has only a minor effect on cerebral glucose uptake which operates at a continuously high rate. Plasma insulin is depressed under hypoglycemic conditions, which reduces the glucose uptake of most tissues and thus allows the brain to take up an increased proportion of the glucose available in the blood.

B. CELLS OF THE BRAIN

The brain contains two specialized cell types, neurons and neuroglia (glia), each of which can further be divided into distinct varieties.

i) Neurons

Although no two neurons are identical, all neurons have several fundamental characteristics. Morphologically, the most striking features of the neuron are its very long processes and its high degree of subcellular differentiation.[6] A schematic diagram of a neuron is shown in Figure 1.2. Many processes arise from the cell body of the neuron. One process, the *axon,* originates from a morphologically distinct area, the *axon hillock,* and is different from the other processes, the *dendrites,* in many ways. The axon is generally longer and straighter than the dendrites and terminates upon the cell which the neuron innervates. This may be the dendritic or perikaryal region of another neuron, or it may be a muscle fiber or other target cell. The junction between the cells is known as a *synapse.* Electrical impulses arise within the axon hillock and travel distally along the axon to the presynaptic area, where they may result in the release of stored neurotransmitter.

There may be many dendritic processes which are often fine and ramify in such an extensive and complex manner that normally the bulk of neuronal processes are dendritic. The dendritic tree varies considerably in size and form and may be extensively branched (Figure 1.3). A more detailed description of axons and dendrites and their differences appears in Chapter 4 (p. 71).

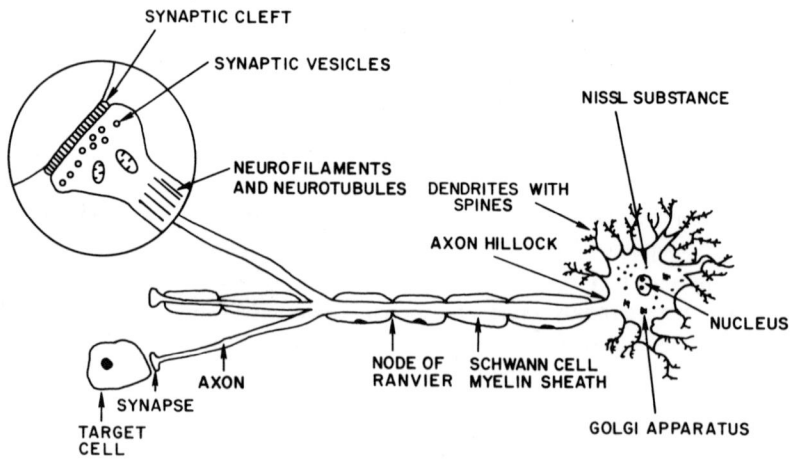

Figure 1.2 Schematic representation of a neuron, showing the interrelationships of its components.

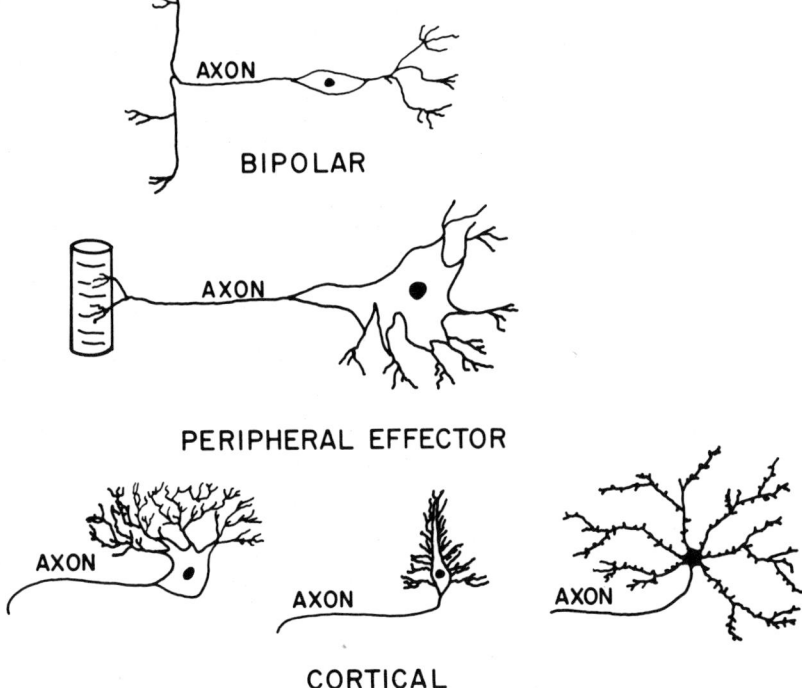

Figure 1.3 Different types of neuron.

The highly asymmetric structure of the neuron has evolved from a primordial, unspecialized ectodermal cell, and many of the chemical and morphological characteristics of the nerve cell are an exaggeration of properties shared by most cells. For example, while many cells are capable of the selective concentration of certain inorganic ions, this ability is much enhanced in the nerve cell. The sodium- and potassium-activated ATPase, which is probably responsible for the transport of sodium ions, is extremely active in nervous tissue. The cell interior contains about ten times as much potassium and only one-tenth as much sodium as the surrounding extracellular fluid, and the resting neuron uses a considerable amount of energy to maintain this unequal distribution of ions across its surrounding plasma membrane. The unequal distribution results in an excess negative charge within the cell and is the basis of the electrical properties of neurons (p. 73).

The function of the brain is to integrate sensory input and to produce an appropriate effector output. The single nerve cell reflects this function in miniature. The dendritic network and the surface of the nerve cell body can be thought of as the sensory data-collecting end of the neuron. Connections from other neurons or from sensory cells impinge upon these regions, forming synapses. Each nerve cell may receive from one to several tens of thousands of synaptic inputs. When activated by the firing of presynaptic nerve cells, the ionic permeabilities of the postsynaptic membrane — and thus the potential across it — may be altered. This changed potential is known as a postsynaptic potential (PSP) and may be positive or negative. Postsynaptic potentials arising in the dendrites are transmitted to the nerve cell body. Here they are summed along with those arising directly in the perikaryon. This summation is an integrative process and results from the cumulative effect of a series of dendritic and perikaryal events. The neuronal perikaryon may be thought of as a processing center where incoming data is quantified, the net magnitude of the potential change determining whether or not the cell will respond. Raising the potential of a nerve cell body to a hyperpolarized state reduces the likelihood of the cell's firing. However, if the potential across the membrane of the nerve cell body falls below a critical value due to a bombardment of excitatory synaptic events, an instability results. This instability results in an *action potential* which arises in the region of the axon hillock. Once initiated, the action potential sweeps down the axon as a transient wave of depolarization.

The action potential travels distally as a chain reaction of constant magnitude until it reaches the presynaptic area, where it may result in the release of a neurotransmitter or neurohumor. Such liberated substances can alter the chemical and membrane properties of the tissue upon which the synapse impinges. Thus the axon is the effector of the neuron.

Synapses may be made upon the nerve cell bodies and dendrites of other neurons or, more rarely, upon their axons or presynaptic regions. As much as 80 percent of the surface of the neuron may be covered with synapses. Axons may also form synapses on effector tissues and, by so doing, may regulate muscle or secretory glands. Certain specialized secretory nerve cells, such as those found within the hypothalamus and neurohypophysis, terminate at blood spaces into which they directly release neurohormones. These hormones may then be transported by the blood to other target cells. However, most brain neurons receive innervation from and innervate other neurons.

The regions of the neuron are morphologically and histochemically distinct. The predominant feature of the nerve cell body is a large nucleus, which normally contains one prominent nucleolus (Figures 1.4, 1.5). The nucleus contains the genetic material and ultimately dictates the types and

I. Anatomical Features of the Brain 9

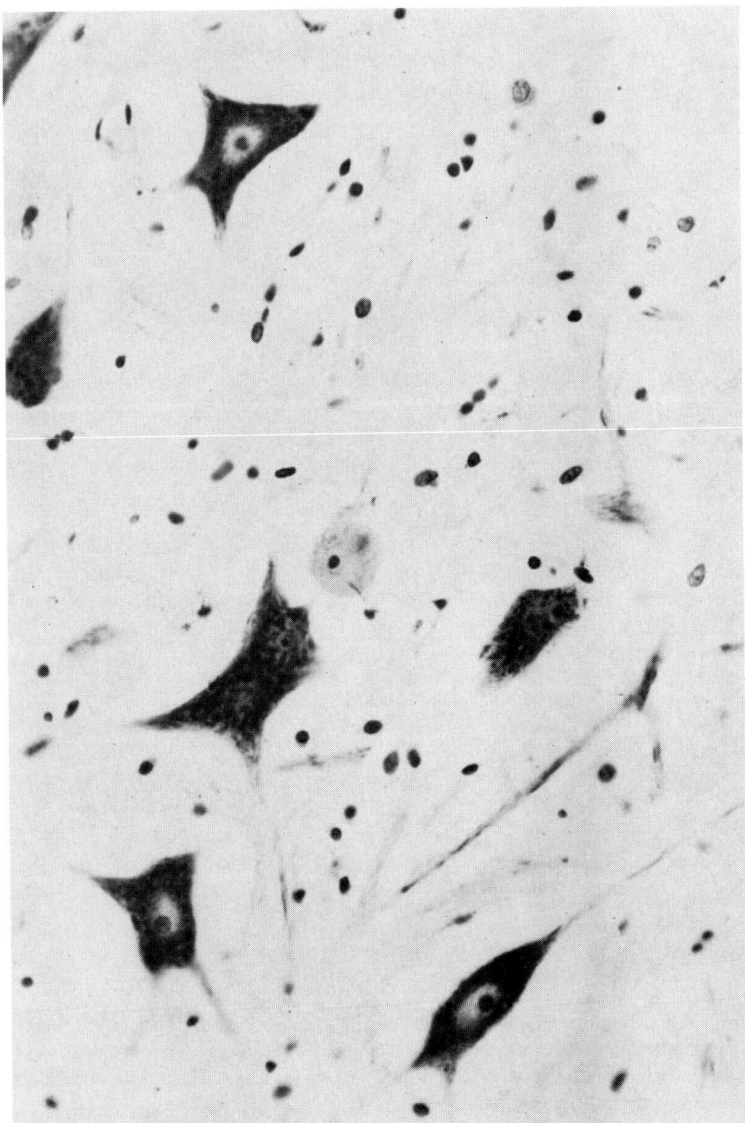

Figure 1.4 Nissl-stained section of spinal cord. In the large motor neuron cells note that the nucleus is pale but with a prominent nucleolus. The Nissl bodies in the perikaryon have a granular appearance. The smaller staining spots are the nuclei of astroglia and oligodendroglia. (Photo courtesy of Dr. R. Foelix).

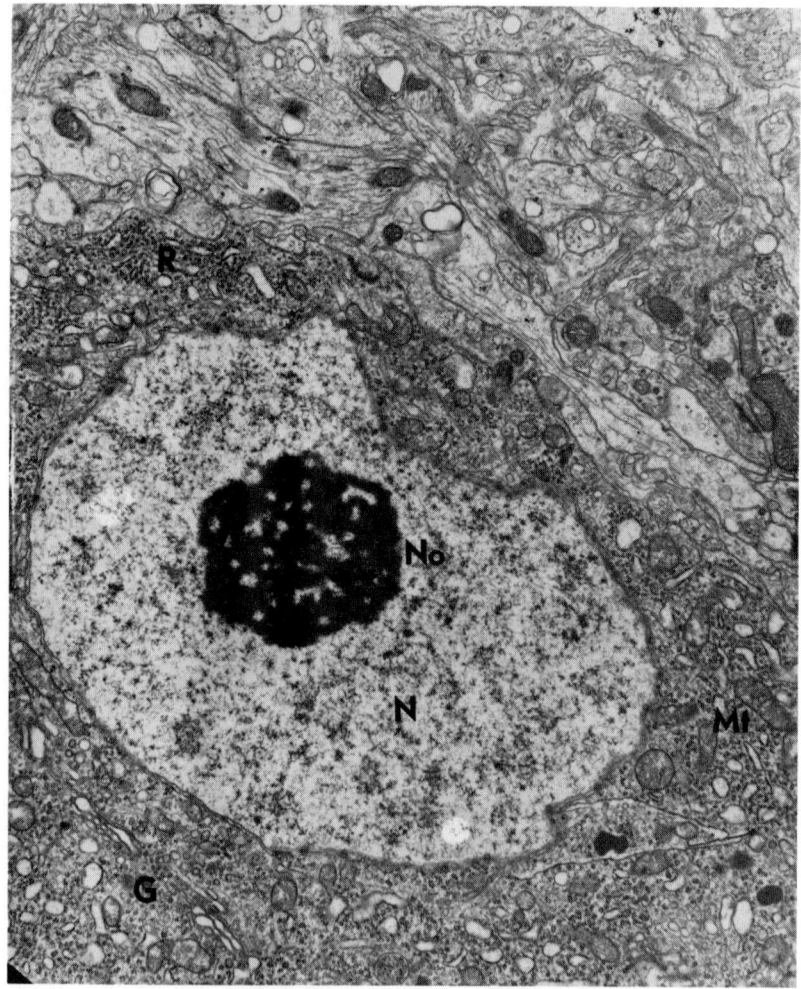

Figure 1.5 Electronmicrograph of the cell body of a neuron. Note the nucleus (N), nucleolus (No), and the large collection of ribosomes (R) which correspond to Nissl bodies in the light microscope. There are also mitochondria (Mt) and vesicles associated with a Golgi apparatus (G). (Photo courtesy of Dr. R. Foelix).

amounts of proteins synthesized. Its morphology may be affected by the degree of activity of the nerve or by neuronal trauma such as section of the axon. The nucleus may thus respond to cytoplasmic events. The central location of the nucleus enables it to react to changes in the chemical composition of the surrounding perikaryal cytoplasm. In this way the genetic

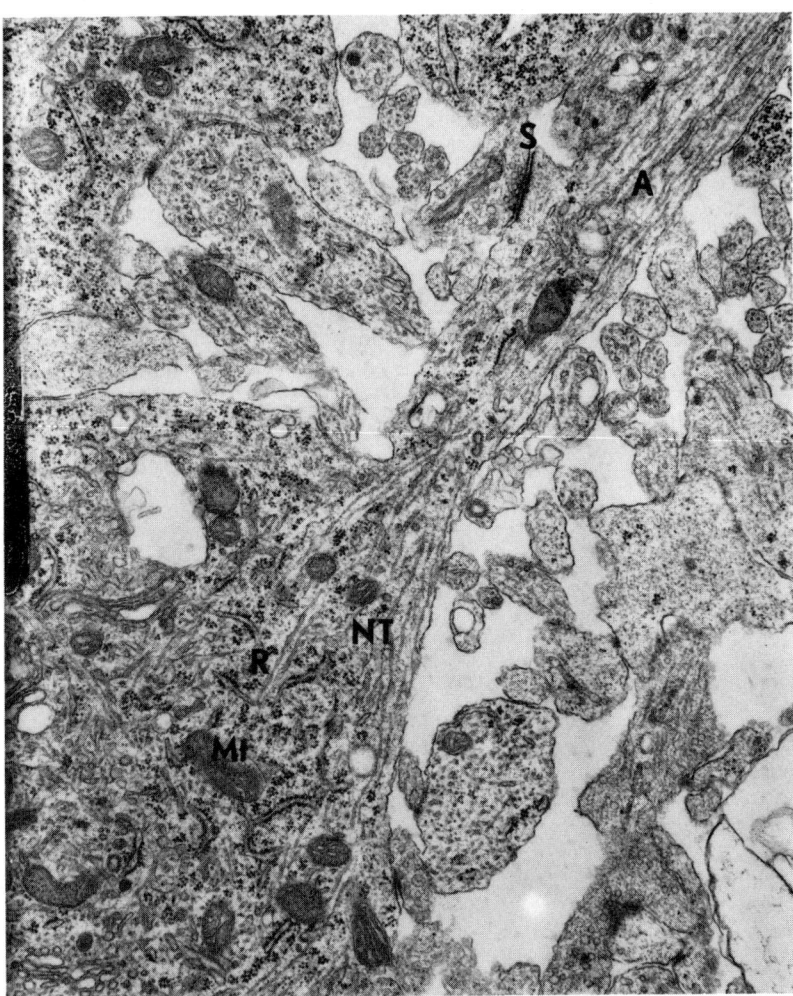

Figure 1.6 Electronmicrograph of the axon hillock of a Purkinje cell (10-day old chick embryo). Note the funnelling of the neurotubules (NT) into the axon (A), and the absence of ribosomes in the axon past the hillock. There is also an axo-axonal synapse (S). (Photo courtesy Dr. R. Foelix).

output of the nucleus may be modified in response to activity in the cell. Once differentiated, neurons do not divide; interdiction is so complete that tumors of differentiated nerve cells are unknown. Immature neurons (neuroblasts) do, however, possess malignant variants such as neuroblastomas and retinoblastomas.

The perikaryon and occasionally the dendrites contain the characteristic

Nissl substance (Figure 1.4). This substance stains intensely with acidophilic dyes and consists of a dense collection of ribosomes loosely associated with folds of the endoplasmic reticulum (Figures 1.5, 1.6).[6] The perikaryon is also packed with other organelles such as mitochondria, lysosomes, neurofilaments, neurotubules and the Golgi apparatus.[6] Some of these features can be seen in the electronmicrographs in Figures 1.4 and 1.5.

The dendrites resemble extensions of the perikaryon and contain similar organelles except for the Golgi apparatus. Unlike axons, dendrites are almost never sheathed in myelin and often have an irregular contour with spines that bear the postsynaptic elements. Dendritic surface area can be very large, often more than ten times that of the perikaryon of a neuron in cells such as the Purkinje cells of the cerebellum. In the sensory dorsal root cells of the spinal cord the remote receptor area is connected to the perikaryon by a single long fiber that is morphologically (and biochemically) an axon. Such cells are called bipolar or pseudo-unipolar neurons.

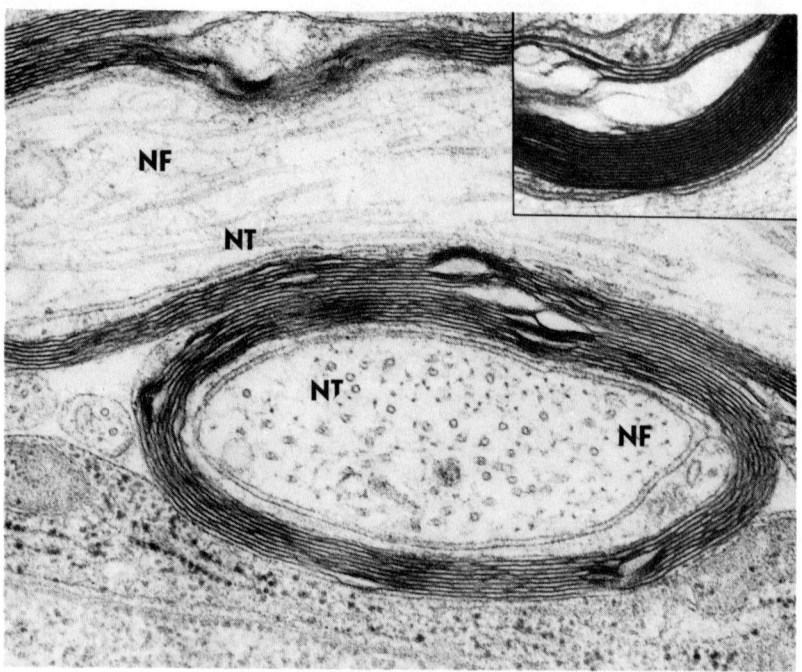

Figure 1.7 Electronmicrograph of two myelinated axons crossing transversely. Note the neurotubules (NT) and neurofilaments (NF) in transverse and cross-section running parallel with the axons themselves. In the magnified inset the different intensities of the inner and outer fusions of the membranes can be seen. (Photos courtesy of Dr. R. Foelix).

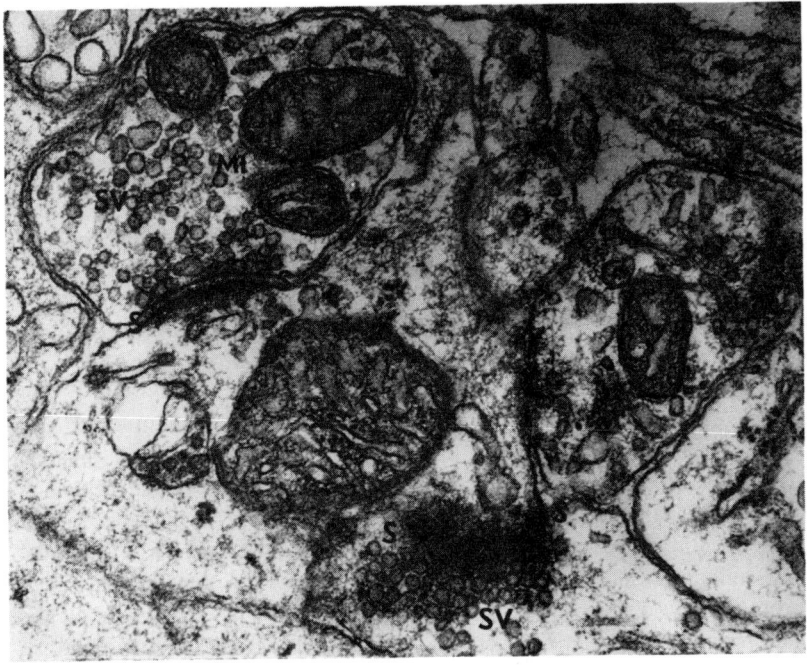

Figure 1.8 Electronmicrograph of two synapses in pigeon spinal cord. Note the presynaptic vesicles (SV), the intraterminal mitochondria (Mt) and the pre- and postsynaptic thickenings of the membranes at the synaptic junction. (Photo courtesy of Dr. R. Foelix).

Ribosomes are rarely seen in the axon and presynaptic areas which thus have a limited capacity for the synthesis of proteins. The axon is rich in longitudinally arranged microtubular structures which closely resemble those found in the dividing cell during mitosis (Figures 1.6, 1.7). Whereas microtubules are associated with the intracellular movement of chromosomes, there is evidence that neuronal microtubules (neurotubules) may function in the transport of proteins and neurotransmitters along the axon (Chapter 4). The axons and dendrites also contain long thin filaments known as neurofilaments (Figure 1.7).

Presynaptic terminals have many forms. They may occur along the length of the axon or at its distal terminus. The presynaptic area is often rich in mitochondria, and also in granules or vesicles which may contain neurotransmitters. These particles are especially concentrated in the region of the synaptic junction (Figure 1.8). The synaptic cleft itself has a characteristic striated appearance in the electron microscope. Selective staining procedures reveal it to be rich in carbohydrate. Another type of junction

— a gap junction, or electrical synapse — is present commonly in lower vertebrates and invertebrates, but also in the brains of chicks and possibly mammals. At these junctions the pre- and postsynaptic membranes are very close to each other and electrically coupled so that electrical impulses may pass from one nerve cell to another without chemical neurotransmitters as intermediates.

ii) Neuroglia

The role of glia in the central nervous system is much less clear than that of neurons.[7] Three major species of glial cell exist: *oligodendroglia* (oligodendrocytes), *astroglia* (astrocytes) and *microglia*.

The oligodendroglia tend to occur packed around axons and cell bodies and are responsible for the formation of the proteolipid myelin sheaths of myelinated nerve fibers (Figure 1.7 and Chapter 4). They are first apparent at the stage of cerebral development immediately preceding myelination. The oligodendroglia are analogous to the Schwann cells which form the myelin sheaths of peripheral nerves. Within the central nervous system the many cell processes of oligodendroglia are completely interwoven. These processes may invest several axons and contain many mitochondria and much rough endoplasmic reticulum. The satellite cells of the neuronal perikarya and of cerebral blood vessels are commonly oligodendroglia.

Astroglia, like oligodendroglia, are of ectodermal origin and have many cytoplasmic processes. There are two distinct types of astroglia: *protoplasmic* and *fibrous*. Protoplasmic astroglia have numerous short processes and are largely confined to gray matter. Fibrous astroglia have fewer, longer processes and are largely confined to white matter. Both types of astroglia send processes to the capillaries, where they form *endfeet*. These endfeet partially surround the blood vessels and are thought to mediate the transport of materials from the bloodstream to the neuron. They may thus constitute part of the blood-brain barrier. Oligodendroglia do not form end feet. Astroglia commonly surround synaptic junctions and may insulate them from one another, ensuring that the junctions act in an independent manner.

Astroglia contain a nonspecific cholinesterase that will inactivate the neurotransmitter acetylcholine should it diffuse into them. Astroglia have been shown to respond to the presence of the neurotransmitter, norepinephrine, increasing the activity of adenyl cyclase.[14] Thus, these cells may participate in and respond metabolically to neuronal events (Chapter 6). Glial cells may also act as regulators of the extracellular concentration of potassium ion (K^+), absorbing that released by nerve cells during the passage of electrical impulses.[15] If the extracellular concentration of K^+ is not buffered in this way, it may rise and cause an elevation of neuronal excitability. Malfunctioning of this K^+ absorbing capacity may be a causative factor in some cases of epilepsy.

Microglia differ from the oligodendroglia and astroglia in that they are of mesodermal rather than ectodermal origin and invade the brain relatively late in development. They are small, dense cells found in both white and gray matter, but more common in the latter. Microglia may appear as perineural or perivascular satellite cells, but are less common than oligodendroglia in this role. They may also serve a macrophagic function.

Unlike nerve cells, glial cells can continue to proliferate throughout the life of an organism. Under various pathological conditions such as nerve cell damage or scrapie (a demyelinating disease of cloven-hoofed animals), the rate of glial turnover may rise,[16] this indicates a repair or phagocytic function for glia. Astroglial cells proliferate and wall off damaged cerebral areas following cortical wounding. Glial proliferation has also been related to increased neuronal function in both motor and sensory areas. Increased glial division has been detected in the brains of mice reared in an environment rich in both sensory stimuli and motor activity (p. 219).

The ratio of glia to neurons within the cerebral cortex has been reported as 0.25 for the frog, 0.45 for the mouse and 1.6 for man.[17] This ratio also rises during the later stages of cerebral development as the major part of gliogenesis follows neuroblast proliferation. These data were at one time taken to signify that the glial-neuronal ratio was directly related to intelligence. However, the whale has a glial-neuronal ratio of about 4.5, which suggests that the proportion of glial cells may be related more to total brain mass. The numbers are explained by the observation that in vertebrates the average size of the neurons increases with the size of the brain, whereas that of the glia remains relatively constant. This is in accord with the original view of glial function: that of a structural matrix supporting the neuronal elements. There is little true connective tissue within the brain, and glia may take on this function to maintain tissue integrity

Hydén has suggested that there is a major exchange of chemicals between neurons and glia during various forms of stimulation, based on the finding of reciprocal changes in a variety of chemicals and enzymes.[8] These include cytochrome oxidase (p. 165), succinic dehydrogenase (p. 165) and RNA (pp. 165, 208).

Summary of glial function:
1. a matrix to physically support neuronal elements and to hold the tissue together;

2. a buffer to maintain the homeostasis of nerve cells — probably forming part of the blood-brain barrier.
3. the electrical insulation of axons and dendrites from one another — especially by the formation of myelin sheaths;
4. the metabolic support of the nerve cell — especially during intense neuronal activity;
5. tissue repair following damage — especially by macrophagic mechanisms.

iii) Separation of cell types

The heterogeneity of cerebral tissue has necessitated the development of methods for the selective isolation or concentration of different cell types in order to determine their respective contributions to the total chemical and enzymic make-up of the brain. Hydén pioneered the microdissection of small numbers of nerve cell bodies and glial cell clumps from fresh brain tissue.[8] This separation is incomplete because the glial clumps also contain neuronal processes torn off during separation of the neuronal perikarya. Nevertheless, useful chemical data have been obtained with these preparations if the contamination is taken into consideration. Swedish workers have developed several very delicate methods for the analysis of RNA and protein. For example, Hydén has reported the RNA base composition of these preparations determined by hydrolysis and electrophoresis of the resulting bases on single cellulose fibers. Protein fractionation has been carried out using electrophoresis on polyacrylamide gel columns within capillary tubes, and protein bands containing as little as 10^{-9} gram have been measured quantitatively by interference microscopy.[8]

Another approach to the separation of neurons and glia has been developed in several laboratories, notably those of Rose, Satake, Norton and Sellinger.[9] These workers attempted the bulk separation of cell types, using their different sedimentation properties. Although there are individual modifications, the fundamental steps in these methods are similar. The first step is the separation of the cells from one another. Despite the small amount of connective tissue in the brain, cells are not readily dissociated in an undamaged state because their numerous long processes are so intricately intertwined. Disaggregation has been achieved using enzymes such as trypsin or collagenase to loosen the intercellular matrix, by mechanical means such as passing tissue through fine nylon mesh or by gentle homogenization. Cell processes are torn away but the nerve cell body apparently seals off effectively at the points of rupture. Centrifugation of the cell suspension in a density gradient of sucrose or Ficoll is then used to separate the cell types. The different sedimentation characteristics of the cells cause them to be selectively concentrated at different regions in the gradient. Ficoll, a high molecular weight polydextran, is used to vary density while maintaining isotonic conditions. This prevents cell lysis (caused by hypotonic media) and the loss of soluble proteins due to cell shrinkage (caused by hypertonic media). The cells obtained in this way accumulate potassium ions and amino acids against a concentration gradient, indicating the integrity of the plasma membrane.

The most controversial aspect of these preparations is their cellular origin. Criteria of purity and integrity include enzyme content and the respiratory capacity of isolated cells. Enzymes predominantly located in neurons or glia have been used as markers to estimate the degree of contamination of one cell type by another. Thus β-galactosidase appears to be several-fold more concentrated in neurons than in glia.[18] Presumably, also, most of the enzymes for the synthesis of neurotransmitters are neuronal. On the other hand, the brain-specific S-100 protein is glial.

Neuronal and glial cells may be studied through the cloning of pure cell lines in tissue culture.[10] Considerable quantities of homogeneous cell types may be prepared in this way. However, a disadvantage is that many of these cell lines are derived from glial tumors or neuroblastomas, which can hardly be considered as closely resembling the normal cell. Also, cells grown in culture over several generations tend to lose their more specialized features. Yet such cultures have helped to resolve certain problems. The glial location of the brain-specific protein S-100 was confirmed when it was shown to be synthesized by astrocytoma cells. Nirenberg and his group have been concerned with neuroblastoma cultures which retain neuronal characteristics such as electrical excitability for many generations. With such cell lines, factors regulating growth, differentiation and the levels of enzymes associated with nerve function can be studied. For example, acetylcholinesterase is elevated in non-dividing neuroblastoma cells and falls when division is induced.

C. CHEMICAL ANALYSIS OF CEREBRAL ANATOMY

The brain is comprised of many different cell types that are adjacent to or superimposed on each other. Although chemical heterogeneity is not readily apparent to the eye, regional assays of various chemicals show them to be very localized with steep concentration gradients over short distances. For instance, the probable neurotransmitter, dopamine, is highly localized in certain areas such as the basal ganglia. Chemical specificity is also revealed by regionally specific viruses such as the poliomyelitis virus, which attacks only the motor neurons within the spinal cord.

The loci and concentrations of substances can be studied by histochemical techniques. This approach has helped to determine the concentration profiles of many substances in brain sections.[11] However, there is the possibility of artifacts due to the diffusion of substances within sections prior to fixation, staining or enzyme assay. Histochemical techniques have now been refined so that they have enormous scope and variety. The range of approaches possible is best illustrated by example:

1. Tissue sections may be examined with stains of known specificity. The specificity of the stains may be determined in appropriate ways. For example, RNA stains should disappear following treatment of a section with ribonuclease. Because of the possibility of degradative artifact, such ribonuclease treatment must be checked by adding a ribonuclease inhibitor, which should prevent the loss of staining material.

2. The distribution of an enzyme may be determined by using carefully designed substrates that form readily detectable products. Thus the enzyme acetylcholinesterase may be located by using acetylthiocholine as a substrate. The thiocholine formed will readily precipitate lead sulfide from soluble lead salts, and the lead precipitate may readily be identified in the light or electron microscope. A similar approach uses inhibitors of the enzyme that bind to it irreversibly. Suitable tags include radioisotopes (which can be detected by radioautography), fluorescent compounds and heavy metals, as well as distinctively colored products. With the use of radioautography some enzyme activities may be studied *in vivo,* using precursors of readily fixed compounds such as proteins, nucleic acids or polysaccharides.

3. Antibodies to specific compounds can be used to immunologically determine the location of such compounds. It is possible to tag or label the antiserum with either a heavy metal, radioisotope or fluorescent chemical group.

4. Techniques are no longer restricted to fixable compounds since by freeze-drying tissue sections, the location of small readily diffusible compounds may be determined by radioautography or with suitable antisera (e.g., for cyclic AMP).[19]

5. A tissue section may be examined for its anatomical components (e.g., synapses and nuclei) and then microchemical analyses performed on the appropriate parts of the section. This technique loses the anatomical resolution of methods that can directly visualize chemicals in sections, but it is useful for chemicals for which staining methods have not been developed. Hess and Pope have used this technique to localize cerebrosides in myelin and gangliosides at synapses.[11]

Altered concentrations of certain chemicals in specific brain regions may be useful in neuropathological diagnosis. In Alzheimer's disease decreased amounts of cerebroside and proteolipid protein are demonstrable by specialized histochemical methods, before major changes are detectable with standard myelin stains.

The classical method for mapping the nervous system has been the tracing of the degeneration of distal fiber paths after nerve section. Using the silver technique of Nauta which selectively impregnates degenerating neurons, the destinations of sectioned nerves can be traced.[20] Electron microscopy may also be used for degeneration studies, but in this case, due to the higher magnification, it is necessary to know the approximate area in which to look for degenerating nerves. The visualization of many biogenic amines at the cellular level has been made possible by sensitive fluorescence microscope methods.[21] This localization of possible neurotransmitters has been used in tracing certain nerve tracts within the brain. Several monoamine pathways have been well charted recently by a combination of nerve section and fluorescence microscopy.[22] Lesions of aminergic nerve bundles cause neurotransmitters such as dopamine to accumulate at the proximal side of the lesion. These accumulations can then be detected by fluorescence techniques. By means of a series of lesions, dopaminergic tracts have been traced from the cell bodies within the substantia nigra, along the nigrostriatal tract to terminations within the caudate nucleus.

Histochemical methods may be used to corroborate electrophysiological data. Stimulation of sensory nerves may produce evoked electrical potentials at their primary terminations and also at regions that are indirectly connected. These evoked potentials may be detected by recording from electrodes implanted in the brain. Electrophysiological methods have the disadvantage that they are relatively insensitive, since evoked potentials will be detected only when there are appreciable numbers of connections to that area. This problem could in theory be solved with intracellular electrodes, but the task of screening all the necessary cells would be impossibly great.

A new and excellent technique for mapping neuronal tracts uses axoplasmic flow. Locally injected radioactive amino acids are incorporated into proteins in the perikarya, and the radioactive proteins formed are transported axoplasmically to the presynaptic terminals. The fiber tracts may then be followed by radioautography[23] or by otherwise estimating the radioactivity in different brain areas. A combination of electron microscopy and radioautography permits the precise identification of the terminal projections of labeled neurons. Since the principal site of protein synthesis in the brain is perikaryal, the background noise in these experiments is low. This technique is capable of very fine resolution, and with careful administration of the isotopes the area of the brain being studied may be relatively undamaged, in contrast to the lesion techniques.

Developments in analyzing cerebral architecture have been paralleled by new ways of examining small numbers of cells chemically, using microtechniques. Lowry isolated nerve cell bodies from freeze-dried (lyophilized) tissue sections and assayed many of their components.[12] He used methods in which a molecular species (enzyme or substrate) participates in a series of sequential reactions so that molecules of a readily measurable product are produced. For example, ATP can be determined in the following way: the sample of ATP is incubated with excess glucose and NADP in the presence of hexokinase and glucose-6-phosphate dehydrogenase. A series of reactions takes place such that for each molecule of ATP, one molecule of NADPH is produced.

```
                 ATP    ADP              NADP⁺   NADPH
glucose ─────────⤻⤻───── glucose-6-phosphate ─────⤻⤻───── 6-phosphogluconate
                HEXOKINASE                   GLUCOSE-6-PHOSPHATE
                                               DEHYDROGENASE
```

NADPH can be assayed fluorimetrically in amounts as low as 10^{-11} mole. By coupling together enzymic reactions, very small amounts of many molecular species can be assayed in this way.

For even further sensitivity, Lowry developed a system of enzymatic recycling. In this the NADPH produced is used to catalyze a two-enzyme system such as glutamic dehydrogenase and glucose-6-phosphate dehydrogenase.

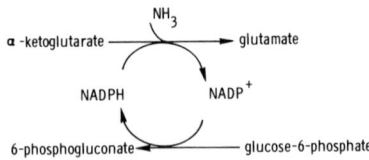

By allowing this system to cycle for a fixed period of time, one molecule of NADPH could result in the production of several thousand molecules of 6-phosphogluconate. These may then be assayed by a further oxidation to ribulose-5-phosphate with the production of NADPH.

6-phosphogluconate + NADP⁺ ──────▶ ribulose-5-phosphate + NADPH

For each original molecule of NADPH there are now about ten thousand molecules. This amplification makes it possible to assay as little as one molecule of an enzyme and very low concentrations of substrates.

There is great need for very sensitive assays of this kind. In conjunction with improved procedures for handling the diverse cell types within the brain, detailed chemical-anatomical data could be obtained. More knowledge of the brain at the cellular level is a prerequisite for a deeper understanding of its complex properties.

CHAPTER I REFERENCES

Reviews and General References

1. Katzman, R. Blood-brain-CSF barriers. In *Basic Neurochemistry* (Ed. R. W. Albers, G. J. Siegel, R. Katzman, and B. W. Agranoff), Little, Brown, Boston, 1972, pp. 327–39.
2. Davson, H. The cerebrospinal fluid. In *Handbook of Neurochemistry*, Vol. 2 (Ed. A. Lajtha), Plenum Press, New York, 1969, pp. 23–48.
3. Csáky, T. Z. Choroid plexus. In *Handbook of Neurochemistry*, Vol. 2 (Ed. A. Lajtha), Plenum Press, New York, 1969, pp. 49–69.
4. Prockop, L. D. Disorders of cerebrospinal fluid and brain extracellular fluid. In *Biology of Brain Dysfunction*, Vol. 1 (Ed. G. E. Gaull), Plenum Press, New York, 1973, pp. 229–63.
5. Dobbing, J. Undernutrition and the developing brain. In *Handbook of Neurochemistry*, Vol. 6 (Ed. A. Lajtha), Plenum Press, New York, 1971, pp. 255–66.
6. Peters, A., Palay, S. L., and Webster, H. de F. *The Fine Structure of the Nervous System*, Harper and Row, New York, 1970.
7. Lasansky, A. Nervous function at the cellular level: glia. *Ann. Rev. Physiol.* 33:241–256, 1971.
8. Hydén, H. Dynamic aspects on the neuron-glia relationship — a study with microchemical methods. In *The Neuron*, Elsevier Press, Amsterdam, 1967, pp. 179–219.
9. Poduslo, S. E., and Norton, W. T. The bulk separation of neuroglia and neuron perikarya. In *Research Methods in Neurochemistry*, Vol. 1 (Ed. N. Marks and R. Rodnight), Plenum Press, New York, 1972, pp. 19–32.
10. Herschman, H. R. Tissue and cell culture as a tool in neurochemistry. In *Proteins of the Nervous System* (Ed. D. J. Schneider), Raven Press, New York, 1973, pp. 95–115.
11. Hess, H. H., and Pope, A. Quantitative neurochemical histology. In *Handbook of Neurochemistry*, Vol. 7 (Ed. A. Lajtha), Plenum Press, New York, 1972, pp. 289–327.
12. Lowry, O. H. The chemical study of single neurons. *Harvey Lectures*, 58.1–19, 1963.

Literature Cited

13. Davies, P. W., and Bronk, D. W. Oxygen tension in mammalian brain. *Fed. Proc.* 16:689–92, 1957.
14. Clark, R. B., and Perkins, J. P. Regulation of adenosine 3′:5′-cyclic monophosphate concentration in cultured human astrocytoma cells by catecholamines and histamine. *Proc. Nat. Acad. Sci., U.S.A.* 68:2757–60, 1971.
15. Henn, F. A., Haljämae, H., and Hamberger, A. Glial cell function: active control of extracellular K^+ concentration. *Brain Research* 43:437–43, 1972.

16. Kimberlin, R. H. Incorporation of [³H]thymidine into the DNA of brain, liver, spleen and submaxillary salivary gland in normal and scrapie-affected mice. *Res. in Veterinary Sci.* 10:392–94, 1969.
17. Jacobson, M. Neuronal-glial ratios. In *Developmental Neurobiology*, Holt, Rinehart and Winston, New York, 1970, p. 69.
18. Sinha, A. K., and Rose, S. P. Compartmentation of lysosomes in neurones and neuropil and a new neuronal marker. *Brain Research* 39:181–96, 1972.
19. Bloom, F. E., Hoffer, B. J., Battenberg, E. R., Siggins, G. R., Steiner, A. L., Parker, C. W., and Wedner, H. J. Adenosine 3',5'-monophosphate is localized in cerebellar neurons; immunofluorescence evidence. *Science* 177:436–38, 1972.
20. Nauta, W. J. H., and Gygax, P. A. Silver impregnation of degenerating axon terminals in the central nervous system. *Stain Techn.* 26:5–11, 1951.
21. Falck, B., Hillarp, N.-Å., Thieme, G., and Torp, A. Fluorescence of catecholamines and related compounds condensed with formaldehyde. *J. Histochem. Cytochem.* 10:348–54, 1962.
22. Livett, B. G., Geffen, L. B., and Rush, R. A. Immunochemical methods for demonstrating macromolecules in sympathetic neurons. *Phil. Trans. Roy. Soc. Lond.* B 261:359–61, 1971.
23. Cowan, W. M., Gottlieb, D. I., Hendrickson, A. E., Price, J. L., and Woolsey, T. A. The autoradiographic demonstration of axonal connections in the central nervous system. *Brain Research* 37:21–51, 1972.

II. The Basic Biochemistry of the Brain

A. THE GENERATION AND USE OF ENERGY[1,2]

The brain is exceedingly dependent upon a constant supply of blood. Consciousness is lost in the human less than ten seconds after interruption of the blood supply, and within a few minutes irreparable damage occurs. Blood flow through the adult human brain is about 750 ml per minute, or some 15 percent of the total bodily blood flow in the resting state. The brain removes approximately 50 ml of oxygen from the blood each minute, reducing the oxygen content by about one-third—rather more than the bodily average. Thus the brain, only 2 percent of the weight of the body, consumes about 20 percent of the total oxygen used, and approximately the same proportion of the energy. However, in the fetal or infant human, more than 50 percent of the total bodily oxygen may be consumed by the brain. When there is intense muscular activity, the oxygen consumption of the body may rise by up to fivefold, whereas that of the brain remains constant. Two processes account for the disproportionately large amount of energy used: the translocation of ions important for the electrical activity, and the extremely active biosynthetic mechanisms operating in the brain. The high metabolic rate of brain is not a characteristic of all neural tissue; peripheral nerves use about 3 percent as much oxygen as an equivalent weight of CNS tissue.

The oxygen consumption of the brain is essentially constant under normal physiological conditions. Cerebral blood flow may fluctuate, but the arteriovenous differences of oxygen and carbon dioxide adjust accordingly so that net oxygen uptake and energy consumption are not changed. Cerebral capillaries are not extensively innervated and their diameter is largely controlled by a local mechanism known as *autoregulation*. Increases in neural activity are presumably associated with increases in oxygen consumption, carbon dioxide production and a fall in pH. These changes, of which CO_2 concentration is probably the most important, cause vasodilation and thus increased blood flow (Figure 2.1). In this way the nutrient supply to specific cerebral areas can be regulated by metabolic demand.

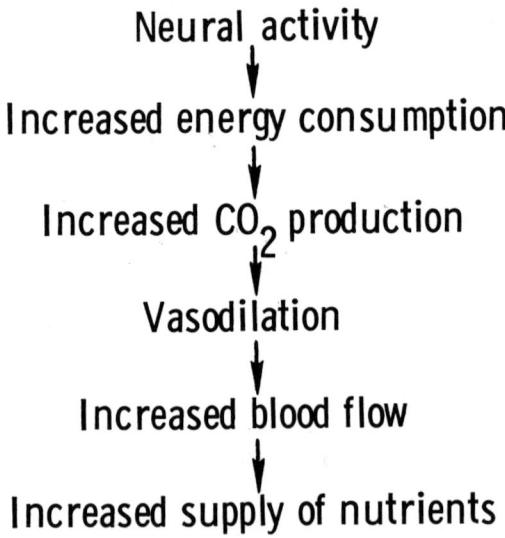

Figure 2.1 Autoregulation.

Measurements of oxygen consumption during arithmetical problem-solving, when increased mental activity might be expected, show no change over apparently less active periods. Similarly, during slow-wave sleep there is no change in cerebral energy utilization. However, cerebral blood flow and oxygen consumption are accelerated during REM sleep (see p. 221). Thus, while minor regional changes may occur, the overall high metabolic rate of the brain is substantially unaltered during normal activity.

When cerebral oxygen falls, as it may do during hypoglycemia and after convulsions, human subjects feel confused. Pronounced falls in oxygen consumption are associated with coma and occur in severe hypoglycemia and during anesthesia. Increases in energy consumption are often (but not always) seen during convulsions when there is a great deal of electrophysiological activity. Thus energy consumption may be closely tied to neural electrical activity, which accounts for the major part of the energy used (Figure 2.2).

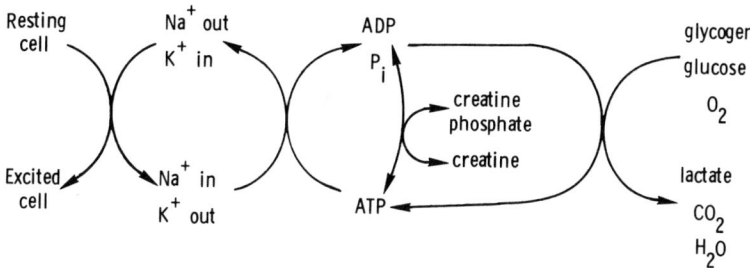

Figure 2.2 The coupling of neural activity to glucose and oxygen consumption.

Studies of the composition of cerebral arterial and venous blood show that the principal chemicals consumed by the brain in the intact animal are glucose and oxygen, with the production of carbon dioxide and water. The 75 mg of glucose consumed by the human brain each minute is more than adequate to account for the 50 ml of oxygen consumed. The discrepancy is exactly balanced by the output of lactate and pyruvate, so that in the normal state the conversion of glucose and oxygen to carbon dioxide, pyruvate and lactate fully accounts for the observed arteriovenous differences. The oxidation of glucose alone is also consistent with the observed respiratory quotient (CO_2 produced/O_2 consumed) of close to 1, which indicates oxidation of carbohydrates only. Except in special circumstances, it has been difficult to demonstrate net utilization of any other carbon source by the brain. Studies with isolated, perfused brain also show its poor ability to use any carbon source other than glucose. However, in the absence of glucose, the perfused rat brain can use mannose (by conversion to mannose-6-phosphate and hence fructose-6-phosphate). Studies using radioactively labeled compounds indicate that, whereas many substances can be taken up and metabolized by the brain, they will not substitute for glucose as an energy source. An exception to this is the metabolism of ketone bodies occurring in fetal and starving animals (see below).

Glucose is metabolized in the brain by the classical biochemical pathways of glycolysis (Figure 2.3) and the tricarboxylic acid cycle (Figure 2.4).

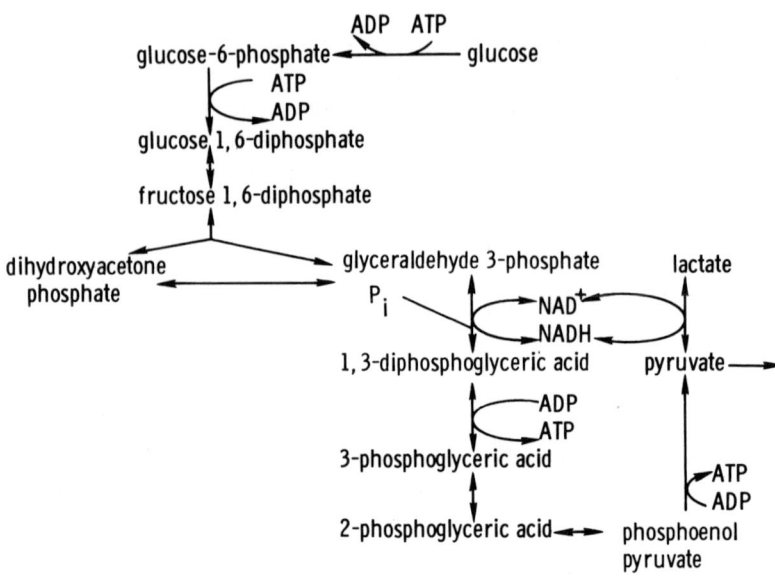

Figure 2.3 The pathway of glycolysis.

Glycolysis is the phosphorylation of glucose and its subsequent conversion to pyruvate. Pyruvate may then be reduced to lactate so that in this case the glycolytic process requires no oxygen and is *anaerobic*. Alternatively, pyruvate may be incorporated into the tricarboxylic acid cycle so that the total catabolism of glucose requires oxygen and is *aerobic*. The lactate excreted from the brain gives a measure of the proportion of glucose catabolized anaerobically. This proportion is equal to:

$$\frac{\text{arteriovenous difference in lactate concentration}}{\text{arteriovenous difference in glucose concentration}}$$

In the brain, as in muscle and many other tissues, the supply of oxygen controls the ratio of anaerobic to aerobic metabolism by a mechanism known as the *Pasteur effect*. In the presence of adequate supplies of oxygen, glycolysis is suppressed (probably because phosphofructokinase is inhibited by ATP). In the mature brain under normal conditions, the proportion of glucose metabolized anaerobically is about 15 percent. This proportion increases in times of high energy demand or low oxygen supply, but anaerobic

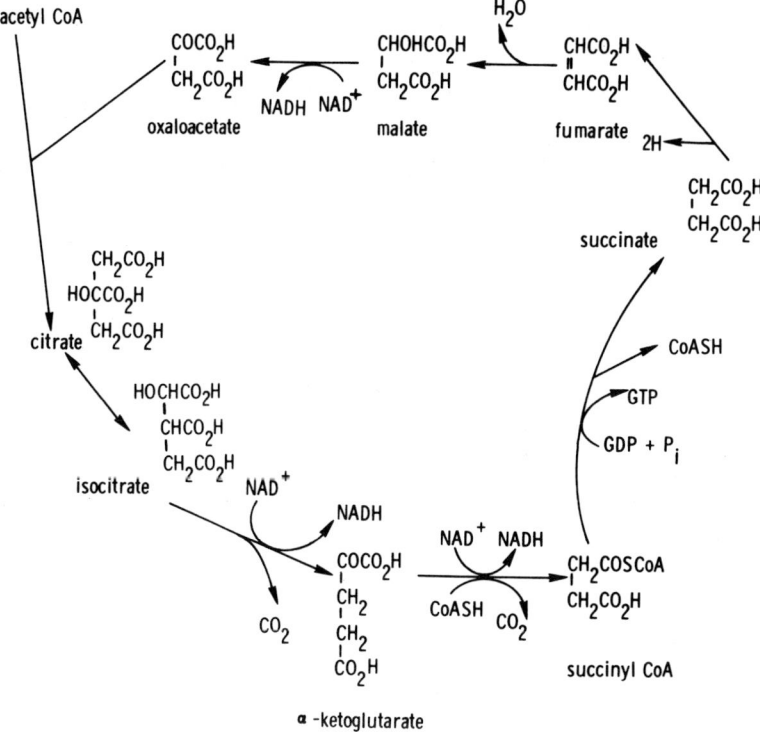

Figure 2.4 The tricarboxylic acid cycle.

glycolysis cannot proceed at a rate adequate to provide the total energy requirements of the conscious brain.

Anaerobic glycolysis yields two energy-rich bonds in the form at ATP for each molecule of glucose consumed, while total aerobic catabolism yields about thirty-eight energy-rich bonds. The difference in energy yield of the two processes thus provides a rationale for the strong orientation of cerebral metabolism to aerobic glycolysis. Because of the low carbohydrate (glycogen) reserves in the brain, the rate-limiting process in the production of energy at times of high demand is the supply of glucose to the cell. This supply may be limited by the large number of membranes to be traversed and the long distances between the blood and the neuron. The limited role of anaerobic glycolysis may also be related to the toxicity of lactate and the difficulty of removing it, caused by its low permeability in brain.

The immature brain is less dependent on aerobic metabolism. During development there is a metabolic transition from anaerobic to aerobic metabolism. Thus the newborn rat can survive for over fifty minutes in a nitrogen atmosphere, while the adult rat can live for only one to two minutes.

Energy stores exist in the brain in the form of glycogen and creatine phosphate. Glycogen is essentially a store of glucose, and creatine phosphate may rapidly transfer its high energy phosphate to ADP to form ATP:

$$\text{creatine} + \text{ATP} \longleftrightarrow \text{creatine phosphate} + \text{ADP}$$

Unlike liver and muscle, the brain contains limited glycogen and creatine phosphate reserves, and these are sufficient for only about thirty seconds of normal brain metabolism. When the energy demands of the brain are increased, as during electroshock-induced convulsions or when the cerebral oxygen supply is cut off, the creatine phosphate is depleted first, followed by the glycogen, and only then do ATP levels fall appreciably. Conversely, during recovery the ATP levels return to normal first, followed by the creatine phosphate and finally the glycogen.

The dependence of the brain on glucose is dramatically demonstrated in hypoglycemia. The fall in blood glucose and consequently in glucose consumption by the brain is coupled to a fall in oxygen consumption. As blood glucose falls, confusion and then coma result. In severe hypoglycemia the close relationship between glucose and oxygen consumption no longer holds, but the respiratory quotient remains unity. In this state the brain oxidizes its own stores of carbohydrate and associated amino acids, especially glutamate and glutamine. In the absence of blood glucose the human brain can survive in the comatose state for twenty to twenty-five minutes. In hypoglycemia the brain is dependent upon supplies of glucose from glycogenolysis and gluconeogenesis in other organs, principally the liver.

Whether or not insulin affects glucose uptake by the brain in the intact animal is unresolved. Insulin does accelerate glucose uptake into slices of brain tissue *in vitro,* but *in vivo* the effect on peripheral tissues seems to predominate and the brain suffers from the consequent hypoglycemia. (But see p. 5). Insulin overdose may result in hypoglycemic coma and possibly convulsions.

The enzymes of the glycolytic pathway, which are predominantly cytoplasmic, are present in greater concentrations in the brain than they are in the liver. This presumably reflects the absolute dependence of brain upon glucose as a carbon source. In contrast, the key enzymes required for gluconeogenesis (the reverse of glycolysis) are present in low or negligible concentrations in the brain, and those for glycogen metabolism are low. Thus these pathways are relatively unimportant in brain.

Acetyl coenzyme A, produced from glycolysis, is incorporated into the tricarboxylic acid cycle located inside the mitochondria. The reduced pyridine nucleotide (NADH) produced by the cycle is then oxidized by the mitochondrial respiratory chain, resulting in the production of ATP. Mitochondria may travel throughout the cytoplasm of the cells and are often particularly concentrated in regions with a high demand for ATP, such as the presynaptic terminal. ATP cannot be transported across the mitochondrial membrane, but the energy-rich bond of the terminal (gamma) phosphate may be transferred through the membrane to an ADP molecule on the outside. The mitochondrion is by far the most important cellular site for the production of ATP.

The tricarboxylic acid cycle in brain is similar to that found in all tissues. The activities of the enzymes are generally slightly lower than those of the

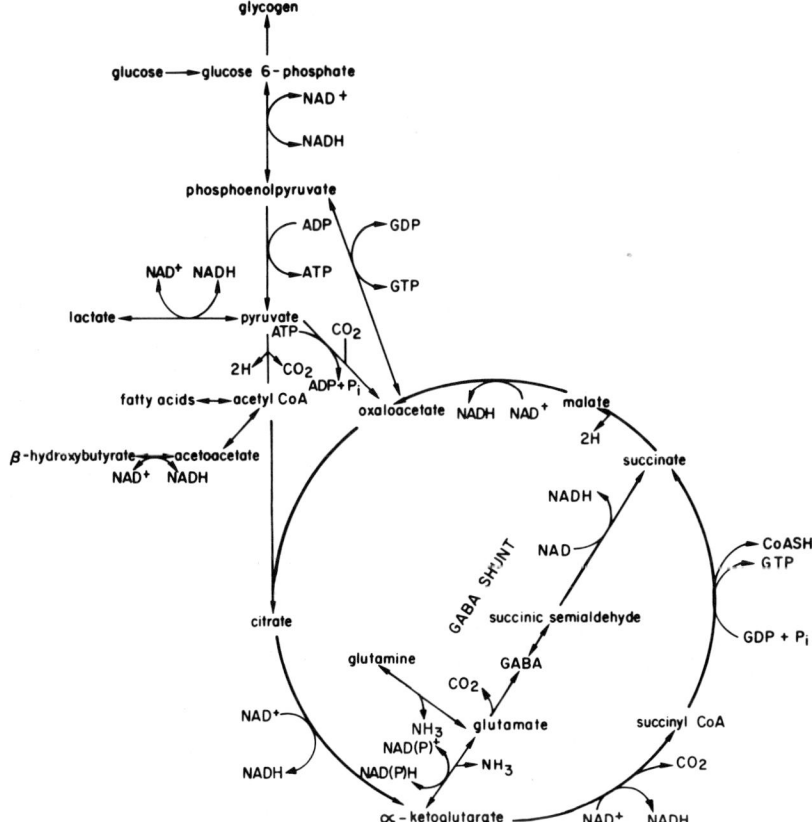

Figure 2.5 Intermediary carbohydrate metabolism and the GABA shunt.

equivalent liver enzymes. The only aspect of specific importance for the brain is the existence of the *GABA shunt* (Figure 2.5). In this pathway gamma-aminobutyric acid (GABA) is produced by decarboxylation of glutamic acid. GABA may then be transaminated to succinic semialdehyde which may be reduced to succinate and reincorporated into the tricarboxylic acid cycle, thus forming an alternative route to a part of the cycle. The shunt is almost certainly concerned with the production of GABA, rather than energy (see p. 36).

It is not obvious why the brain normally prefers carbohydrates rather than fatty acids, which theoretically would produce a higher energy yield by aerobic catabolism. It may be that there is no way of rapidly transporting fatty acids throughout the brain. Fatty acid and aliphatic amino acid oxidation does occur, but this is not significant in the overall energy metabolism. However, under certain conditions cerebral fatty acid oxidation becomes important. During starvation the body mobilizes its fat stores and becomes ketotic due to the circulation of ketone bodies (β-hydroxybutyrate and acetoacetate). In this state, ketone bodies are oxidized by the brain by metabolism to acetyl coenzyme A and incorporation into the tricarboxylic acid cycle (Figure 2.5). Nevertheless, glucose is still required, and the oxidation of ketone bodies accounts for only about half the total oxygen consumption.[1,2,6]

The fetal brain also oxidizes significant quantities of fatty acids. The activity of the enzyme β-hydroxybutyrate dehydrogenase, which is responsible for the conversion of β-hydroxybutyrate to acetoacetate, falls sharply during development. In the adult, activity of this enzyme increases after two to three days' starvation, at the same time as the increase in the catabolism of ketone bodies. This effect appears to be due to the synthesis of new enzyme molecules.[6]

Fatty acid catabolism occurs by degradation to acetyl CoA which enters the tricarboxylic acid cycle (Figure 2.5). It has long been somewhat puzzling that this catabolism cannot occur in the body in the absence of carbohydrate metabolism. The most likely explanation is that the concentrations of the intermediates of the tricarboxylic acid cycle limit the oxidative process. Use for the biosynthesis of more complex compounds depletes these intermediates which may only be regenerated from glycolytic metabolites. Thus in the absence of glycolysis the tricarboxylic acid cycle slows down.

B. NUTRITIONAL REQUIREMENT

The brain can synthesize most necessary chemicals from a nutritionally adequate diet and requires very few materials that are not essential for the entire body. It can also use certain preformed compounds such as fatty acids, cholesterol and nucleosides if they are present in the blood, whether derived from the diet or from other tissues. In common with other tissues, the brain requires vitamins, essential fatty acids, certain amino acids and inorganic materials.

Studies with the perfused brain suggest that only glucose and oxygen are required to maintain an electrically active brain for several hours. Geiger reported that the normal electroencephalogram of cat brain could be further prolonged in the perfused preparation when the liver was left in circulation. The presence of the liver could be substituted for by the addition to the perfusate of the pyrimidine nucleosides, uridine and cytidine.[7] Recently, however, in perfusion experiments using rats, no requirement for these compounds was shown.[8]

All necessary sugars and other carbohydrates can be synthesized in the brain from glucose, although several sugars are actively taken up and utilized (e.g., fucose and glucosamine). Most lipid components and all complex lipids are synthesized by the brain. Fatty acid and cholesterol synthesis is very active in the brain and incorporation of the exogenous compounds is low.

Brain has the same amino acid requirements as the whole body, with the exception that it also requires tyrosine — a nonessential amino acid. Tyrosine is extremely important as a precursor of the catecholamine neurotransmitters, dopamine and norepinephrine, in addition to its use for the synthesis of protein. In the liver and several other tissues, tyrosine can be produced from phenylalanine by phenylalanine hydroxylase.

$$\text{phenylalanine} \xrightarrow[\text{reduced pteridine} \quad \text{pteridine}]{O_2 \quad H_2O} \text{tyrosine}$$

Remarkably, this enzyme is absent from brain which thus relies on the diet and the liver for its tyrosine supply. The related enzyme, tyrosine hydroxylase (p. 131), has a low phenylalanine hydroxylating activity but this is insufficient for the needs of the brain.

Phenylketonuria is a genetic disease characterized by a reduced phenylalanine hydroxylase activity. This results in high blood and brain concentrations of phenylalanine. If such a condition is not corrected by a diet low in phenylalanine, severe mental retardation occurs. The mechanism of this effect is unknown but it seems likely that the phenylalanine acts as an analogue of tyrosine and competitively interferes with its metabolism. Thus in phenylketonuria, tyrosine uptake by the brain and its use for the synthesis of protein (p. 61) and possibly catecholamines are impaired. In addition, phenylalanine may have toxic effects on general metabolism, since physiological concentrations inhibit pyruvate kinase.[9] Phenylketonuria occurs commonly (1 birth in 10,000) and screening of newborn infants for this disease is now routine.

Essential amino acids are taken up by the brain to a greater extent than nonessential amino acids. This is effected by the specificity of the uptake systems.[10] The metabolism of tryptophan, a precursor of the neurotransmitter serotonin, is of especial interest. The brain concentration of serotonin, which exhibits a diurnal rhythm, is related to the brain concentration of free tryptophan. This is in turn related to the plasma concentration of tryptophan. Tryptophan shares a common uptake mechanism with certain other neutral amino acids (phenylalanine, tyrosine, leucine, isoleucine and valine). Brain tryptophan concentration reflects not so much that of plasma tryptophan but the relative concentration of the competing amino acids in the plasma. Furthermore, in plasma, tryptophan exists both free and bound to serum albumin, the bound form predominating under normal conditions. Thus brain tryptophan, and consequently serotonin concentration, are dependent on the plasma levels of amino acids which in turn depend on the diet. This phenomenon may play a role in the control of appetite.[11]

The requirement of the brain for exogenous nucleic acid precursors is uncertain. Both purine and pyrimidine nucleosides are actively taken up from the blood. However, whereas the purines may be synthesized *de novo* in the brain, cerebral synthesis of pyrimidines has not been demonstrated (see p. 43).

C. CHEMICALS OF SPECIAL SIGNIFICANCE FOR THE BRAIN

Neural tissue contains a large number of chemical components that are either unique or present in very much higher concentrations than in nonneural tissue. Approximately half the dry weight of the brain is lipid. Many lipids are unique to the brain, notably cerebrosides, sulfatides, plasmalogens and some gangliosides (Chapter 4). The other major constituent is protein,

BIOCHEMICAL COMPOSITION OF BRAIN

	Whole brain	*Gray matter*	*White matter*
Water	78	83	70
Lipid	11	6	15
Protein	8	7.5	8.5
Soluble organic substances	2	–	–
Inorganic salts	1.1	1.0	1.3
Nucleic acids	0.3	–	–

and there are many proteins specific to neural tissue (Chapter 3). Cerebral polysaccharides and nucleic acids are quantitatively minor constituents. Complex macromolecules such as glycoproteins, lipoproteins and proteolipids are common because of the large number of membranes present in cerebral tissue. Other special biochemicals include the neurotransmitters, dopamine, norepinephrine, epinephrine, serotonin and acetylcholine, which will be discussed in Chapter 5.

i) **Amino acids**

The total free amino acid concentration of the brain is some six to eight times higher than that of plasma, and higher than that of other body tissues. The composition of this free amino acid pool is very distinctive. High concentrations of unusual amino acids such as N-acetylaspartic acid, GABA, taurine and cystathionine occur (see following table). Glutamate, glutamine,

FREE AMINO ACIDS OF BRAIN
(Adapted from McIlwain & Bachelard[12])

Amino Acid	Concentration
	(μmoles/100 g wet weight)
Glutamate	780 – 1250
N-acetylaspartate	470 – 974
Glutamine	215 – 560
Taurine	125 – 535
Aspartate	153 – 272
γ-aminobutyrate	83 – 227
Serine	39 – 177
Glycine	55 – 146
Alanine	14 – 94
Lysine	11 – 22
Threonine	9 – 29
Arginine	7 – 16
Valine	12 – 18
Asparagine	11
Cystathionine	4 – 18
Leucine	7 – 14
Methionine	8 – 10
Proline	6 – 12
Isoleucine	6 – 9
Histidine	6 – 9
Phenylalanine	5 – 9
β-alanine	7
Tyrosine	3 – 11
Cystine	4
Tryptophan	2.5

aspartate, glycine and serine are present in large amounts relative to the other amino acids used for the synthesis of protein. The pattern of cerebral amino acid concentrations is remarkably similar in all species and differs little between brain regions. An exception to this is a progressive decrease in glutamate and an increase in GABA concentrations from rostral to caudal areas in the brain. This may be due to the larger number of inhibitory, GABA-containing neurons in the cerebellum and hindbrain. Embryonic and fetal brains have a free amino acid composition similar to that of other tissues, and most distinctive features of the free amino acid pool of brain such as the high concentrations of glutamic and aspartic acids, and of the less usual amino acids, appear during maturation of the brain.[13] The free amino acid pattern is also comparatively refractory to nutritional state. However, it is possible to alter cerebral free amino acid concentrations by loading the plasma, especially with leucine and phenylalanine.[14] In such cases, and in others where the amino acid pattern is disturbed, the *total* amount of free amino acids remains relatively constant.

What is the significance of the remarkable constancy and stability of the concentration pattern of the free amino acids of the brain? It is in part due to the probable role of some amino acids as neurotransmitters (glutamate, taurine, GABA and glycine, and possibly aspartate and serine), although the concentrations of other neurotransmitters (acetylcholine, the catecholamines) are very much lower. However, some amino acids that have no known or suspected neurotransmitter role are also present in high concentration (glutamine, N-acetylaspartate and cystathionine).

Glutamate

Glutamate is synthesized either by glutamic dehydrogenase or by one or other of the transaminases from α-ketoglutarate, a component of the tricarboxylic acid cycle. These enzymes are cytoplasmic and the reactions are reversible.

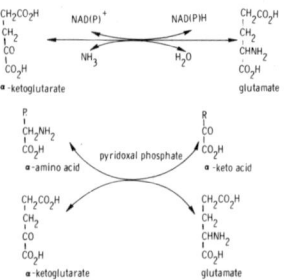

The concentration of glutamate in brain is exceedingly high (10mM) and this is probably only partially explained by its neurotransmitter role. It functions as a biosynthetic precursor of numerous compounds and is also concerned with controlling the levels of free ammonia, which is very toxic in brain. In addition, the high concentration of glutamate may reflect its possible role in the maintenance of cerebral homeostasis, as an energy reservoir and as a pH buffer. Free glutamate and aspartate levels may also be related to the large quantity of acidic proteins that characterize the mature nervous system and that contain many glutamic and aspartic residues (e.g., S-100 protein [p. 61]).

Glutamate may be a general excitatory substance, and the overall activity state of the brain may be controlled by the balance between glutamate and the inhibitory GABA (see p. 179).

Glutamine

Glutamine is synthesized from glutamate by glutamine synthetase.

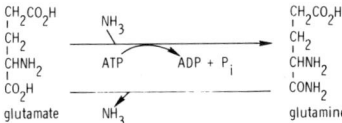

Glutamine has no detected neurotransmitter function, but is used in the synthesis of protein. Its principal function may be to control free ammonia levels in brain. The conversion of α-ketoglutarate to glutamate, and thence to glutamine, requires two ammonia molecules. Thus these reactions may be used to rapidly remove free ammonia released from other reactions. Methionine sulfoximine irreversibly inhibits glutamine synthetase, resulting in an increase of cerebral ammonia and also producing convulsions.

Aspartate

Aspartic acid is produced by transamination reactions from oxaloacetate, which is an intermediate in the tricarboxylic acid cycle.

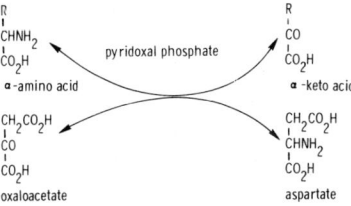

Aspartate is a precursor in the biosynthesis of asparagine, protein and pyrimidines, but has no established neurotransmitter role. It plays a central

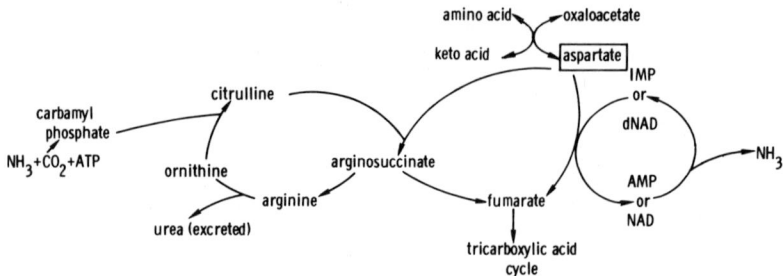

Figure 2.6 Ammonia production and the urea cycle.

role in the transfer of amino groups because it is a substrate for all cellular transaminases. Significantly, there is a large increase in the aspartate transaminase activity in the brain during maturation (twenty-fold in the rat).[15] All brain nitrogen catabolism may be channeled through aspartate as a final common pathway (Figure 2.6). Amino nitrogen from aspartate may be catabolized to urea in two ways: aspartate can transfer its amino group to citrulline forming arginosuccinate, a constituent of the urea cycle; or it can aminate inosine monophosphate (IMP) to adenosine monophosphate (AMP). A parallel reaction converts nicotinamide inosine dinucleotide (deamino-NAD, dNAD) to nicotinamide adenine dinucleotide (NAD). Simple deamination of these adenine nucleotides probably represents the principal source of free ammonia in the brain.[16]

N-acetylaspartate

N-acetylaspartate is formed by acetylation of aspartic acid by acetyl CoA. The high concentration of N-acetylaspartate in brain is an enigma. It has no known function, and radioactive tracer studies suggest that it is metabolically inactive with a very slow turnover of both aspartate and acetyl moieties. Its role may be that of an inert, passive anion balancing the high intracellular K^+ concentration of neurons.

Gamma-aminobutyric acid

Gamma-aminobutyric acid (GABA) is formed by α-decarboxylation of glutamate by glutamic decarboxylase (GAD).

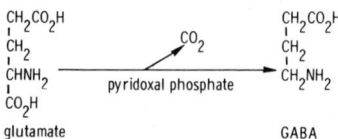

GAD and GABA are largely confined to the nervous system, which suggests a unique neural function for GABA. Breakdown of GABA starts by transamination with α-ketoglutarate to succinic semialdehyde.

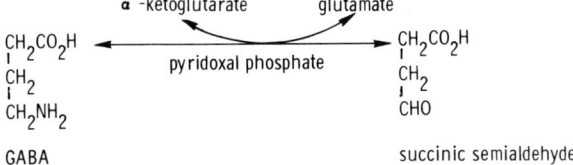

The succinic semialdehyde may be further metabolized by a dehydrogenase to succinate, which can enter the tricarboxylic acid cycle. This series of four reactions then forms an alternative route to part of the tricarboxylic acid cycle (Figure 2.5). Radioactive tracer studies suggest that as much as 8 percent of the cycle in the brain may be channeled through this *GABA shunt*. Metabolism by this route produces only three energy-rich bonds as opposed to four by the conventional tricarboxylic acid cycle route. The shunt is therefore probably more important in GABA production than in energy production. In agreement with this, GAD is only found in those motor neurons in the lobster, which use GABA as a neurotransmitter (p. 142).

GABA is an inhibitory neurotransmitter in several invertebrate systems and probably also in the vertebrate brain. Moreover, it has been implicated in a general inhibitory role in brain (p. 179).

Taurine and cystathionine

Taurine and cystathionine are two sulfur-containing amino acids present in relatively high concentrations in brain. They are both derived from methionine (Figure 2.7). Taurine may have a neurotransmitter function especially in the retina, but no such function has been suggested for cystathionine. Cystathionine is more concentrated in white than in gray matter and may merely be an intermediary metabolite in sulfur metabolism, important in the synthesis of taurine, sulfatides and sulfated mucopolysaccharides.

N-acetylhistidine

N-acetylhistidine is found in the brains of fishes, reptiles and amphibia, but not in birds or mammals. It is formed by direct acetylation of histidine by acetylCoA. Its function is unknown.

Urea

Urea is present in high concentration in brain. It is the end product of catabolism of most nitrogenous compounds and is produced by operation of the urea cycle (Figure 2.6). However, while brain tissue can convert citrul-

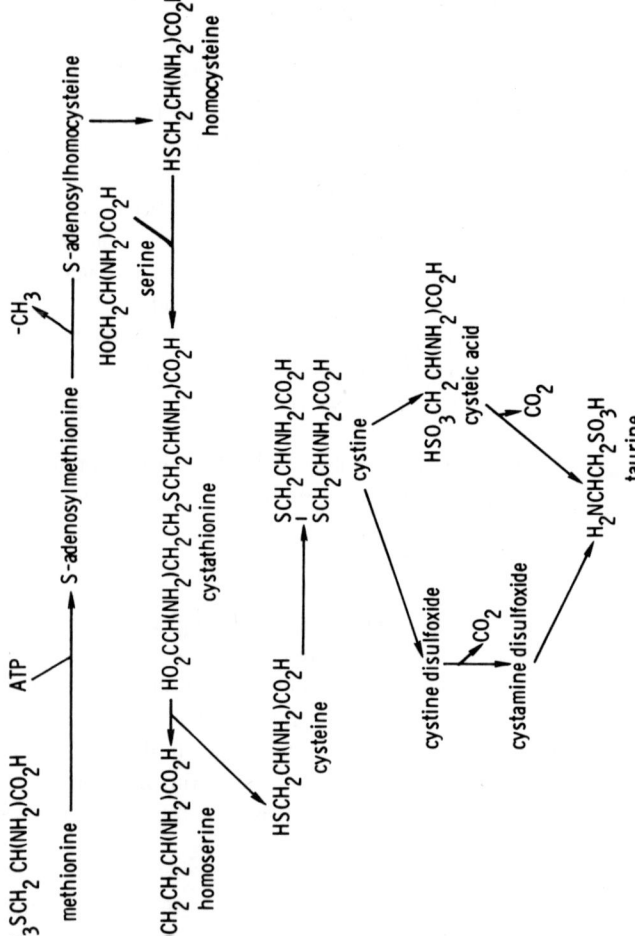

Figure 2.7 Synthesis of the sulfur-containing amino acids, cystathionine and taurine.

line to arginine and split the latter to yield urea and ornithine, the synthesis of citrulline has not been demonstrated in brain. Nor has ornithine transcarbamylase, the enzyme responsible for the synthesis of citrulline, been detected in the brain. Furthermore, the activity of carbamyl phosphate synthetase is exceedingly low. It is possible that in the brain urea synthesis operates not as a complete cycle, but as part of a cycle in which plasma citrulline is converted to ornithine. If this is so, there is no obvious reason for it.

ii) Peptides

Glutathione (GSH)

The tripeptide glutathione accounts for up to one-third of nonmacromolecular (acid-extractable) nitrogen and about 95 percent of the sulfhydryl groups of brain. It is synthesized as follows:

$$\text{glutamate} + \text{cysteine} + \text{ATP} \xrightarrow{Mg^{2+}} \gamma\text{-glutamylcysteine} + \text{ADP} + P_i$$

$$\gamma\text{-glutamylcysteine} + \text{glycine} + \text{ATP} \xrightarrow{Mg^{2+}} \gamma\text{-glutamylcysteinylglycine (GSH)} + \text{ADP} + P_i$$

Glutathione is ubiquitous and has several known functions. An important role in amino acid transport has recently been demonstrated.[17] It had been known for a number of years that the γ-glutamyl group of glutathione could be transferred to amino acids to form γ-glutamyl peptides.

glutathione + amino acid ↔ γ-glutamylamino acid + cysteinylglycine

Many different amino acids could participate in this reaction.

The γ-glutamyl peptides had been isolated from a number of sources but were particularly prominent in brain. Meister has now demonstrated that the γ-glutamyl transfer is part of a cycle concerned with amino acid transport in the kidney and probably also in the brain. The sequence of reactions involved is known as the γ-glutamyl cycle (Figure 2.8).

All these reactions have been demonstrated in the kidney, and the cycle has been shown to operate with all the physiological amino acids except

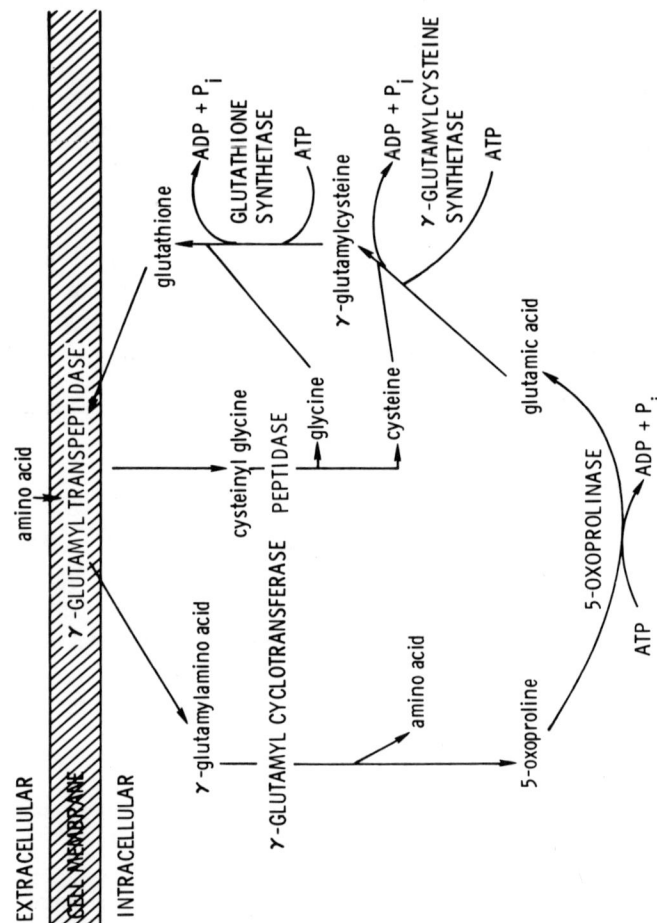

Figure 2.8 The γ-glutamyl cycle for the intracellular uptake of amino acids. (After Meister[17]).

proline. Most of the reactions have also been demonstrated in brain. The key feature is the ability of the membrane-bound enzyme γ-glutamyl transpeptidase to transfer γ-glutamyl groups to amino acids on the outside of the cell membrane and release the resulting dipeptide inside the cell. This dipeptide is then hydrolyzed, releasing the free amino acid inside the cell. Thus the particular location of this enzyme enables it to translocate amino acids from the outside to the inside of the cell. The rest of the cycle is concerned with the resynthesis of glutathione. Operation of the γ-glutamyl cycle requires three ATP molecules per amino acid taken up. This seems extraordinarily high, but other biochemical processes such as urea formation and protein synthesis are also "expensive" in terms of ATP. The high energy requirement does, however, explain the energy dependence of the amino acid uptake systems.

It remains to be determined whether the transport of all amino acids occurs by this mechanism, and what the role of Na^+ is in this process. To reconcile this new cycle with the known multiple systems for amino acid uptake, γ-glutamyl transpeptidases with different specificities have been proposed. Alternatively the specificity may occur in receptor sites on the membrane from which the amino acids could be transferred to a common transpeptidase.

Other roles of glutathione include that of an oxidation reduction buffer. Disulfides can be reduced by glutathione to thiols with a resulting oxidation of glutathione to the disulfide form (GSSG):

$$RSSR' + 2GSH \longleftrightarrow RSH + R'SH + GSSG$$

The oxidized glutathione may then be reduced again by reduced NADP.

$$GSSG + NADPH + H^+ \longleftrightarrow 2GSH + NADP^+$$

Glutathione also binds heavy metals and reduces hydrogen peroxide.

$$2GSH + H_2O_2 \longrightarrow GSSG + 2H_2O$$

Finally, glutathione is a cofactor in a number of reactions of enzymes such as glyoxylase and DDT-dehydrochlorinase in which no oxidoreduction occurs.

Substance P

In 1933 Von Euler and Gaddum discovered a substance in brain extracts that caused contraction of the gut and was a powerful vasodilator. They named the active principal *substance P*. It is found in nervous tissue and intestine of all vertebrate species. Substance P is a peptide which has now been purified from bovine hypothalamus, and the inferior and superior colliculi. The sequence of its 11 amino acids has been determined and confirmed by synthesis.[18] In the nervous system, substance P is probably neuronal since it is absent from glial tumors and disappears when nerves degenerate. The degradation of substance P is specifically inhibited by LSD. There is some evidence that substance P has a neurohumoral function in spinal cord, and it is likely to exert similar effects elsewhere.[19]

Other peptides

Several peptides unique to the brain have been characterized (other than those found in the pituitary, Chapter 6). Two related brain-specific peptides are *homocarnosine* (γ-aminobutyrylhistidine) and *homoanserine* (γ-aminobutyryl-l-methylhistidine). *N-acetylaspartylglutamate* and *N-acetylglutamylglutamate* are also exclusive to the central nervous system. Some phosphopeptides have been detected, as well. The phosphate in these peptides is esterified with serine and has a very rapid turnover. Undoubtedly many uncharacterized peptides exist in brain and these may have neurohumoral functions.

iii) Nucleotides[3]

There are no special nucleotides prominent in brain but the concentrations of several, including cytidine and uridine diphosphate derivatives and cyclic GMP, are relatively high compared with other tissues. The adenine nucleotides predominate, with lesser quantities of the guanine and uracil nucleotides, and still smaller quantities of the cytosine nucleotides (see following table). This pattern of nucleotides is characteristic of all species and brain regions and develops during maturation. The high concentration of all adenine nucleotides may be related to the great need for ATP in the active metabolism of brain. Guanine nucleotides are also used as energy sources for several reactions, notably peptide bond formation in protein synthesis. They also participate in the transfer of fucose and mannose to glycoproteins (p. 97) and in the formation of cyclic GMP. Uracil nucleotides are used extensively in glycoprotein, glycolipid and polysaccharide synthesis, and cytosine nucleotides for the transfer of alcohols in lipid biosynthesis (p. 82).

Most of the free nucleotides in brain are present as the triphosphate derivatives, but the proportion of cytidine triphosphate is relatively low. Since the nucleotide triphosphates are the immediate precursors of RNA, it has been suggested that the level of cytidine triphosphate may limit the rate of cerebral RNA synthesis.[3]

Since the metabolic rate of brain is so high, the nucleoside triphosphates

FREE NUCLEOTIDES OF BRAIN (35-day-old rat)
(from Mandel and Edel-Harth[20])

Nucleotide	Concentration	
	(μmoles/100 g wet weight)	
ATP	223.0	⎫
ADP	16.0	⎬ Total adenine 67.1%
AMP	–	⎭
CTP	3.1	⎫
CMP	0.3	⎬ Total cytosine 3.1%
CDPcholine + CDPethanolamine	7.7	⎭
GTP	33.7	⎫
GDP	9.0	⎬ Total guanine 12.8%
GMP	3.0	⎭
IMP	3.9	
NAD	7.6	
UTP	26.7	⎫
UDP	1.9	⎬ Total uracil 13.9%
UMP	1.0	⎪
UDPglucose + UDPglucosamine	19.9	⎭
Total nucleotides	356.8	

are very rapidly degraded to di- and monophosphates following death or anoxia. In order to extract the nucleotides from brain in their *in vivo* state of phosphorylation, the tissue must be very rapidly frozen. In practice this is done by immersing the live animal in liquid nitrogen or some other low-temperature coolant. Even then it may take thirty seconds or so before the center of the brain becomes cooled to 0°C. Fortunately, it appears that the blood circulation continues in the unfrozen central regions of the brain while the outer regions are being frozen, since the ratio of ATP to ADP obtained is similar for inner and outer regions. Also, freezing of severed heads produces lower ATP values. Recently a new technique for obtaining samples of frozen brain tissue very rapidly has been devised. This technique uses a jet of compressed air to blow the entire brain out of the skull and into a liquid nitrogen-cooled chamber.[21] It is estimated that in this way brain samples can be frozen in one second or less, permitting more accurate estimates of metabolism to be made, albeit with some loss of anatomical definition.

The nucleotides may be synthesized *de novo* in the brain, or nucleosides may be taken up from the plasma and phosphorylated by the so-called *salvage* pathways. The *de novo* synthesis of purines,[3] but not pyrimidines, has been demonstrated in brain.[22] However, pyrimidines may be syn-

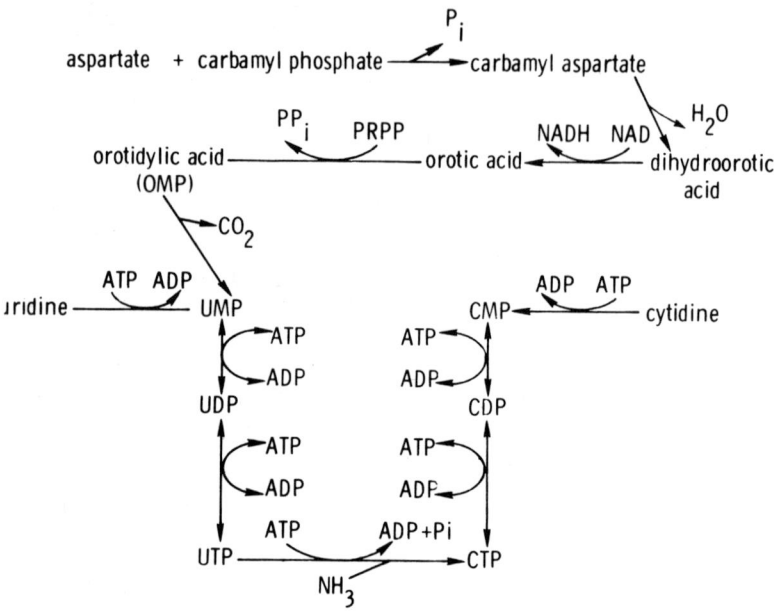

Figure 2.9 The synthesis of pyrimidine nucleotides.

thesized in brain, since all the enzymes in the pathway have been detected in brain extracts (although the activity of carbamylphosphate synthetase is very low). The biosynthetic pathways are similar to those of other tissues (Figures 2.9, 2.10).

Nucleosides are readily taken up by the brain from the blood, whereas bases and nucleotides are not. Uridine, cytidine or thymidine can be phosphorylated to mononucleotides by pyrimidine nucleoside kinase.

$$\left.\begin{matrix} \text{cytidine} \\ \text{thymidine} \\ \text{uridine} \end{matrix}\right\} + \text{ATP} \rightarrow \left\{\begin{matrix} \text{CMP} \\ \text{TMP} \\ \text{UMP} \end{matrix}\right. + \text{ADP}$$

A second enzyme performs a similar function for adenosine and probably guanosine.

$$\left.\begin{matrix} \text{adenosine} \\ \text{guanosine} \end{matrix}\right\} + \text{ATP} \rightarrow \left\{\begin{matrix} \text{AMP} \\ \text{GMP} \end{matrix}\right. + \text{ADP}$$

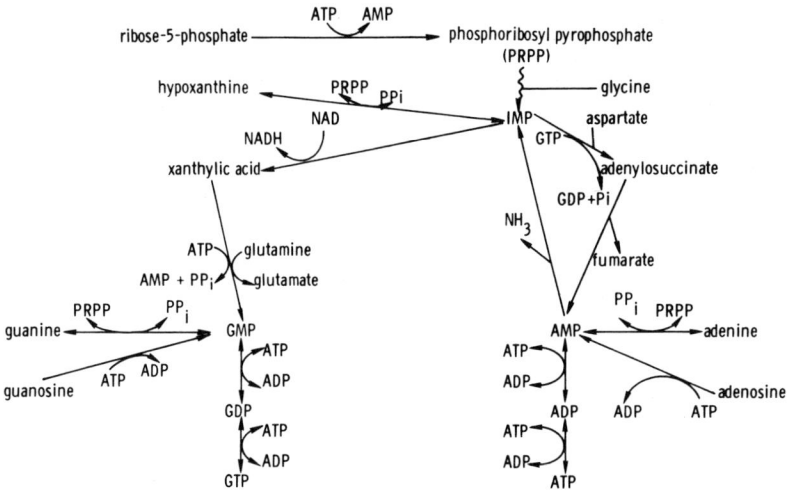

Figure 2.10 The synthesis of purine nucleotides.

In addition the purine bases may be converted to the corresponding mononucleotides by using phosphoribosyl pyrophosphate (PRPP) and the enzyme phosphoribosyl pyrophosphate transferase.

$$\left.\begin{array}{l}\text{adenine}\\ \text{guanine}\\ \text{hypoxanthine}\end{array}\right\} + \text{PRPP} \longrightarrow \left\{\begin{array}{l}\text{AMP}\\ \text{GMP}\\ \text{TMP}\end{array}\right. + \text{PP}_i$$

There are two enzymes which perform this reaction, one for adenine and one for hypoxanthine and guanine. Both enzymes are very active in the brain. However, they cannot be involved in cerebral uptake since the free bases are virtually absent from plasma. It has been suggested that the enzymes are used for the transfer of free bases, either between subcellular compartments or between cells. Adenine is selectively incorporated into adenine nucleotide pools that are immediate precursors of cyclic AMP, whereas adenosine is not. Thus, adenine phosphoribosyl transferase may be associated with a specific brain compartment (p. 188).

The relative importance of the *de novo* and salvage pathways is controversial. Inhibitors of both purine and pyrimidine synthesis affect nucleotide metabolism and cause neurological defects. 6-azauridine, an inhibitor of orotic acid decarboxylase, depresses free uridine nucleotide levels 30 to 60 percent, and causes abnormalities of the EEG and a lack of motor coordination.[23] Genetic defects in the pathways of purine and pyrimidine metabolism cause neurological disorders in man. One such disease, orotic aciduria, is characterized by excretion of orotic acid. This occurs because the enzymes orotidylic acid pyrophosphatase and decarboxylase, essential for pyrimidine synthesis, are absent. The defect in orotic aciduria may be corrected by oral uridine, so that an exogenous supply of pyrimidine will suffice in this case. This suggests that in man the *de novo* pathway for pyrimidine synthesis is unnecessary in the presence of sufficient preformed compounds. Further evidence for the importance of the salvage pathway is that the absence of hypoxanthine-guanine phosphoribosyl transferase causes severe neurological defects (Lesch-Nyhan syndrome, Chapter 9).

Cyclic Nucleotides[4]

The only naturally occurring 3′,5′cyclic nucleotides are cyclic 3′, 5′AMP and cyclic 3′,5′GMP. The concentration of cyclic AMP in brain is about 1 to 2 nmoles/gram tissue and that of cyclic GMP about 0.2 nmoles/gram tissue. The concentrations of the cyclic nucleotides are thus about one thousandth of the total for each purine base. While the brain concentration of cyclic AMP is typical for most tissues, that of cyclic GMP is the highest observed for any tissue. The concentration of cyclic AMP in the brain rises very rapidly after death and, as in the case of the nucleoside triphosphates, brain tissue must be frozen very rapidly to obtain accurate estimates. A rather unusual alternative fixation procedure has recently been developed for the cyclic nucleotides. The enzymes for both the synthesis and the degradation of cyclic AMP are unstable to heat, but cyclic AMP itself is not. Thus the cyclic AMP can be "fixed" in the intact animal with the use of microwave irradiation. Using this procedure, the fixation time can be considerably reduced and better cyclic AMP values obtained.[24]

Cyclic AMP and cyclic GMP are formed by separate enzymes from their respective nucleoside triphosphates.

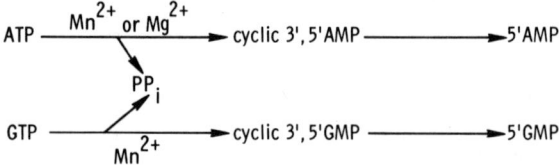

Adenyl cyclase is associated with plasma membranes, whereas guanyl cyclase is soluble. Subcellular fractionation studies suggest that adenyl cyclase is partially concentrated in synaptosomes, and that guanyl cyclase may be neuronal and perhaps synaptosomal. The adenyl cyclase from brain requires

Mg^{2+} or Mn^{2+} and is inhibited by Ca^{2+}. Guanyl cyclase, however, requires Mn^{2+} for which Mg^{2+} will not substitute. Brain adenyl cyclase is stimulated by a variety of neurotransmitters including norepinephrine, dopamine, serotonin and histamine. It is also markedly stimulated by adenosine, and it has been suggested that it is this stimulation which may be responsible for the rise in brain cyclic AMP observed following decapitation or during convulsions. It is presumed that small amounts of adenosine may be released subsequent to the mass degradation of adenine nucleotides which occurs during anoxia.

The cyclic nucleotides are degraded by hydrolysis to 5'mononucleotides by cyclic nucleotide phosphodiesterases. There are separate enzymes for cyclic AMP and cyclic GMP, and at least three distinct cyclic AMP phosphodiesterases have been detected in brain. The phosphodiesterases are both particulate and soluble. Cyclic AMP phosphodiesterase is concentrated in synaptosomal fractions and has been shown histochemically to be associated with postsynaptic membranes. All the phosphodiesterases are inhibited by the methyl xanthines, theophylline and caffeine.

The enzymes for the synthesis and degradation of cyclic AMP are present in brain in greater amounts than in any other tissue. This suggests a very active metabolism and probably an important role for cyclic nucleotides in the brain — possibly in synaptic transmission; the evidence for this will be discussed in Chapter 7. Both cyclic nucleotides stimulate the phosphorylation of proteins by protein kinases, and this may be the unitary mechanism underlying their activity. Each of the two cyclic nucleotides stimulates distinct kinases. In the brain, cyclic AMP does not accelerate glycogen and lipid breakdown, and decrease glycogen synthesis, as it does in other tissues.

D. METABOLIC COMPARTMENTATION [5]

Several studies have indicated that certain low molecular weight compounds are not homogeneously distributed in the brain, but appear in distinct compartments or pools, with differing rates of turnover. This compartmentation appears during cerebral maturation and reflects the fact that plasma membranes and those of subcellular organelles are not freely permeable to many metabolites. Compartmentation may thus occur between cells or between different subcellular compartments of the same cell. Because similar types of cells are likely to have similar metabolic properties, a biochemical compartment may encompass many thousands of cells and thus be composed of very many microcompartments.

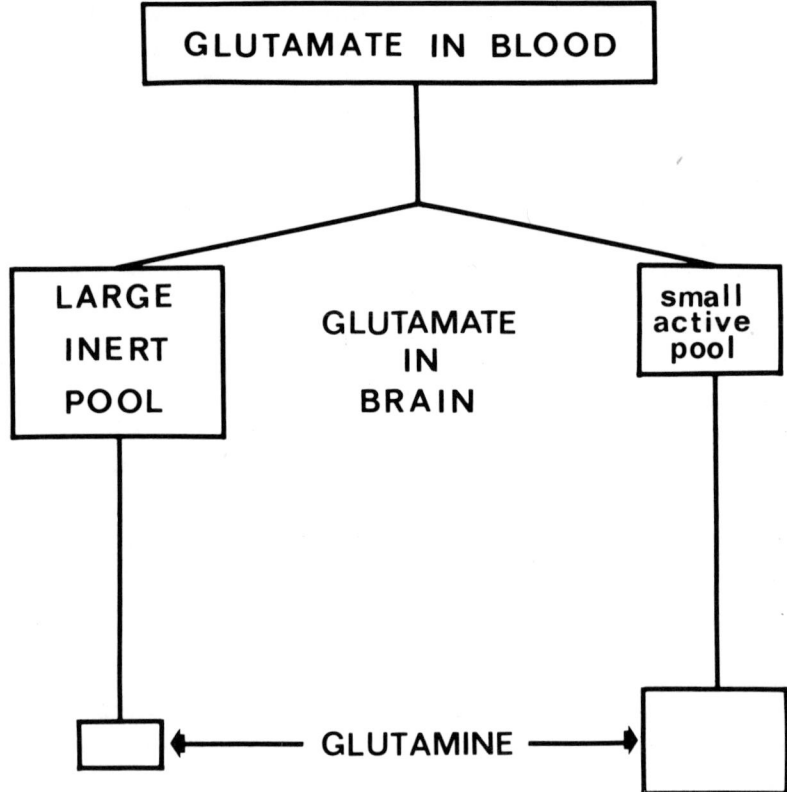

Figure 2.11 The compartmentation of brain glutamate and glutamine.

The results that indicate compartmentation arise from studies where radioactive isotopes are administered and the specific radioactivities* of the administered precursor and various products examined. In the case of [^{14}C]glutamate, following either intravenous or intracisternal injection, the specific radioactivity of the glutamine isolated from the brain is considerably higher than that of the glutamate isolated from the same tissue.[15] The simplest explanation of this phenomenon is that there is a large compartment of glutamate that contains relatively little glutamine, and a smaller compartment of glutamate that contains relatively greater quantities of glutamine. If the exogenously administered glutamate readily penetrates the smaller compartment but not the larger one, then the *net* specific radioactivity of glutamine could be higher than that of glutamate (Figure 2.11).

*Specific radioactivity = radioactivity/molar or gram amount.

Rose has studied the distribution and metabolism of glutamate between neuronal perikarya and "neuropil" fractions separated by centrifugal methods.[25] The neuronal perikarya contained less glutamate and more glutamine than the neuropil, but only the neuropil showed a specific activity of glutamine greater than that of glutamate following the injection of [^{14}C]glutamate. Since the neuropil fraction contains a mixture of nerve terminals and glial cells, the results are consistent with the interpretation that the large glutamate compartment is glial or in the nerve terminals, and the small glutamate compartment in the neuronal cell bodies. A complete kinetic analysis of cerebral glutamate metabolism suggests the existence of at least three compartments, the third of which could reasonably be mitochondrial.

Similar kinds of phenomena have been observed for other radioactive precursors, especially those closely related to the tricarboxylic acid cycle or to neurotransmitter metabolism. Compartments for the latter may be confined to neurons that use the particular neurotransmitter and could be presynaptic. Apparent compartmentation of adenine nucleotides used for the synthesis of cyclic AMP has been mentioned above (see p. 188).

The existence of compartmentation, which appears to be much more highly developed in brain than in other tissues, poses serious problems in the interpretation of isotope data from *in vivo* studies. For example, it is difficult to know the real specific radioactivity of a precursor for the synthesis of macromolecules because it may be distributed among several compartments, yet only a net specific radioactivity for the whole brain may be measured. This limitation severely handicaps the interpretation of data on the rates of synthesis and the half-lives of molecular species.

CHAPTER 2 REFERENCES

Reviews and General References

1. Sokoloff, L., Circulation and energy metabolism of the brain. In *Basic Neurochemistry* (Ed. R. W. Albers, G. J. Siegel, R. Katzmann and B. W. Agranoff), Little, Brown and Company, Boston, 1972, pp. 299–325.
2. Maker, H. S., and Lehrer, G. M. Carbohydrate chemistry of brain. In *Basic Neurochemistry* (Ed. R. W. Albers, G. J. Siegel, R. Katzmann, and B. W. Agranoff), Little, Brown and Company, Boston, 1972, pp. 169–89.
3. Mandel, P. Free nucleotides. In *Handbook of Neurochemistry*, Vol. 5. (Ed. A. Lajtha), Plenum Press, New York, 1971, pp. 249–82.
4. *Advances in Cyclic Nucleotide Research*, Vol. I. (Ed. P. Greengard, R. Paoletti and G. A. Robinson), Raven Press, New York, 1972, pp. 317–477.
5. *Metabolic Compartmentation in the Brain* (Ed. R. Balázs and J. E. Cremer), John Wiley, New York, 1972.

Literature Cited

6. Sokoloff, L. Changes in enzyme activities in neural tissues with maturation and development of the nervous system. In *The Neurosciences, Third Study Program* (Ed. F. O. Schmitt and F. G. Worden), M.I.T. Press, Cambridge, Mass., 1974, pp. 885–98.
7. Geiger, A., and Yamasaki, S. Cytidine and uridine requirement of the brain. *J. Neurochem.* 1:93–100, 1956.
8. Krieglstein, G., Krieglstein, J., and Urban, W. Long survival time of an isolated perfused rat brain. *J. Neurochem.* 19:885–86, 1972.
9. Miller, A. L., Hawkins, R. A., and Veech, R. L. Phenylketonuria: Phenylalanine inhibits brain pyruvate kinase *in vivo*. *Science* 179:904–06, 1973.
10. Neame, K. D. A comparison of the transport system for amino acids in brain, intestine, kidney and tumour. *Prog. Brain Res.* 29:185–96, 1968.
11. Wurtman, R. J., and Ferstrom, J. D. Nutrition and the brain. In *The Neurosciences, Third Study Program* (Ed. F. O. Schmitt and F. G. Worden), M.I.T. Press, Cambridge, Mass., 1974, pp. 685–93.
12. McIlwain, H., and Bachelard, H. S. *Biochemistry and the Central Nervous System*, 4th ed., Churchill-Livingstone, London, 1971.
13. Davis, J. M., and Himwich, W. A. Amino acids and proteins of developing mammalian brain. In *Biochemistry of the Developing Brain*, Vol. I. (Ed. W. Himwich), Marcel Dekker, New York, 1973, pp. 55–110.
14. Roberts, S. Influence of elevated circulating levels of amino acids on cerebral concentrations and utilization of amino acids. *Prog. Brain Research* 29:235–43, 1968.
15. Berl, S. Metabolic compartmentation in developing brain. In *Biochemistry of the Developing Brain*, Vol. I. (Ed. W. Himwich), Marcel Dekker, New York, 1973, pp. 219–52.
16. Buniatian, H. C. Deamination of nucleotides and the role of their deamino forms in ammonia formation from amino acids. In *Handbook of Neurochemistry*, Vol. 3. (Ed. A. Lajtha), Plenum Press, New York, 1970, pp. 399–413.
17. Meister, A. On the enzymology of amino acid transport. *Science* 180:33–39, 1973.
18. Chang, M. M., Leeman, S. E., and Niall, H. D. Amino-acid sequence of substance P. *Nature, New Biology* 232:86–87, 1971.
19. Krivoy, W., and Zimmerman, E. A possible role of polypeptides in synaptic transmission. In *Chemical Modulation of Brain Function* (Ed. H. C. Sabelli), Raven Press, New York, 1973, pp. 111–21.
20. Mandel, P., and Edel-Harth, S. Free nucleotides in the rat brain during post-natal development. *J. Neurochem.* 13:591–95, 1966.
21. Veech, R. L., Harris, R. L., Veloso, D., and Veech, E. H. Freeze-blowing: a new technique for the study of brain *in vivo*. *J. Neurochem.* 20:183–88, 1973.
22. Bourget, P. A., and Tremblay, G. C. Pyrimidine biosynthesis in rat brain. *J. Neurochem.* 19:1617–24, 1972. See also addendum, *J. Neurochem.* 19:2472, 1972.
23. Koenig, H. Neurobiological action of some pyrimidine analogs. *Int. Rev. Neurobiol.* 10:199–229, 1967.
24. Schmidt, M. J., Schmidt, D. E., and Robison, G. A. Cyclic adenosine monophosphate in brain areas: microwave irradiation as a means of tissue fixation. *Science* 173:1142–43, 1971.
25. Rose, S. P. R. The compartmentation of glutamate and its metabolites in fractions of neuron cell bodies and neuropil; studied by intraventricular injection of $[U^{-14}C]$ glutamate. *J. Neurochem.* 17:809–16, 1970.

III. Genetic Expression in the Brain

A. GENOME TO PROTEIN

i) Nuclei

The genetic apparatus of brain cells is largely confined to the nucleus, but as in other cells there is a small amount of genetic autonomy in mitochondria. Although nuclei of brain cells vary greatly in size, neuronal nuclei are generally larger than glial (especially oligodendroglial and microglial). Nuclei can be separated on the basis of size and thus to some extent of cell type by sucrose gradient centrifugation.[8] Neuronal nuclei from the mature animal usually contain only a single prominent nucleolus (a small, particularly dense-staining spot within the nucleus), but those from the immature animal may contain multiple nucleoli. In contrast, nucleoli are not obvious in glial cells, though they can be demonstrated in both astroglia and oligodendroglia. Astroglial nuclei are large and pale, while oligodendroglial nuclei contain clumps of aggregated chromatin associated with the limiting membrane. The nucleus comprises the major part of the neuronal cell body, and neurons with large cell bodies such as pyramidal cells, Purkinje cells or the giant motor neurons of the anterior horn of the spinal cord have the largest nuclei.

Nuclear metabolism has not been studied extensively because pure preparations are not easy to obtain. Neuronal nuclei are frequently deeply invaginated with cytoplasm, and tissue homogenization may result in the inclusion of cytoplasmic organelles within the nuclei. Separation procedures are based on the high density of nuclei, and require hypertonic media which result in the loss of soluble components.[8] Other components may be lost through the large pores in the nuclear membrane. Nuclei may also be separated by procedures using nonaqueous media which allow study of the soluble components.[8] Using these methods, nuclear nucleotide metabolism has been studied and nuclei have been shown to contain 10 percent of the free nucleotides of brain. The relative proportions of the four principal bases in nuclear nucleotides are indistinguishable from those found in the cytoplasm.[9]

ii) Deoxyribonucleic Acid (DNA)

Although brain cells vary greatly in size, they all apparently contain approximately the same amount of DNA (about 7 picograms per cell in rats). This is the same as in other diploid nondividing cells in the body. The cerebellum contains the highest concentration of DNA, which may be due to the greater concentration of cells in this region. However, cytospectrophotometric observations in several laboratories suggested that the large nuclei of cerebellar Purkinje cells and hippocampal pyramidal cells contained twice the diploid amount of DNA, and it was suggested that these cells might be tetraploid. More recent observations, including direct chemical analyses, show that the earlier results concerning Purkinje cells were an experimental artifact and that the cells are after all diploid.[10,11] However, in this latter study some cerebellar glial cells were found to be tetraploid.[11] The giant neurons of invertebrates (notably those in the *Aplysia* abdominal ganglion) contain large quantities of DNA, up to more than one thousand times the diploid amount.[12] Since in these neurons the DNA content is always an exact power of 2 times the diploid amount, it seems likely that this is genuine ploidy rather than selective gene amplification. Such multiploidy may reflect the greater demands on the genetic material of the large-sized cells.

Brain DNA is indistinguishable from that of other cells in the body by the criteria of base-composition or DNA-DNA hybridization.*[13]

---

*Hybridization techniques exploit the complementarity of sequences inherent in the double-stranded structure of DNA. The separated strands have a high affinity for their complements and may thus be hybridized together in the test tube. Such tests are sensitive measures for the similarity of base sequences in DNA or RNA.

Differentiated neurons never divide, although neuroblast division may occur postnatally in some species.[1] Thus most neurons have the same life span as the animal. Since DNA in non-dividing cells is not renewed, neuronal DNA molecules must be remarkably stable, especially in long-lived animals. In view of this longevity it is likely that DNA repair mechanisms operate in neurons. The interdiction of neuronal DNA synthesis may be regulated by cytoplasmic factors since DNA synthesis can be induced in neuronal nuclei by transplanting them into the cytoplasm of embryonic cells.[14] Glial cells of all types divide, though their rate of division is generally not great. However, in certain pathological states such as mechanical injury to the brain, astroglia and microglia may proliferate extensively.

The data concerning neuronal death are conflicting.[15] In humans, studies of post-mortem material suggest strongly that there is a decline in the number of neurons in the brain after about twenty years of age, and there are some indications that the rate of loss accelerates after about the age of sixty. The neurons are to a certain extent replaced by oligodendroglia or astrocytes, but there may also be an increase in extracellular space. Several careful studies in mice and rats have not shown detectable changes in the total number of cells or amount of DNA in aged animals, while other studies have noted declines in both. A recent study suggests that there is no decline in the number of neurons in mouse brain up until about two years, after which there is a sharp decline preceding death.[16] This decline may be a consequence of other physiological manifestations of senility. The disparity between the human and animal studies may only reflect the greater time span of human lives. If mature neurons cannot divide, some loss is to be expected in sixty years.

Brain mitochondria, like those of other tissues, contain small amounts of DNA. Despite the large numbers of mitochondria, mitochondrial DNA accounts for less than 0.1 percent of the total DNA in the brain. This is because the DNA content of mitochondria is very low.

DNA is synthesized by the enzyme DNA polymerase from the deoxyribonucleotide triphosphates of adenine, cytosine, guanine and thymine. These precursors are at such low concentrations that they are not easily detectable in normal nucleotide analyses of brain. Two different DNA polymerases from rat brain have been distinguished. In several species the total DNA polymerase activity falls dramatically with development. In the rat the decrease in the two polymerases is disproportionate.[17] This may reflect different cellular origins, but it is also possible that one enzyme is used for DNA replication and the other for DNA repair. In rat brain, mitochondrial DNA polymerase is distinguishable from the nuclear enzymes by its sedimentation coefficient. Its activity also decreases markedly with development, accounting for 9 percent of the total in the ten-day-old but less than 1 percent in the adult.[17]

iii) Chromosomal Protein

Chromosomes contain protein and RNA closely associated with the DNA. The proteins have been classified into two types: *histones,* which are soluble in dilute mineral acids, and *non-histone* (sometimes *acidic*) proteins. Histones are basic proteins by virtue of their high content of arginine and lysine. They are thought to be nonspecific repressors of gene expression which act by binding ionically to the acidic DNA. There are a rather limited number of different histones and most of these are not tissue-specific, and are present in the brain in the same proportions as in other tissues. The histones are very stable, with half-lives of the order of weeks, but may turn over more rapidly than the DNA.[18] They may be modified by acetylation or methylation of the lysine groups and by phosphorylation of the serine and threonine groups. These reactions may modify the affinity of the histones for the DNA and thus have significance for genetic derepression.

In contrast, there are many diverse non-histone proteins in brain, many of which are tissue-specific.[19] Some of these may regulate the precise expression of the cerebral genome, blocking or unblocking distinct regions of the DNA by directing the binding positions of the histones. Exposed DNA segments can then be transcribed into messenger RNA and hence the genes expressed. Nuclear acidic proteins may also be reversibly phosphorylated on serine residues, and changes in the phosphorylation have been observed in animals exposed to various behavioral treatments (p. 216).

iv) Ribonucleic Acid (RNA)

Four major types of RNA may be characterized in eukaryotic cells: ribosomal RNA (rRNA), transfer RNA (tRNA), messenger RNA (mRNA) and heterogeneous nuclear RNA (hnRNA).

By far the most predominant of these is ribosomal RNA, accounting for approximately 70 percent of the total in brain cells. Most of this is present as part of the structure of ribosomes in the cytoplasm, though small amounts may be present in the nucleus as ribosomal precursors. Ribosomal RNA is of three types: 28S, 18S and 5S, characterized by their sedimentation coefficients in a centrifugal field, roughly related to their size. 28S and 18S rRNA's are derived from a single 45S precursor in the nucleolus according to the scheme of Figure 3.1. 45S RNA is transcribed from DNA by RNA polymerase I. This transcription is particularly sensitive to inhibition by ac-

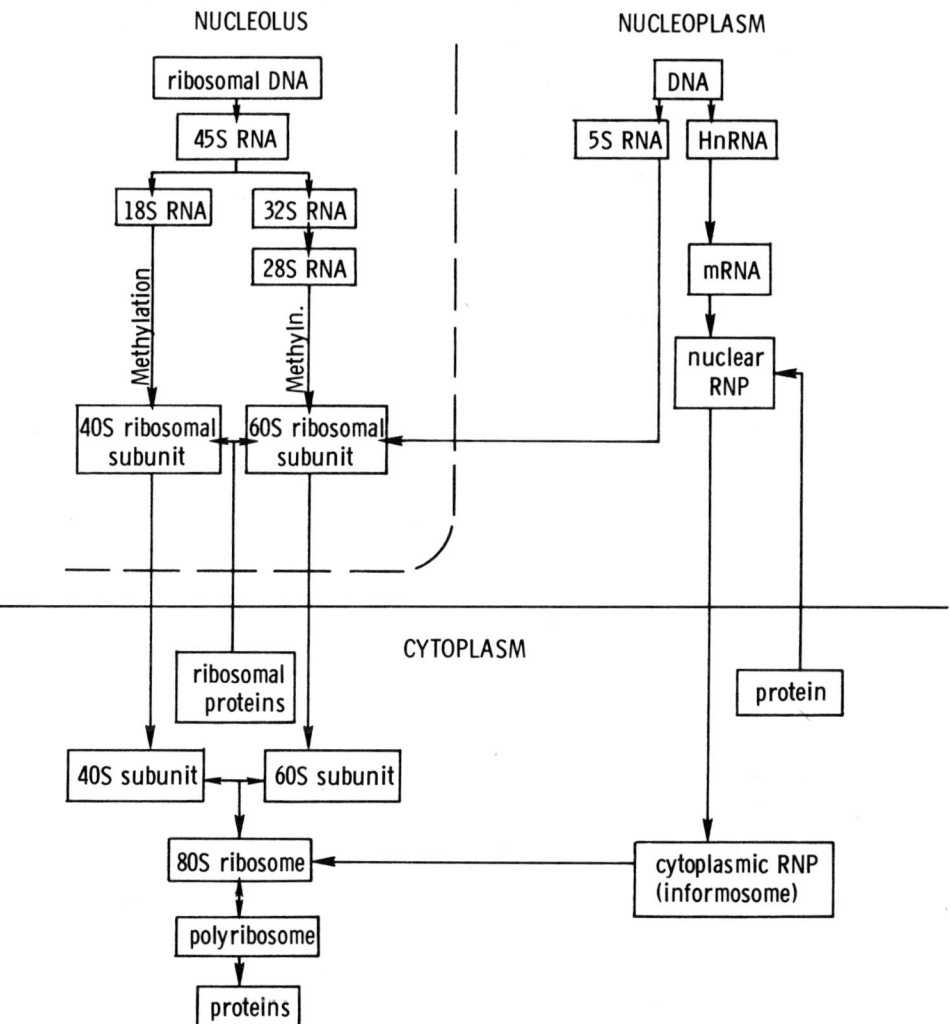

Figure 3.1 The synthesis of RNA, ribosomes and proteins in animal cells.

tinomycin D, a drug which acts by binding to guanine bases in double-stranded DNA. The selective inhibition of rRNA synthesis may thus be due to the high content of guanine and cytosine bases (60 percent) in DNA regions responsible for rRNA synthesis. Before being incorporated into the ribosomal structure, rRNA is methylated on specific ribose residues (forming 2'O-methylribose).

The addition of many different basic ribosomal proteins in a precise sequence results in the formation of ribosomes. 5S RNA is synthesized elsewhere in the nucleus, probably by a different polymerase, and is added to the larger ribosomal subunit at a late stage in its assembly. Precursors of rRNA are observed in sucrose gradients or electropherograms of cerebral nuclear RNA, but they are not as prominent as they are in similar preparations from other tissues.[20] This may be because the turnover of ribosomes in brain is relatively slow, and because there is a greater preponderance of other RNA's in brain tissue (see below). Ribosomal RNA's of all tissues are indistinguishable,[21] and the multiple genes producing them seem to be a sequence of identical copies.

Transfer RNA comprises some 15 percent of brain RNA and is predominantly cytoplasmic in location. In brain it has not been extensively characterized but performs the usual function of transfer of amino acids to ribosomes for polymerization into proteins. Transfer RNA's specific for most of the twenty amino acids directly incorporated into protein have been detected in brain. They have a sedimentation coefficient of about 4, and a molecular weight of 25,000 to 30,000. The amount of tRNA in brain increases markedly during the course of brain development, but there do not appear to be changes in the relative amounts of individual tRNA's.[22] Transfer RNA is probably synthesized in the nucleus by RNA polymerase III, but this is uncharacterized in the brain.

The best criterion for messenger RNA is its translation by ribosomes into a functional protein. According to the classical model, genes on the chromosomes are transcribed into mRNA's, which are transported to the cytoplasm, attached to ribosomes and translated into the amino acid sequence of a protein. Several ribosomes could attach to the same mRNA, forming a polyribosome. It was originally believed that all RNA that was not rRNA, or tRNA, was mRNA. In particular, RNA labeled rapidly in the presence of radioactive precursors (rapidly labeled RNA) was identified as mRNA because:

1. It is heterogeneous in size, as would be expected for a collection of messengers for different-sized proteins.

2. Its base composition is like that of DNA and it hybridizes specifically to parent DNA.

3. It contains no methylated or other unusual bases, and lacks secondary structure (unlike rRNA and tRNA).

4. It apparently associates with ribosomes and polyribosomes active in protein synthesis.

5. Treatment with low concentrations of ribonuclease, at low temperatures and for short times, simultaneously destroys the rapidly labeled RNA,

the polyribosomal structure and the protein synthetic activity of polyribosomes.

However, the identification of rapidly labeled RNA with mRNA has come into question. Centrifugal and electrophoretic techniques show that most of the RNA in the nucleus (about 10 percent of that of the whole cell) is heterogeneous in size. In brain, as in other tissues,[23] this RNA (hnRNA) is synthesized and degraded very rapidly, and much of it probably has a mean half-life of only a few minutes.[24] Because the appearance of labeled RNA in the cytoplasm is relatively slow, it follows that much of the hnRNA never enters the cytoplasm and therefore does not perform a classical mRNA function. RNA-DNA hybridization studies also suggest that most nuclear RNA's do not appear in the cytoplasm. In addition, much of the cytoplasmic rapidly labeled RNA is not attached to polyribosomes, but is complexed with proteins forming ribonucleoprotein particles (RNP's) that cosediment with ribosomes in sucrose gradients. These RNP's have been called informosomes and may be cytoplasmic stores of mRNA's or may perform other, unknown functions.

hnRNA is synthesized in the nucleoplasm (extranucleolar nucleus) by RNA polymerase II. This enzyme is specifically inhibited by α-amanitin obtained from the mushroom *Amanita phalloides*. DNA-RNA hybridization studies indicate that part of hnRNA is a precursor to mRNA in the cytoplasm. The role of the remainder is unknown, but it may be involved in the regulation of gene transcription or in the transfer of RNA from the nucleus to the cytoplasm. About 10 to 11 percent of cerebral DNA appears to be transcribed into RNA.[13,25,26] This degree of genetic expression appears greater than values for other body tissues such as liver, kidney and spleen (2 to 5 percent*). A concurring observation is that there is more non-ribosomal RNA, other than tRNA, in brain as determined by gel electrophoresis.[24] The greater extent of gene expression in brain may reflect the great diversity of cell types. This diversity is so marked that Hahn has suggested that genes required for brain cells may account for most of the large amount of DNA found in higher animals.

The mRNA is probably transported from the nucleus to the cytoplasm in ribonucleoprotein particles distinct from ribosomes. These RNP's, or informosomes, may then interact with free single ribosomes to form polyribosomes active in protein synthesis. Recently, sequences of polyriboadenylic acid (poly A) containing 100 to 200 adenine residues have been found attached to the 3' end of some hnRNA's and all cytoplasmic mRNA's. It has

---

*These figures refer to hybridization of the so-called unique sequences of DNA, that is to say, whole-cell DNA from which the repetitive (rapidly hybridizing) sequences have been removed.

thus been suggested that this poly A sequence acts as a tag for mRNA.[27] An enzyme synthesizing poly A from ATP has long been known in brain nuclei[28] and has now been discovered in nuclei of other cells. This enzyme is distinct from the RNA polymerases in that it does not require a DNA template. The role of this poly A terminal sequence is unknown but could, for example, play a role in identifying the RNA as a messenger for nucleocytoplasmic transport. Other homopolyribonucleotide-synthesizing enzymes specific for poly C, poly G and poly U have been found in brain nuclei. Mandel has shown that nuclear nucleotides are synthesized in the cytoplasm and has hypothesized that the homopolyribonucleotides are the nuclear stores of nucleotides for RNA synthesis.[4]

The principal species of radioactive RNA after labeling periods of less than one hour is hnRNA (about 90 percent). Since the turnover of hnRNA is so rapid, rates of RNA synthesis cannot be estimated by pulses of radioactive precursors of fifteen minutes or longer because considerable turnover occurs in this time. In fact, the radioactivity in nucleotides is essentially in equilibrium with that in the hnRNA. The slower rate of accumulation of radioactive RNA in brain is due to the appearance of more stable cytoplasmic species (mRNA, rRNA and tRNA) transported from the nuclear pool. This accumulation in the cytoplasm is thus sensitive to changes in nuclear nucleotides as well as nucleic acid metabolism. Many observations formerly ascribed to changes in rates of RNA synthesis have later been shown to be changes in precursor metabolism and pool size (p. 184 and 209–210).

The overall rate of RNA synthesis in brain is high. However, despite the high mRNA content, there is no reason to suspect that brain RNA metabolism differs in any qualitative respect from that of other tissues. Theories of memory involving specific RNA's, other than as classical messenger RNA's, thus have little empirical foundation. This particularly applies to the studies that claimed the transfer of memories or learned experiences by RNA extracts. Many of these are now acknowledged to be erroneous; most of the effects observed are now ascribed to peptide contaminants of the RNA (p. 217). The earlier reports that dietary RNA improves brain function may have been due to the correction of nutritional deficits, though some nucleic acid components may have psychoactive effects.

v) **Mitochondria**

Cerebral mitochondria are morphologically and biochemically diverse, as might be expected in a heterogeneous tissue such as brain. Following sedimentation of mitochondria on sucrose gradients, differing profiles are obtained for several different mitochondrial enzymes.[29] This heterogeneity of mitochondria may reflect their various locations, in different types of neurons and glia, and in various specialized neuronal regions. In particular, astroglial mitochondria are very small. The high rate of cerebral oxidative metabolism is accounted for by the large numbers of mitochondria which constitute 10 to 20 percent of cerebral protein.

Brain mitochondria resemble those of other tissues in that they contain small amounts of DNA and appear to be self-replicating. However, their DNA content is limited and sufficient for only a few genes (about twenty to thirty). Ribosomal and transfer RNA's of mitochondria are of the prokaryotic (bacterial) type, and the genes for the ribosomal and some transfer RNA's are included in the mitochondrial DNA. Consequently, mitochondrial protein synthesis is sensitive to antibiotics such as chloramphenicol, but not to those such as cycloheximide which inhibit eukaryotic systems. (Reports to the contrary have now been shown to be erroneous.[30]) The proteins that are synthesized by mitochondria are insoluble and probably of the membrane type. Soluble mitochondrial proteins appear to be synthesized on cytoplasmic ribosomes and transported into the mitochondria. The genes for the proteins synthesized by mitochondria probably reside in the mitochondrial DNA, but there may also be transport of mRNA from the nucleus. Since mitochondria synthesize about 15 percent of their protein, mitochondrial protein synthesis amounts to less than 2 percent of total brain protein synthesis.[31]

vi) Ribosomes

Ribosomes are the only known sites of protein synthesis. In the nerve cell they are the basophilic components of Nissl substance, where they are loosely associated with, but not predominantly bound to, folds of endoplasmic reticulum. Ribosomes in neurons are not exclusively associated with Nissl bodies but are also distributed fairly densely in the cytoplasm surrounding the nucleus and in the dendrites. They are, however, hardly ever seen in axons or presynaptic regions. This is consistent with the very low amounts of RNA detected in axons and synaptosomes, much of which seems to be mitochondrial or of low molecular weight (4S to 5S).[32]

Brain ribosomes contain approximately equal proportions of RNA and protein, and morphologically and physically closely resemble those of other tissues. However, differences in ribosomal proteins, especially those of the smaller subunit, have been observed between different strains of mice, as well as between ribosomes from brain and other tissues.[33]

The half-life of both the protein and RNA components of ribosomes of rat and mouse brain is about ten to twenty days, which is longer than that of liver.[34] Since ribosomes are synthesized exclusively in the nucleus, they must be transported considerable distances proximodistally in dendrites and perhaps in axons. This, along with the low rate of cell division, may explain the relative stability of ribosomes in nervous tissue. Proximodistal flow of ribosomes in dendrites has been demonstrated radioautographically in cultured isolated neurons.[35]

Most of the ribosomes in brain are aggregated into polyribosomes, some of which may be very large.[2] They are not predominantly bound to the membranes of the endoplasmic reticulum. Their properties *in vitro* are generally similar to those of ribosomes from other tissues, but the cell-free incorporation of amino acids and the stability of cerebral polyribosomal structure are especially sensitive to cation concentrations.[5,24]

vii) Protein Synthesis

While the synthesis of proteins in brain occurs predominantly on cytoplasmic ribosomes, there have also been reports of synthesis in nuclei, mitochondria and synaptosomes. The protein synthesis observed in isolated brain nuclei has now been largely attributed to bacterial contamination.[36] Furthermore, cytoplasmic inclusions within the nucleus (see above) may be fully capable of protein synthesis.

Synaptosomal protein synthesis is in part due to synaptosomal mitochondria. Recent radioautographic studies have shown that ribosomes contaminate many synaptosomal preparations, and this may account for much of their protein synthetic capacity. There may, however, be a limited synthesis of proteins within the membrane. (See p. 148 for a fuller discussion.)

The capacity of the brain for protein synthesis is high and comparable to that of tissues that actively secrete protein such as the liver and pancreas. A large proportion of the proteins synthesized in the neuron are transported along the axon (Chapter 4). This export from the perikaryon may be considered a secretory process and may account for the high rate of cerebral protein synthesis.

During development, the rate of protein synthesis reaches a peak early in myelination and thereafter declines.[37] This finding is not an artifact due to greater brain penetration by amino acids in younger animals but a real phenomenon reflected in a greater proportion of ribosomes in polyribosomal aggregates,[38] indicating that more ribosomes are actively engaged in polymerizing amino acids. At the peak period of myelination a large fraction of the proteins synthesized are insoluble, and are probably the structural proteins of myelin.[37]

Brain protein synthesis is affected by treatments that disturb normal ATP levels such as electroshock,[39] and by abnormal amino acid concentrations, as in phenylketonuria.[40]

viii) Brain Proteins

Brain contains a preponderance of proteins not easily solubilized in aqueous media at neutral pH. These are thought to be structural membrane proteins. Separation of brain proteins by chromatography or electrophoresis reveals the presence of several acidic, low-molecular-weight proteins. The most studied of these is the S-100 protein discovered by Moore.[41] This protein, so named because of its solubility in 100 percent saturated ammonium sulfate, contains 190 amino acids of which 36 are glutamic acid and 21 are aspartic acid. It is found throughout the nervous system, to which it is also confined. Proteins cross-reacting with S-100 antiserum have been found in all vertebrate species studied and some nonvertebrates, including lobster, octopus, cockroach and *Drosophila*. S-100 comprises about 0.4 percent of the total soluble protein of mammalian brain. Studies using fluorescent antisera or neural degeneration indicate that it is confined to glia.[41] The protein turns over relatively slowly with a mean half-life of sixteen days. Despite a strong calcium binding activity, its function is unknown.

A similar protein, 14.3.2, has also been described by Moore.[41] There is twice as much of this protein in brain as there is of S-100. Studies using fluorescent antisera indicate that it is neuronal, found in the perikaryal and nucleolar regions, but its function also is unknown.

Very many other brain-specific proteins have been described, including other acidic proteins and actin and myosin-like proteins (see p. 119). Important also are the myelin proteins (p. 99). The most predominant brain protein is the structural subunit of neurotubules, tubulin (p. 108). Other brain proteins may be regionally specific; one such has been described in the olfactory lobe, to which it is transported axoplasmically from the cell bodies of neurons located in the olfactory epithelium.[42] The protein components of separated neurons and glia are quite different as judged by chromatographic and electrophoretic analyses.[43]

Recently it has become possible to examine the protein components of individual nerve cells, such as those of the abdominal ganglion of *Aplysia*, by polyacrylamide gel electrophoresis. The several cells that have been examined reveal quite distinct profiles, though common components exist.[44] These observations underline the extreme biochemical heterogeneity that we may expect from brain tissues at the cellular level.

Specific proteins also occur in sensory organs. Dastoli has purified a glycoprotein from the tips of bovine tongue that complexes with sweet-tasting compounds,[45] thereby undergoing a configurational change. This glycoprotein is rich in lysine and also contains neuraminic acid. Porcine tongues have yielded a protein that complexes with bitter-tasting compounds. The basis of chemoreception may be the conversion of such a structural change to an electric impulse.

ix) Protein Catabolism

Several enzymes (proteases) that will break down protein have been detected in brain.[46] However, not much is known about the control of this process. Recent studies from rat liver suggest that for both soluble and membrane proteins the rate of degradation is related to size: the larger the protein, the faster it is degraded.[47] The results are entirely consistent with random protease action. Larger proteins with more peptide bonds in effect have more substrates for the enzymes. Protein conformation and presumably cellular location are also important, so that the generalization with respect to size should not be taken too far. It does appear, however, that no special mechanisms for the control of protein degradation need be present.

Estimates of the half-life of brain proteins depend on the method of measurement. Such estimates may be made either by observing the rate of synthesis from a radioactive precursor or by following the decay of the radioactively labeled protein. The former method tends to favor the proteins that turn over rapidly, and the latter those with slow turnover. In addition, the decay method tends to overestimate half-lives because of recycling of radioactive amino acids from degraded proteins. The half-life of total brain protein in the adult rat is about fifteen days, but the range for individual proteins is enormous.[46] Myelin proteins and histones have half-lives of many months, while certain unstable enzymes may have half-lives on the order of a few minutes.

B. REGULATION

i) Degeneration and Regeneration of Neurons; Chromatolysis

When the axon of a peripheral nerve is cut, degeneration on the proximal side of the cut is limited and only occurs for a short distance toward the cell body (retrograde). However, the distal, severed part of the axon degenerates completely along with its myelin sheath if it has one. This process of myelin degeneration is known as Wallerian degeneration. The degeneration processes are acccompanied by cytological changes in the cell body, notably nuclear swelling and *chromatolysis*. The nucleus is displaced to one side and the cell body appears vacuolated, staining only on the periphery. Chromatolysis involves the dissolution of the Nissl bodies. The ribosomes and cisternae are not destroyed but the dense aggregations which account for the Nissl staining are dispersed. If the nerve has not been damaged too badly (which normally means that the axonal cut is not close to the cell body), the nerve will regenerate. This commences with the formation of a growth cone where the retrograde degeneration ceased. Neurites grow out from this cone and penetrate the scar at the site of the wound. Eventually new fibers grow into the tracts left by the old ones, reform the synaptic contacts and become myelinated. This whole process may take several months to complete.

Chromatolysis precedes the regeneration and appears to be a rearrangement of the cisternae and their associated ribosomes, which probably synthesize the protein for axoplasmic transport (especially since they appear to be oriented around the axon hillock). Nissl bodies reappear as regeneration commences and the cell body returns to its former appearance. During this period the RNA content of the nucleolus approximately doubles and this is followed by a similar increase in the cell body.[48] These changes are accompanied by an increased incorporation of $[^3H]$uridine into RNA, an increased transfer of RNA from the nucleus to the cytoplasm and an increased incorporation of $[^3H]$lysine into protein. The perikaryal RNA concentration returns to normal slowly, over a period of about ten to thirty days. It seems likely that these biochemical observations indicate an accelerated production of new ribosomes which are used to synthesize the components of the new axons.

The mechanism of the chromatolytic response is not understood. The presence of the axonal lesion is rapidly communicated to the cell body since changes are seen in the cell body within hours of the lesion. The closer the lesion to the cell body, the more rapidly chromatolysis occurs. While it is likely that a chemical messenger is transported axonally by reverse axoplasmic flow (p. 108), a glial role has also been suggested.[49] Because prostaglandins are normally produced following membrane damage, they are good candidates for such a chemical messenger.

Degeneration also occurs when central nervous system neurons are damaged, but until recently it was thought that, at least in mammals, regeneration did not occur. Limited regeneration is now known to occur, though it is unusual for full function to be restored. In the spinal cord, partial functional regeneration has been observed in rats. In several regions of the brain, neurite growth indicative of regeneration has been observed following lesions. The poor functional regeneration may be because the central nervous system develops in a more complicated way, and its structure depends upon a precise sequence of growth and development of individual cells which can rarely be emulated following tissue damage.

ii) Enzyme Induction

The activity of an enzyme may be altered in a number of ways. Rapid changes may be produced by alterations in the concentrations of cofactors and by allosteric effectors* which may activate or inhibit the overall processes. Longer-term changes may result from the synthesis of more enzyme molecules (enzyme induction). This synthesis occurs on ribosomes using an mRNA template. In cells of the prokaryotic type, mRNA's are short-lived. Their translation into protein commences before their synthesis is complete, and mRNA's are only translated a few times before degradation. This whole process occurs within a few minutes. Thus in the prokaryotic cell enzyme induction requires the synthesis of new mRNA. However, in animal cells, mRNA's may be much more stable and translated very many times over. Following synthesis, the mRNA's may be stored in the cytoplasm and activated at a later time by the attachment of ribosomes. Thus in the animal cell enzyme induction may require synthesis of new mRNA or merely involve the activation of a preexisting mRNA, stored either in the nucleus or in the cytoplasm.

In differentiated animal cells the enzyme complement is relatively stable. However, the induction of more or different enzymes or proteins may occur in response to changing conditions. These conditions include tissue damage, changes in the supply of nutrients, the presence of drugs or hormones, and changes in physiological activity.[50]

The normal test for the induction of an enzyme is to examine the effect of inhibitors of protein synthesis. If inhibition of protein synthesis prevents the increase in activity of an enzyme, then the increase was probably due to new synthesis rather than to the activation of preexisting molecules. Since inhibitors are not totally specific, such data are not completely conclusive and other explanations may be possible. (See p. 205 for a discussion of these points in relation to learning studies.) If the induction of the protein requires new mRNA synthesis, then it will be blocked by inhibition of RNA synthesis. Antibiotic inhibitors of protein and RNA synthesis have been used extensively as diagnostic tools to implicate gene activation and/or enzyme induction in complex processes. Thus it has been reported that the development of tolerance to, and dependence on, morphine in rats requires both new mRNA and protein synthesis.[51] Inhibitors of either of these processes block the appearance of both tolerance and dependence.

An example of an enzymic response to a nutritional change is the induction of the enzymes necessary for the metabolism of ketone bodies under

---

*Small molecules that affect the activity of an enzyme by binding to sites distinct from the substrate binding sites.

starvation conditions (p. 30). Hormone action is often mediated by the induction of specific proteins. The brain is generally considered to be relatively inert to the action of most hormones. However, thyroid hormone is an important factor during its development, and the steroid sex hormones bind to specific sites in the brain and influence sexual behavior (Chapter 9).

The corticosteroids secreted from the adrenal cortex may also act directly on the brain, their effect being detectable behaviorally and electrophysiologically. There is considerable evidence that steroid hormones in general act at the nuclear level. On entering the target cell they rapidly bind to specific cytoplasmic proteins and are transported into the nucleus, where they become attached to different proteins. Steroid hormone action is generally associated with effects on RNA metabolism, and it seems likely that new mRNA's mediate the response of the tissue. In the brain, corticosteroids are known to alter the activity of tyrosine-α-ketoglutarate transaminase, tryptophan pyrrolase, glycerol phosphate dehydrogenase and Na^+, K^+-ATPase.[50]

A particularly interesting case of enzyme induction is that provoked by neural activity. In several systems, enzymes involved in catecholamine metabolism may be induced by increased neural stimulation (p. 181).

There is thus considerable evidence that gene induction, in some cases involving new mRNA synthesis, occurs in the brain in response to changes in its environment.

C. GENETIC APPROACHES TO BRAIN FUNCTION

Mutants which have defective enzymes are particularly useful for determining the importance or function of biochemical pathways. A good example is orotic aciduria in man. In this disease orotidylic acid decarboxylase, required for the synthesis of pyrimidines, is absent. This defect is accompanied by severe neurological disorders, but patients can live normally if maintained on oral uridine. The *de novo* synthesis pathway for pyrimidine synthesis is thus not essential but is normally used.[52]

In other cases animals live normally up to a certain age, then develop disorders. One such class is the myelin mutants, of which several are known in mice.[53] These mutants are normal until the period when myelination should occur. They then develop neurological disorders such as shaking in the Jimpy and tremor in the Quaking strains. Histological studies show that little or no normal myelin is made. These strains have been used extensively in the study of myelin synthesis. The maturation of the visual system has been similarly studied using mutant mice that develop retinal degeneration and blindness.

Premature death may occur in other mutants in which there are defects in degradative pathways. Such defects frequently lead to the abnormal accumulation of substances that cannot be broken down. Several gangliosidoses are known in which an enzyme necessary for ganglioside degradation is absent (p. 93). The best-known example of this is Tay-Sachs disease, which affects 1 in 500,000 of the human population and is especially prevalent in Jews of East European origin (where the incidence may be 1 in 6,000). In this autosomal recessive disease a particular ganglioside (Tay-Sachs ganglioside, G_{M2}) accumulates in the brain, from which it cannot apparently be mobilized. Severe mental disturbance and eventual death are the result.

Genetic defects with neurological symptoms do not necessarily indicate a defect in a brain enzyme. In phenylketonuria (p. 31) a defect in a liver enzyme results in a mental disorder. Animal mutants are also known where blindness is caused by a defect in the uptake of vitamin A by the gut.

Benzer has used a novel approach to determine the site of action of a gene.[54] Using certain techniques, it is possible to breed mutant *Drosophila* as mosaics, in which only some body parts have the mutation and the rest has a normal gene complement. The variety of these mosaics is enormous, and by studying many different ones it is possible to determine which part of the body contains the gene defect that gives rise to the mutant phenotype. Using this technique, the location of the activity of the defective gene can be ascertained, avoiding much guesswork and often many years of work.

Population genetic studies of particular neurological diseases or psychoses may suggest the number of genes involved, and whether they are dominant or recessive. Behavior geneticists are also interested in breeding animals with particular behavioral characteristics such as intelligence, aggression or a tendency to depression. By studying the morphology and biochemistry of these mutants, the basis of the behavioral characteristics may be revealed. However, this approach is fraught with difficulties, perhaps best illustrated by the studies on inbred strains of mice. It was originally reported that mice of the C3H/He strain never learned to perform well in a shuttle-box conditioned-avoidance task. In contrast, DBA/2J mice learned somewhat more slowly but soon achieved a higher level of performance.[55] However, C3H/He mice have a severe retinal defect which might account for their poor performance.[56] To complicate matters further, while it has been claimed that the visual defect is not responsible for the differences in learning,[56] these differences have more recently been ascribed to a differential response of the two strains to stress.[57] Clearly, genetic lesions in any of the physiological processes associated with behavior will appear as behavioral defects, and it will generally be difficult to prove that they are associated with learning *per se*.

Brenner, working with nematodes, has chosen to study the morphology of the nervous system of behaviorally abnormal worms.[58] Since the neuromuscular system contains only 250 neurons and 96 muscles, it is feasible to completely analyze the system in individual mutants. Having characterized neuroanatomical differences between behaviorally distinguishable mutants, he can then study the way in which the genome dictates the structure of the nervous system and how this structure dictates behavior. Hopefully, these genetic approaches will bring to neurobiology the distinctive power they formerly brought to molecular biology.

CHAPTER III. REFERENCES

Reviews and General References

1. Altman, J. DNA metabolism and cell proliferation. In *Handbook of Neurochemistry*, Vol. 2. (Ed. A. Lajtha), Plenum Press, New York, 1969, pp. 137–82.
2. Hydén, H. RNA in brain cells. In *The Neurosciences, A Study Program* (Ed. G. C. Quarton, T. Melnechuk and F. O. Schmitt), Rockefeller University Press, New York, 1967, pp. 248–66.
3. Mandel, P., and Jacob M. RNA Metabolism. In *Handbook of Neurochemistry*, Vol. 5. (Ed. A. Lajtha), Plenum Press, New York, 1971, pp. 165–98.
4. Mandel, P. Problems of genetic expression in the nervous system. In *The Future of the Brain Sciences,* (Ed. S. Bogoch), Plenum Press, New York, 1969, pp. 197–215.
5. Roberts, S. Protein Synthesis. In *Handbook of Neurochemistry*, Vol. 5. (Ed. A. Lajtha), Plenum Press, New York, 1971, pp. 1–48.
6. Lajtha, A. *Protein Metabolism of the Nervous System.* Plenum Press, New York, 1970.
7. Schneider, D. Johnson. *Proteins of the Nervous System.* Raven Press, New York, 1973.

Literature Cited

8. McEwen, B. S., and Zigmond, R. E. Isolation of brain nuclei. In *Research Methods in Neurochemistry*, Vol. 1. (Ed. N. Marks and R. Rodnight), Plenum Press, New York, 1972, pp. 139–61.
9. Mandel, P. Free Nucleotides. In *Handbook of Neurochemistry*, Vol. 5. (Ed. A. Lajtha), Plenum Press, New York, 1971, pp. 249–82.
10. Mann, D. M. A., and Yates, P. O. Polyploidy in the human nervous system. *J. Neurol. Sci.* 18:183–96, 1973.
11. Cohen, J., Moreš, V., and Lodin, Z. DNA content of purified preparation of mouse Purkinje neurons isolated by a velocity sedimentation technique. *J. Neurochem.* 20:651–57, 1973.
12. Lasek, R. J., and Dower, W. J. Aplysia californica: analysis of nuclear DNA in individual nuclei of giant neurons. *Science* 172:278–80, 1971.
13. Hahn, W. E., and Laird, C. D. Transcription of nonrepeated DNA in mouse brain. *Science* 173:158–61, 1971.
14. Gurdon, J. B., and Woodland, H. R. On the long-term control of nuclear activity during cell differentiation. *Current Topics in Developmental Biology* 5:39–70, 1970.

15. Howard, E. DNA content of rodent brains during maturation and aging and autoradiography of postnatal DNA synthesis in monkey brain. *Prog. Brain Res.* 40:91–114, 1973.
16. Johnson, H. A., and Erner, S. Neuron survival in the aging mouse. *Exptl. Gerontol.* 7:111–17, 1972.
17. Chiu, J. F., and Sung, S. C. Intracellular distribution of DNA polymerase activities in developing and adult rat brain. *J. Neurochem.* 20:617–20, 1973.
18. Bondy, S. C. Synthesis and decay of histone fractions and of deoxyribonucleic acid in developing avian brain. *Biochem. J.* 123:465–69, 1971.
19. Wu, F. C., Elgin, S. C. R., and Hood, L. E. Nonhistone chromosomal protein of rat tissues: a comparative study by gel electrophoresis. *Biochemistry* 12:2792–97, 1973.
20. Judes, C., Jacob, M., and Mandel, P. Demonstration of the precursors of ribosomal RNA in brain cells by polyacrylamide-gel electrophoresis. *J. Neurochem.* 18:170–72, 1971.
21. Mohan, J., Dunn, A., and Casola, L. Ribosomal DNA in the rat. *Nature* 223:295–96, 1969.
22. Johnson, T. C., and Chou, L. Level and amino acid acceptor activity of mouse brain tRNA during neural development. *J. Neurochem.* 20:405–14, 1973.
23. Soeiro, R., Vaughn, M. H., Warner, J. R., and Darnell, J. E. The turnover of nuclear DNA-like RNA in HeLa cells *J. Cell Biol.* 39:112–18, 1968.
24. Dunn, A. Unpublished observations.
25. Brown, I. R., and Church, R. B. RNA transcription from nonrepetitive DNA in the mouse. *Biochem. Biophys. Res. Commun.* 42:850–56, 1971.
26. Grouse, L., Chilton, M. D., and McCarthy, B. J. Hybridization of ribonucleic acid with unique sequences of mouse deoxyribonucleic acid. *Biochemistry* 11:798–805, 1972.
27. Darnell, J. E., Philipson, L., Wall, R., and Adesnik, M. Polyadenylic acid sequences: role in conversion of nuclear RNA into messenger RNA. *Science* 174:507–10, 1971.
28. Dravid, A. R., Pete, N., and Mandel, P. An enzyme system in rat brain nuclei incorporating AMP into polyadenylate. *J. Neurochem.* 18:299–306, 1971.
29. Blokhuis, G. G. D., and Veldstra, H. Heterogeneity of mitochondria in rat brain. *FEBS Letters* 11:197–99, 1970.
30. Deanin, G. G., and Gordon, M. W. Chloramphenicol- and cycloheximide-sensitive protein synthetic systems in brain mitochondrial and nerve-ending preparations. *J. Neurochem.* 20:55–68, 1973.
31. Mahler, H. R., Jones, L. R., and Moore, W. J. Mitochondrial contributions to protein synthesis in cerebral cortex. *Biochem. Biophys. Res. Commun.* 42:384–89, 1971.
32. Lasek, R. J., Dabrowski, C., and Nordlander, R. Analysis of axoplasmic RNA from invertebrate giant axons. *Nature. New Biol.* 244:162–65, 1973.
33. MacInnes, J. W. Differences between ribosomal subunits from brain and those from other tissues. *J. Mol. Biol.* 65:157–61, 1972.
34. Von Hungen, K., Mahler, H. R., and Moore, W. J. Turnover of protein and ribonucleic acid in synaptic subcellular fractions from rat brain. *J. Biol. Chem.* 243:1415–23, 1968.
35. Kreutzberg, G. W., and Schubert, P. Neuronal activity and axonal flow. In *Metabolic Regulation and Functional Activity in the Nervous System* (Ed. H. Herkin and E. Genazzani), Springer, Berlin, 1974. In press.
36. Dravid, A. R., and Wong, E. Studies on the incorporation of [^{14}C]amino acids into protein by isolated rat brain nuclei. *J. Neurochem.* 19:2709–25, 1972.
37. Lim, L., and Adams, D. H. Microsomal components in relation to amino acid incorporation by preparations from the developing rat brain. *Biochem. J.* 104:229–38, 1967.
38. Fellows, A., Francon, J., Nunez, J., and Sokoloff, L. Protein synthesis by highly aggregated and purified polyribosomes from young and adult rat brain. *J. Neurochem.* 21:211–22, 1973.

39. Dunn, A. Brain protein synthesis after electroshock. *Brain Research* 35:254–59, 1971.
40. MacInnes, J. W., and Schlesinger, K. Effects of excess phenylalanine on *in vitro* and *in vivo* RNA and protein synthesis and polyribosome levels in brains of mice. *Brain Research* 29:101–10, 1971.
41. Moore, B. W. Brain-specific proteins. In *Proteins of the Nervous System* (Ed. D. J. Schneider), Raven Press, New York, 1973, pp. 1–12.
42. Margolis, F. L., and Tarnoff, J. F. Site of biosynthesis of the mouse brain olfactory bulb protein. *J. Biol. Chem.* 248:451–55, 1973.
43. Packman, P. M., Blomstrand, C., and Hamberger, A. Disc electrophoretic separation of proteins in neuronal, glial and subcellular fractions from cerebral cortex. *J. Neurochem.* 18:479–87, 1971.
44. Gainer, H. Patterns of protein synthesis in individual identified molluscan neurons. *Brain Research.* 39:369–85, 1972.
45. Dastoli, F. R., Taste receptor proteins. *Life Sciences.* 14:1417–26, 1974.
46. Lajtha, A., and Marks, N. Protein turnover. In *Handbook of Neurochemistry,* Vol. 5 (Ed. A. Lajtha), Plenum Press, New York, 1971, pp. 551–629.
47. Schimke, R. T. Principles underlying the regulation of synthesis and degradation of protein in animal tissues. In *The Neurosciences, Third Study Program* (Ed. F. O. Schmitt and F. G. Worden), M.I.T. Press, Cambridge, Mass., 1974, pp. 813–25.
48. Watson, W. E. Observations on the nucleolar and total cell body nucleic acid in injured nerve cells. *J. Physiol.* 196:655–76, 1968.
49. Cragg, B. G. What is the signal for chromatolysis? *Brain Research* 23:1–21, 1970.
50. McIlwain, H. Metabolic adaptation in the brain. *Nature* 226:803–06, 1970.
51. Cox, B. M., and Osman, O. H. Inhibition of the development of tolerance to morphine in rats by drugs which inhibit ribonucleic acid or protein synthesis. *Brit. J. Pharmacol.* 38:157–70, 1970.
52. Nyhan, W. L. Disorders of nucleic acid metabolism. In *Biology of Brain Dysfunction,* Vol. I. (Ed. G. E. Gaull), Plenum Press, New York, 1973, pp. 265–300.
53. Sidman, R. L., Green, M. C., and Appel, S. H. *Catalog of the Neurological Mutants of the Mouse,* Harvard University Press, Cambridge, Mass., 1966.
54. Benzer, S. Genetic dissection of behavior. *Scientific American* 229:24–37, Dec. 1973.
55. Bovet, D., Bovet-Nitti, F., and Oliviero, A. Genetic aspects of learning and memory in mice. *Science* 163:139–49, 1969.
56. Henry, K. R., Buckholtz, N. S., Bowman, R. E., Bovet, D., Bovet-Nitti, F., and Oliviero, A. Genetics of memory. *Science* 165:1148, 1969.
57. Duncan, N. C., Grossen, N. E., and Hunt, E. B. Apparent memory differences in inbred mice produced by differential reaction to stress. *J. Comp. Physiol. Psychol.* 74:383–89, 1971.
58. Brenner, S. The genetics of behaviour. *Brit. Med. Bull.* 29:3, 1973, pp. 269–71.

IV. Neuronal Processes

A. AXONS AND DENDRITES[1]

Cells of the brain are characterized by large numbers of extensions, or processes, that are often very long. This feature is not confined to neurons, being also true of glial cells, but only the neurons have processes that extend more than one cell layer and may reach several feet in length. The surface area and the volume of these extensions is often much greater than that of the nerve cell body, and most of the metabolic activity of the neuron may occur in these processes. Neuronal processes are of two fundamental types: axons and dendrites. The physiological role of these is reflected in their specialized structure and chemistry. The differences between these two types of processes are as follows:

1. One single axon emerges from each neuronal perikaryon but there may be several dendrites. Axons are generally longer and straighter than dendrites, though both processes may terminate at considerable distances from the cell body. Both axons and dendrites grow outward from the cell body from their point of origin on the perikaryal surface, but the final direction

and morphology are greatly influenced by contacts with other cells. The point of emergence of the axon from the cell body is called the axon hillock and has a characteristic morphology (Figure 1.6). Dendrites tend to have irregular contours, with spines and thorns protruding from their surfaces, whereas axonal contours are generally smooth.

2. The membranes of both dendrites and axons are electrically polarized. However, the axon is excitable and transmits a wave of reversed polarity known as an *action potential.* Dendrites may also transmit electrical depolarizations but do not display action potentials. The wave of depolarization may travel in either direction, but under physiological conditions depolarizations generally travel proximodistally in axons (from the cell body) and distoproximally in dendrites (to the cell body). In an axon a proximodistal impulse is termed *orthodromic,* and one in the reverse direction *antidromic.*

3. Axons are frequently surrounded by oligodendroglia or, in the case of peripheral nerve, by Schwann cells. These may enclose the axon within a myelin sheath. This sheath chemically and electrically insulates the axon from the milieu that it traverses. Dendrites are not surrounded by myelin and are more readily influenced chemically and electrically by the surrounding cells, which are normally astrocytes.

4. Neuronal processes are characterized by the conspicuous presence of neurotubules and neurofilaments. These structures are also present in the perikaryon, but their longitudinal arrangement in the processes is more striking, especially in axons because of the lack of other organelles. Both structures are tubular, but neurotubules are of larger diameter (200Å to 260Å) than neurofilaments (100Å). Neurofilaments are comparatively rare in dendrites. The ratio of neurofilaments to neurotubules decreases as axons decrease in diameter, so that it may be difficult to distinguish dendrites from small axons in this respect.

5. Dendrites contain ribosomes and are capable of more local protein synthetic activity than axons, which contain few if any ribosomes. The low capacity of axons to synthesize proteins requires the existence of specialized mechanisms for the transport of protein from its perikaryal synthetic site. It is likely that the highly organized neurotubular and neurofilamentous array plays some role in this process (p. 107).

6. Axonal function is the distal transmission of action potentials, neurotransmitters and neurohumors. Axons may synapse on receptor cells or may secrete neurohumors into the bloodstream, thus affecting remote cells. Dendritic function is the reception of chemicals liberated by the presynaptic neuron. These chemical neurotransmitters may locally alter the permeability of the postsynaptic membrane to ions, and thus the membrane potential may

change. Dendritic potentials are transmitted to the cell body where summation occurs.

Biochemical studies of neuronal processes have been hampered by the unavailability of pure preparations of axons or dendrites. Many invertebrates contain giant axons which can be dissected out and used for biochemical study. A persistent problem with these preparations has been the presence of small axonal collaterals and tightly bound myelin sheaths, but soluble axoplasm in pure form may be extruded from these giant axons. An axolemmal-rich preparation from squid retina has been described. DeVries and Norton have prepared axons from bovine white matter, but these lack visible axolemmae and neurotubules.[21]

B. NEURONAL CONDUCTION

i) Mechanism

The axonal membrane exhibits a differential permeability to ions. The resting squid axon is about 100 times as permeable to potassium ions as it is to sodium ions.[2] There is also an asymmetrical distribution of charged ions across the membrane. The extracellular fluid surrounding the squid axon contains about 460 mM Na^+ and 20 mM K^+, while the axoplasm contains 50 mM Na^+ and 400 mM K^+. This difference in the concentration of Na^+ and K^+ across the axonal membrane is maintained by pumping Na^+ out of the axon and K^+ into it.[2] Many cells have the capacity to concentrate potassium ions, but to a lesser extent. Anions are also asymmetrically distributed, chloride ion being approximately 560 mM externally and 40 mM internally. The internal anionic deficit is made up by anionic groups on structural proteins and anions such as glutamate and N-acetylaspartate, to which the nerve cell membrane is rather impermeable. The differential permeabilities of the ions result in diffusion potentials across the membrane. The magnitude of these potentials is defined by the Goldman equation.[1] Since in the resting state the axonal membrane is much more permeable to K^+ than to Na^+ or Cl^-, the most important diffusion potential is that due to K^+. In fact, the resting potential of the axon (commonly about -40 to -80 mV) is almost entirely due to K^+.

Depolarization of the axonal membrane may occur at the axon hillock as a result of depolarization of the cell body, or it may be induced by direct electrical stimulation. When the axon is depolarized, the membrane characteristics alter, probably because of conformational changes in the membrane proteins.[22] The permeability of sodium increases and Na^+ diffuses into the cell. The entry of this positive ion decreases the voltage across the axonal membrane, which is further depolarized. (This is equivalent to a diffusion potential in the opposite direction.) What happens then depends on the extent of the depolarization.

If the initial depolarization exceeds a certain *threshold voltage*, the permeability of the membrane to Na^+ further increases so that the Na^+ influx eventually reverses the resting potential, thus producing an action potential. If the initial depolarization is below threshold, the membrane will be repolarized and thus restored to its original Na^+-impermeable state.

Once the membrane polarity is reversed, a dramatic change in membrane character again occurs and it becomes once more impermeable to Na^+ and more permeable to K^+. The K^+ conductance increases tenfold and K^+ diffuses down the concentration gradient out of the axon. This loss of cations to the exterior once again polarizes the axon, the inside of which then reverts to being negatively charged with respect to the exterior. Once repolarized, the Na^+ and K^+ permeabilities return to their resting values.

The potential of the axon is now back to its resting state. However, two changes have occurred during the transient depolarization: the axon has lost K^+ and gained Na^+, and the depolarizing spike has partially depolarized the neighboring axonal membrane segment. The total ionic change is very minor relative to the K^+ content of the axon, and the sodium pump soon expels the excess Na^+ from the axoplasm and restores the original K^+. The axon contains sufficient reserves of K^+ so that even if the sodium pump cannot function, the axon will be able to conduct many thousands of impulses before the loss of K^+ and gain of Na^+ is so great that an action potential can no longer be elicited.

The depolarization of the adjacent segments of the axonal membrane triggers exactly the same sequence of events in it as has been described above. In this way the depolarization spreads along the axon. The instability caused by the depolarization is transient, and ceases because during restoration the axon membrane becomes repolarized and then temporarily slightly hyperpolarized. This hyperpolarization increases the threshold voltage in this area enough so that it is refractory to the adjacent depolarization and the disturbances in that segment are terminated. The overall result is a unidirectional wave of depolarization moving away from the site of the disturbance. In the normal situation, where the depolarization is initiated at the axon hillock, it travels in only one direction — toward the synaptic terminal.

The magnitude and velocity of the action potential are constant and characteristic for a given axon. In unmyelinated fibers the velocity is proportional to the square of the diameter.

The permeability properties of the axonal membrane are not well understood but must be related to its structure. Nervous excitation results in changes of the fluorescent light-scattering and the birefringence of nerves. This suggests that neuronal activity involves conformational changes of the molecular components of the nerve membrane.[3] Circular dichroism and nuclear magnetic resonance studies have led to similar conclusions.

ii) Models

Ca^{2+} is important in the Na^+ transport process but its precise role is uncertain. The axon is less permeable to Na^+ in the presence of Ca^{2+}, and during stimulation Ca^{2+} accumulates in the axoplasm. Tasaki and others have suggested that Ca^{2+} is bound on the outer membrane surface of the resting axon.[3] Upon initial depolarization, internal K^+ displaces the Ca^{2+} and the membrane becomes permeable to Na^+, initiating the action potential. Subsequently Ca^{2+} is restored to its former binding site. This binding site may be glycoprotein or ganglioside sialic acid, which has a strong affinity for Ca^{2+}. Hawthorne has suggested that Ca^{2+} binds to di- or triphosphoinositide within the resting nerve membranes.[4] Activation of specific phosphomonoesterases hydrolyzes the di- and triphosphoinositides to monophosphoinositides, which do not bind Ca^{2+} strongly and thus permit its release. This hypothesis is supported by the finding that phospholipases that degrade phosphoinositides inactivate Na^+ carrier systems. It is of interest that the relative potency of cationic local anesthetics correlates with their capacity to inhibit Ca^{2+} binding by phosphatidylserine and phosphatidylethanolamine. This suggests that the binding of Ca^{2+} to lipids is required for the generation of the action potential.

The models described above include as a common feature the displacement of Ca^{2+} from the membrane as a step between the initial depolarization and the effect on Na^+ transport. Nachmansohn has suggested that variations in membrane permeability are regulated by acetylcholine.[23] He proposed that acetylcholine is bound to a storage protein during rest and is released by the initial depolarization. Free acetylcholine then binds to a membrane receptor protein, altering its conformation. This changes the membrane permeability to Na^+, thus causing the action potential. The acetylcholine is then broken down by acetylcholinesterase, allowing the receptor protein to resume its original conformation and the membrane its original permeability. Evidence for this model is the presence of acetylcholine, choline acetylase and acetylcholinesterase within nerve fibers. Acetylcholine depolarizes axons, but only when non-physiological concentrations are used. In some experimental systems, neuronal stimulation increases acetylcholine release from the axon.

Certain other compounds in low concentrations depolarize axons by increasing Na⁺ permeability. These include glutamic and aspartic acids which may physiologically increase axonal excitability by lowering threshold voltages. However, the most potent compounds are the nonphysiological D-homocysteic and N-methyl-D-aspartic acids. All these compounds have features structurally analogous to membrane phospholipids. It has been proposed that they fit into the membrane structure causing conformational changes similar to those that normally initiate the action potential. The carboxyl groups of these compounds may be intimately concerned with the increased Na⁺ permeability, since GABA, which lacks the α-carboxyl of glutamate, has the reverse effect on Na⁺ conductance. Thus glutamate and asparate may physiologically increase axonal excitability by lowering threshold voltages (p. 141).

Tetrodotoxin, a potent neurotoxin isolated from the puffer fish, has a very specific effect on Na⁺ transport. Twenty nM to 50 nM tetrodotoxin blocks excitation and Na⁺ uptake by electrical stimulation of cortical tissue.[24]. It has been calculated that 100 molecules or less are active per square micron of membrane surface, and that each molecule blocks a site at which 10 or more Na⁺ enter per impulse. Tetrodotoxin blocks the effect of glutamate and related cerebral excitants on Na⁺ transport. Since tetrodotoxin is also structurally analogous to the membrane phosphatides, it is possible that it may occupy the same site as glutamate but have the reverse effect on Na⁺ permeability by preventing the appropriate conformational change. Protoveratrine and DDT both extend the period of Na⁺ permeability following excitation, and this is believed to be the mechanism of their neurotoxicity.

iii) The Sodium Pump

Axonal and dendritic membranes are major components of the microsomal pellet obtained from cell homogenates by centrifugal methods. Certain enzymes such as the Na⁺, K⁺-stimulated ATPase that appear to be associated with these membranes are found in the microsomal pellet.[5] This ATPase is sensitive to the concentrations of Na⁺ and K⁺ and has kinetic parameters that closely resemble those of the Na⁺ pump in the intact nerve. The microsomal ATPase is considered to be the vestigial sodium pump, especially since both the pump and the ATPase are inhibited by cardiac glycosides such as ouabain.

Na⁺, K⁺-stimulated ATPases are widely distributed. In addition, to both Na⁺ and K⁺, Mg²⁺ is required for optimal activity. The hydrolysis of ATP is believed to occur by way of a phosphorylated enzyme intermediate, and phosphopeptide fragments have been isolated from preparations of this enzyme. In common with other phosphorylation reactions, Mg²⁺ is required for this phosphorylation.

$$\text{ATP} + \text{Enzyme} \xrightarrow{\text{Na}^+, \text{Mg}^{2+}} \text{Enzyme} \sim \text{P} + \text{ADP}$$

The phosphate is linked to a glutamic acid residue by an acyl phosphate bond. A phosphate may also become bound to a nearby serine residue but this is now known to be related to a phosphate-exchange reaction which is no longer considered to be a part of the ion transport function. The turnover of the phosphate groups attached to the enzyme is accelerated by K^+, thus the dephosphorylation of the enzyme may be K^+-dependent.

$$\text{Enzyme} \sim \text{P} \xrightarrow{K^+} \text{Enzyme} + P_i$$

These reactions may be combined in the membrane to exchange intracellular Na^+ for K^+, and the scheme of Figure 4.1 best explains the available data.[25]

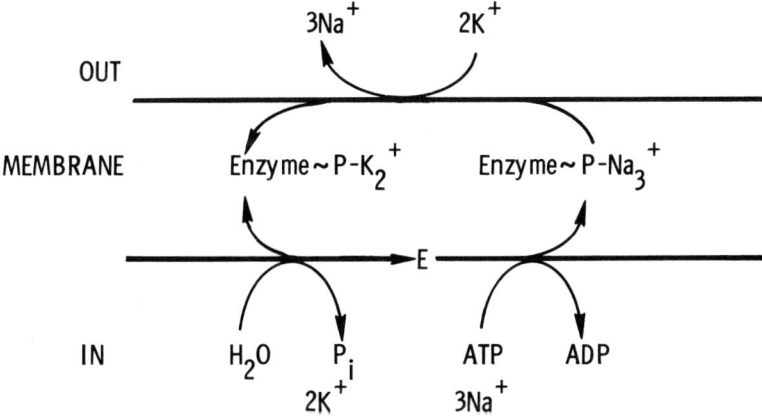

Figure 4.1 The possible mechanism of the Na^+-K^+ pump. The phosphorylated enzyme carries three sodium ions from the interior to the exterior of the cell membrane. There the three sodium ions are exchanged for two potassium ions which are conveyed to the inner surface of the membrane. The protein is then dephosphorylated, releasing the K^+ and is ready to be phosphorylated again.

There are two distinct protein subunits in the enzyme which is thought to have an $\alpha_2\beta_2$ subunit structure. The larger of these (α) becomes phosphorylated physiologically. When the lipids are removed from preparations of the Na^+, K^+-ATPase, activity is lost. The activity of the residual proteins may be restored specifically by the addition of phospholipids, notably phosphatidylserine. Addition of phosphatidylserine also restores the ouabain binding capacity. Thus it seems very likely that this phospholipid plays an important role in the activity of the sodium pump.[26]

Mitochondrial respiratory activity is dependent on and stimulated by ADP, so that cellular respiration is related to ADP levels. Since the activity of the sodium and other ion pumps generates ADP from ATP, the cerebral respiratory rate is to a great extent determined by the activity of the pumps. These pumps (Figure 2.2) have been estimated to consume 25 to 50 percent of total cerebral energy metabolism.[27]

Two pathological conditions have been attributed to impairment of the sodium pump. Epilepsy may be due to a deficient sodium pump in the glia, which would normally remove excess extracellular K^+. Interference with the sodium pump by ouabain causes convulsions in experimental animals.[6] Epileptic brain tissue has depressed K^+ and elevated Na^+ levels. Thus, the threshold voltage required to cause an action potential is reduced so that these axons are very excitable. The cerebral edema that results from traumatic or toxic conditions is also associated with elevated Na^+ and depressed K^+ in brain tissue and with an abnormally high level of K^+ in cerebrospinal fluid. This too may be related to a malfunction of the sodium pump.

C. THE STRUCTURE OF MEMBRANES

The principal chemical constituents of membranes are proteins, phospholipids, cholesterol and glycolipids. The relative proportions of these molecules may vary greatly (see following table) but the major ones are proteins and phospholipids. For a number of years, theories of membrane structure have been dominated by the *Unit Membrane Hypothesis* of Robertson based on the bimolecular lipid layer of Davson and Danielli (Figure 4.2).[7] The essential features of this model are a phospholipid bilayer arranged in such a way that the aliphatic fatty acid tails are directed inwards, with the proteins forming a coat on both surfaces. This arrangement was suggested by the staining properties of membranes seen in the electron microscope, which have a trilaminar appearance. The stains bind to the inner and outer protein layers of the membrane, and are excluded from the lipid core.

It is known that phospholipids will arrange themselves in monolayers at the interphase of aqueous and organic solvents, with the polar phosphate heads in the aqueous phase and the hydrophobic fatty acid tails in the organic phase. The physical properties of the monolayer and considerations of

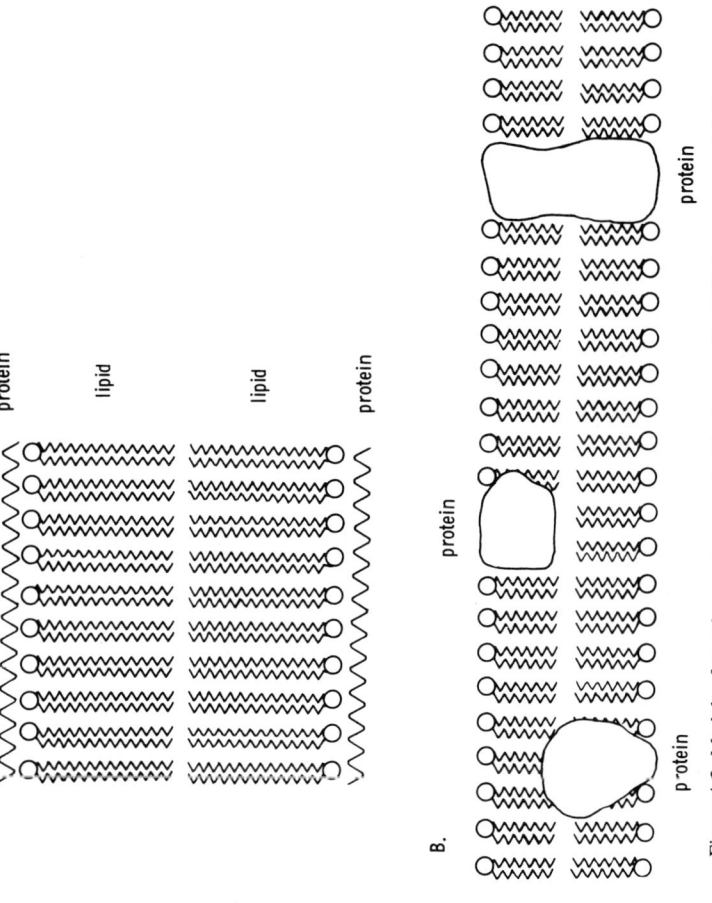

Figure 4.2 Models of membrane structure. A. The Davson-Danielli-Robertson model. B. The fluid mosaic model of Singer.

Chemical Composition of Membranes

	Liver Plasma	Myelin	Axolemma
		(% dry weight)	
Protein	58	21	37
Phospholipids	16	30	29
Cholesterol	6	20	9
Glycolipids	–	20	–
		%Total Phospholipids	
Phosphatidylcholine	42	30	–
Phosphatidylethanolamine	18	40	–
Phosphatidylserine	9	17	–
Phosphatidylinositol	9	2	–
Sphingomyelin	21	13	–

molecular size suggest that the phospholipids are closely packed. With two aqueous surfaces a bilayer may be formed with the fatty acid chains interdigitating. The physical and electrical properties which would be predicted from this structure are consistent with those of real and artificial membranes. The phospholipid content of most membranes is exactly enough to form a lipid bilayer of the required surface area. The essential features of this structure have been verified by X-ray diffraction for myelin.

The state of the membrane proteins is less clear. It was originally conceived that the polar heads of the phospholipids would interact with polar groups on the proteins, and that these in turn would hydrogen-bond with the water giving the membrane its stability. In support of this, up to 95 percent of the lipid can be extracted from mitochondrial membranes without altering their appearance in the electron microscope. However, several predictions based on this model have not been verified. First, it was predicted that the amount of protein would be in a constant ratio to that of phospholipid for all membranes. This was not found to be true (see table above). Second, in order to cover both membrane surfaces adequately, the proteins would have to be in an open conformation known as the β-conformation or pleated sheet. However, the characteristic infrared absorption band of this conformation was not detected in membranes, and optical rotatory dispersion and circular dichroism studies indicate that as much as 60 percent of the protein may be in the α-helical conformation. In this conformation there is not enough protein available to cover both surfaces of the lipid bilayer. (The low protein content of myelin would be insufficient to cover the lipids even in the β-conformation.) In fact, membrane proteins tend to be globular with extensive internal hydrophobic bonding.

The postulated interaction of the polar phosphate heads of the phospholipids with polar groups of the protein is also erroneous. If this interaction were important, membranes would be disrupted by high ionic strength, which would weaken the polar interactions of the membrane constituents. Media of high ionic strength, however, do not cause membrane disruption but stabilize them. Yet membranes are easily disrupted by organic solvents and detergents. These facts suggest that it is the hydrophobic, nonpolar forces rather than the hydrophilic, polar forces that are the most important in the interaction between the proteins and the lipids.

More modern models of the structure of membranes retain the phospholipid bilayer, but the proteins are inserted into this layer and may float on it or pass right through it (Figure 4.2). This is the *Fluid Mosaic Model* in which Singer has described the proteins as icebergs floating over a lipid sea.[28] Proteins that pass right through the membrane could have obvious functions in transport processes. Both the lipids and the proteins of the membranes are in a fluid state. Measurements with spin-labeled* proteins and lipids suggest that both components are highly mobile and travel rapidly in all directions within the membrane. The lipids have a high mobility within the monolayer but do not readily exchange between layers. The axonal membrane is among the most fluid of the membranes studied with this technique.

The position of cholesterol, which appears in all membranes, has not been clearly defined, but it is probably associated with the phospholipid components of the membrane. The glycolipids may be inserted into the lipid bilayer with their carbohydrate parts protruding into the aqueous surround. Some membrane proteins are not simple proteins but have covalent carbohydrate and lipid attachments. Lipoproteins would clearly stabilize membrane structure by linking hydrophobic and hydrophilic regions. Glycoproteins, like glycolipids, could have their hydrophilic carbohydrate parts protruding outwards from the membrane to interact with the aqueous environment.[29]

D. MEMBRANE MOLECULES

i) Fatty Acids

The free fatty acid content of brain is very low, but considerable quantities of fatty acid residues are contained within the more complex lipids that make up membranes: namely phospholipids, cerebrosides, sulfatides and

---

*Molecules containing substituted groups with unpaired electrons that give electron spin resonance (ESR) signals. Motion of the molecule changes the ESR spectrum.

gangliosides. Most of the fatty acids in the brain contain an even number of carbon atoms, usually from sixteen to twenty-four, but fatty acids containing odd numbers of carbon atoms have been detected. The fatty acids are unbranched chains and may be partially unsaturated or hydroxylated. The brain has a high capacity for the synthesis of fatty acids, but there is also some utilization of plasma fatty acids. This is indicated by the way in which the dietary composition of fatty acids may influence the nature of the fatty acids found within the brain. For example, increased intake of arachidonic and linolenic acids results in a high content of these fatty acids in cerebral lipids. Variation in the fatty acid composition of cerebral lipids gives rise to a form of microheterogeneity in these compounds. While this has been the subject of numerous studies, no clear structure/function relationships have emerged.

Fatty acids are synthesized in the brain by separate systems both in mitochondria and in the microsome fraction. The routes are similar to, if not identical with, those of other tissues and involve the polymerization of the 2-carbon units of acetyl coenzyme A via malonyl coenzyme A. There may also be separate systems for chain elongation. As in other tissues, catabolism ocurs by β-oxidation.

ii) Phospholipids

The most important group of phospholipids is the phosphatides, the major components of the lipid bilayer. The phosphatides are derivatives of phosphatidic acid (diesterified glycerol phosphate).[4] To form a phosphatide, the phosphate of phosphatidic acid must be esterified with serine, ethanolamine, choline or inositol (Figure 4.3). This esterification is not simple, but involves derivatives of cytidine nucleotides as intermediates. In the case of ethanolamine and choline, this occurs as follows:

$$CTP + \begin{Bmatrix} ethanolamine \\ choline \end{Bmatrix} phosphate \rightarrow CDP \begin{Bmatrix} ethanolamine \\ choline \end{Bmatrix} + PP_i$$

$$CDP \begin{Bmatrix} ethanolamine \\ choline \end{Bmatrix} + diglyceride \rightarrow phosphatidyl \begin{Bmatrix} ethanolamine \\ choline \end{Bmatrix} + CMP$$

Phosphatidylinositol is formed in a somewhat different way, but one which also involves cytidine nucleotide derivatives. The phosphatidic acid is linked to the cytidine nucleotide and then transferred to inositol:

$$CTP + phosphatidic\ acid \rightarrow CDPdiglyceride + PP_i$$

$$CDPdiglyceride + inositol \rightarrow phosphatidylinositol + CMP$$

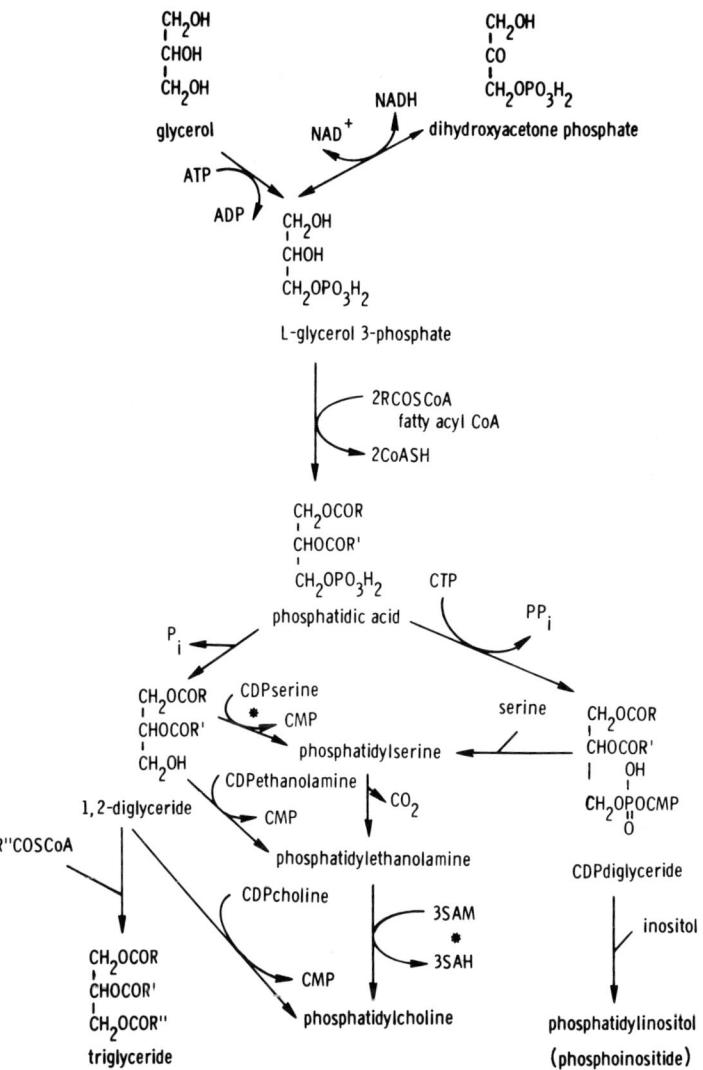

Figure 4.3 The synthesis of phospholipids. *Denotes a reaction which probably does not occur in brain.

Phosphatidylserine is probably synthesized by a similar route in brain. Phosphatidylserine may be directly converted to phosphatidylethanolamine by decarboxylation, and thence by methylation to phosphatidylcholine (Figure 4.3). This is the major route of choline synthesis in mammals, but the methylation step probably does not occur in brain.

Cytidine nucleotides are very important in the brain as cofactors in the biosynthesis of lipids. In fact, more than half of the soluble cytidine nucleotides in the brain are in the form of derivatives, of which the major one is CDPcholine. Because of the high activity of lipid biosynthesis in brain, and since cytidine nucleotides are also required for sialic acid transfer and nucleic acid synthesis, it is surprising that their concentration in brain is the lowest of the four major nucleotide species. Mandel has suggested that cytidine nucleotides may be rate-limiting for RNA synthesis; the same may be true for lipid synthesis.

Phosphatidylinositol (monophosphoinositide [MPI]) may be further phosphorylated to di-, tri- and possibly tetraphospho-derivatives. Monophosphoinositide kinase adds a phosphate from ATP to the 4-position of the inositol ring forming diphosphoinositide (DPI). This requires a divalent ion (Ca^{2+}, Mg^{2+}, Mn^{2+} or Cu^{2+}) and a thiol compound for full activity, and is inhibited by Na^+ or K^+ and thiol-oxidizing reagents. Diphosphoinositide kinase further phosphorylates the DPI, this time on the 3-position of the inositol ring. Unlike the MPI kinase it is a soluble enzyme, prefers Mg^{2+} over Ca^{2+} or Mn^{2+}, and is not inhibited by thiol-oxidizing reagents. Separate soluble enzymes dephosphorylating all three phosphoinositides have been found in brain. The TPI and DPI phosphomonoesterases require Mg^{2+}, but the MPI phosphomonoesterase requires Ca^{2+} for activity.

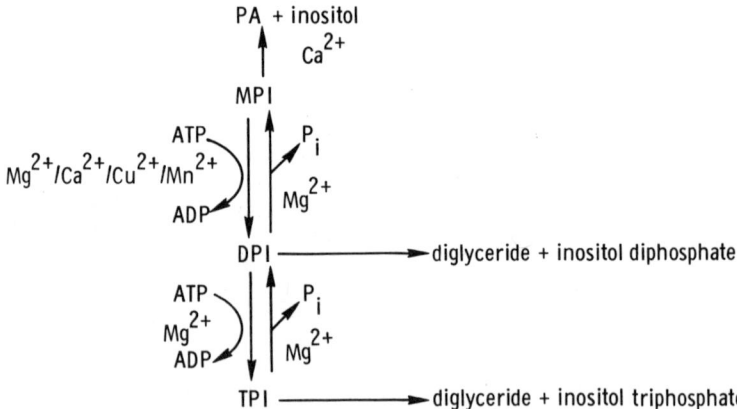

The function of the phosphoinositides is reflected in the very rapid turnover of their phosphate groups, associated with neurotransmission. There is evidence that this turnover specifically requires postsynaptic activation (p. 189).

Lecithin (phosphatidylcholine) may be hydrolyzed by phospholipase A to

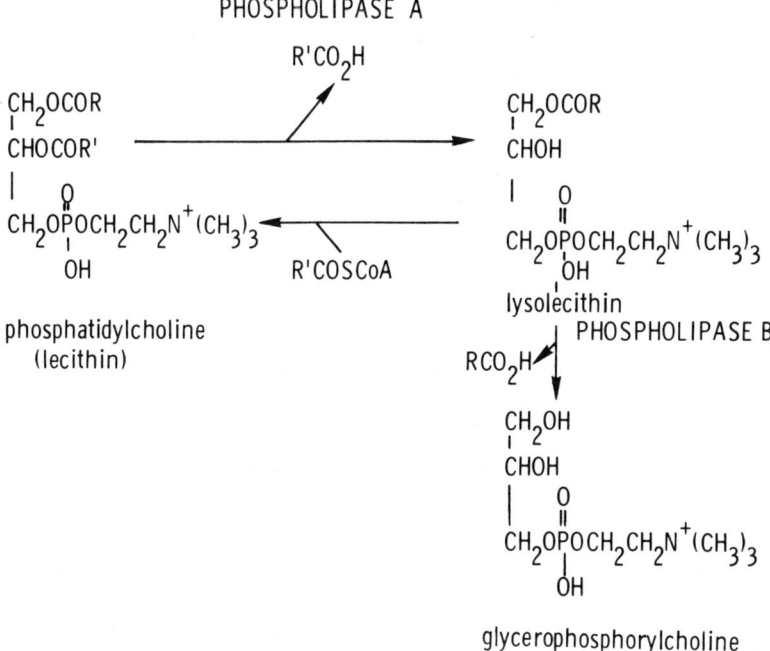

Figure 4.4 Actions of phospholipases A and B.

lysolecithin (lecithin lacking its β-fatty acid) (Figure 4.4). The lysolecithin may then be acylated back to lecithin. Thus the fatty acids of lecithin may turn over independently of the whole molecule. The activity of the acylation reaction is considerably greater than overall lecithin synthesis. Lysolecithin has cytolytic properties including hemolysis, which is probably due to a detergent-like activity. Some of the effects of snakebites may be mediated by phospholipase A in the venom producing lysolecithin in the tissue. The emulsifying properties of lysolecithin may also play an important role in demyelinating conditions.

Acylation and deacylation reactions are not confined to phosphatidylcholine but also occur with the serine and ethanolamine phosphatides. The lysophosphatides are part of a degradative route. Following phospholipase A action, phospholipase B may remove the second (α) fatty acid producing glycerophosphoryl derivates (Figure 4.4). Lecithin and the other phosphatides may also be catabolized by hydrolysis to diglyceride and phosphorylcholine by phospholipase C. (See figure on page 84 for its activity on DPI and TPI.)

A closely related class of phospholipids found in brain is the glyceryl ether phospholipids. The stable ether bond is substituted for the ester bond with the α-carbon of glycerol. The phosphatidal (or plasmalogen) derivatives have an unsaturated double bond adjacent to the ether linkage, thus forming a vinyl ether:

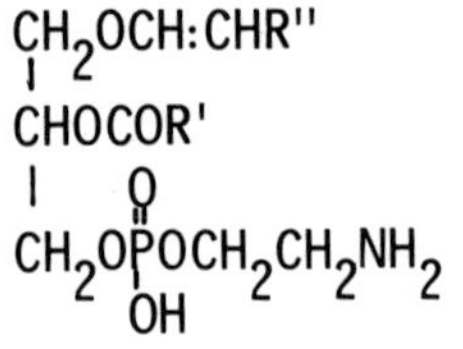

$$\begin{array}{l} CH_2OCH{:}CHR'' \\ |\\ CHOCOR' \\ |\quad\; O \\ CH_2O\overset{\|}{P}OCH_2CH_2NH_2 \\ \quad\;\; OH \end{array}$$

ethanolamine plasmalogen

(phosphatidalethanolamine)

Plasmalogens constitute 18 to 30 percent of total brain phospholipids, and are even more concentrated in myelin. They may be synthesized by reduction of the corresponding phosphatide, and probably also by pathways similar to those of the phosphatides, but starting with a diglyceride in which the reduction to a vinyl ether has already been performed. A plasmalogenase which preferentially cleaves the vinyl ether linkage has been found in brain predominantly in non-myelin membrane fractions of white matter. This may be the degradative route.

The only major sphingolipid containing phosphorus is sphingomyelin, discussed below along with the other sphingolipids.

iii) Sphingolipids[8]

The sphingolipids are derived from the long-chain lipid base sphingosine (see following table). In the synthesis of sphingosine, palmityl coenzyme A and serine are condensed to form 3-ketodihydrosphingosine in a reaction that requires pyridoxal phosphate (Figure 4.5). The keto-derivative may be reduced to dihydrosphingosine (sphinganine), and then oxidized to sphingosine (sphingenine). While these two reactions will occur separately, there is the possibility of an internal oxido-reduction reaction.

Sphingosine may be N-acylated with a fatty acyl CoA derivative to form ceramide. In sphingomyelin the terminal hydroxyl of ceramide is linked by a phosphodiester bond to choline. On the basis of recent metabolic data, ceramide is considered to be the *in vivo* intermediate in sphingomyelin synthesis. The other possible route, in which sphingosine reacts with

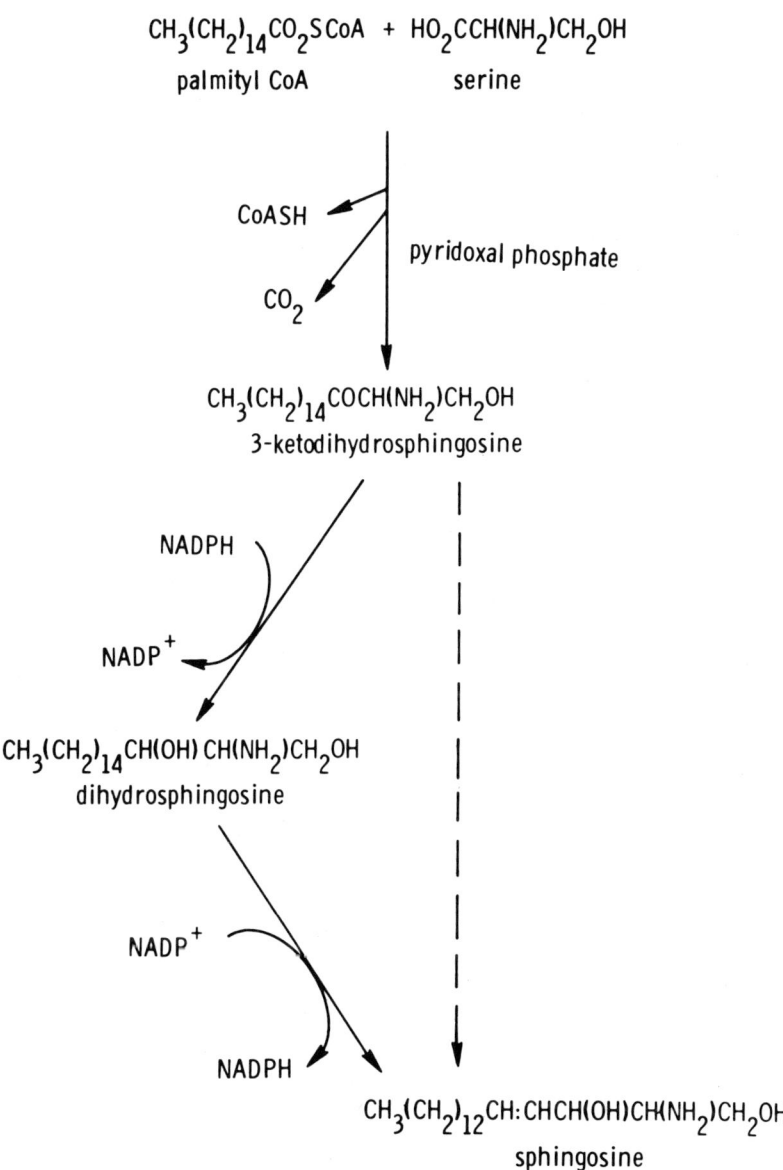

Figure 4.5 Synthesis of sphinogosine.

STRUCTURE OF SPHINGOLIPIDS

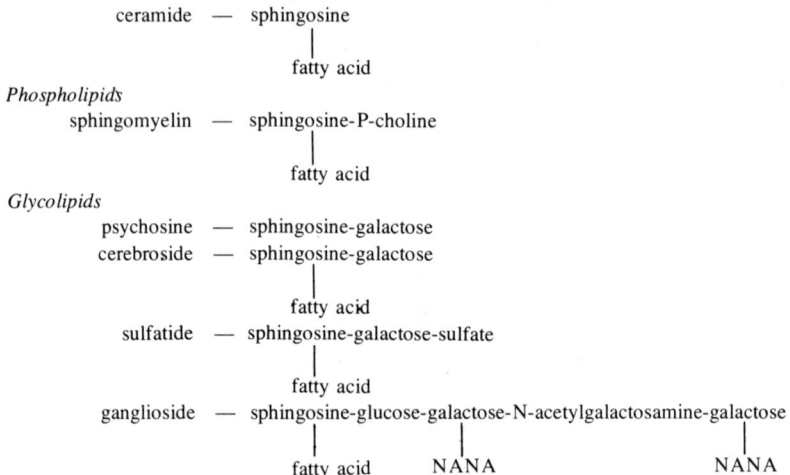

CDPcholine to form sphingosine phosphorylcholine which is then acylated to form sphingomyelin, is probably not functional *in vivo*.

When galactose is added to the terminal hydroxyl group of sphingosine, psychosine is formed. This glycosylation is performed by a uridine diphosphate derivative, as in the case of glycoprotein biosynthesis (see below). Theoretically, cerebroside may be formed by N-acylation of psychosine with a fatty acid, or by glycosylation of ceramide, but the *in vivo* pathway appears to be by way of ceramide. This glycosylation is performed by a specific galactosyl transferase from the appropriate UDPhexose. Galactocerebroside is the principal cerebroside in brain, and neither cerebroside nor sulfatide is present prior to myelination. Unlike the other cerebral lipids, cerebroside contains a high concentration of fatty acids hydroxylated on the α-carbon (60 to 80 percent).

Cerebroside sulfate (sulfatide) is formed by sulfation of the 3-position of the galactose of cerebroside by 3'phosphoadenosine-5'phosphosulfate (PAPS, or "active sulfate"). The human autosomal recessive disease, metachromatic leucodystrophy, is caused by a deficient activity of sulfatidase, the enzyme responsible for sulfatide catabolism. This deficiency leads to sulfatide accumulation in the glial and nerve cells and consequent breakdown of the myelin sheath. Sphingolipid metabolism is summarized in Figure 4.6.

IV. Neuronal Processes   89

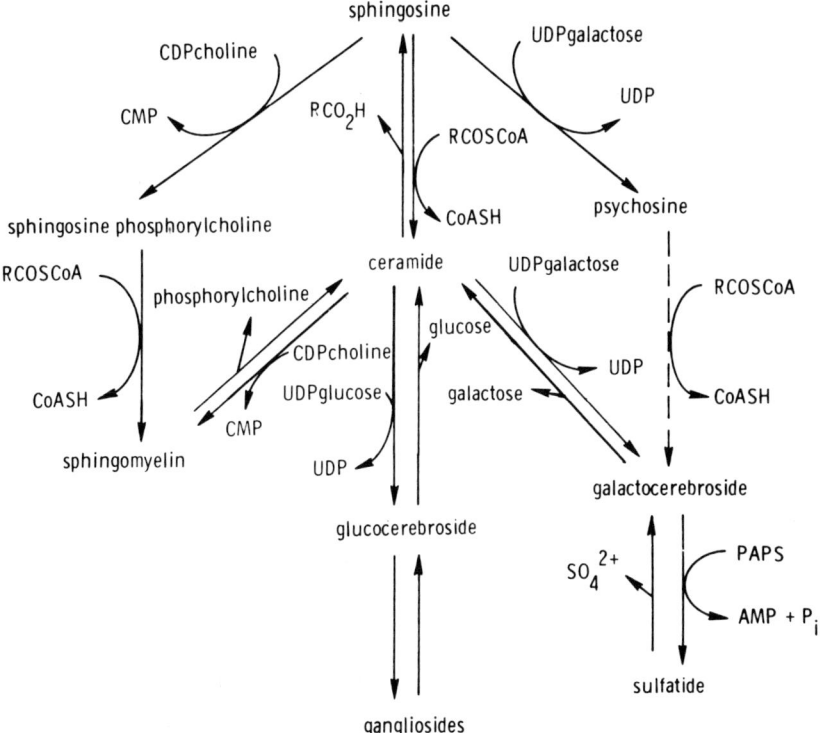

Figure 4.6 Metabolism of sphingolipids.

iv) Gangliosides[9]

Gangliosides are glycosphingolipids containing sialic acid. The structures of the principal brain gangliosides are shown in Figure 4.7. Several others are found, especially in invertebrates. The essential features of the structure are a lipid part, ceramide, and a carbohydrate part consisting of a chain of hexoses and hexosamines to which variable amounts of sialic acid (N-acylneuraminic acid [NANA]) are attached. In the common brain gangliosides the sugar backbone is invariant, with changes only in the number and position of the sites of attachment of the NANA. The sialic acids attached to the main carbohydrate chain markedly alter the character of the molecules so that, unlike any of the other lipids, gangliosides are soluble in

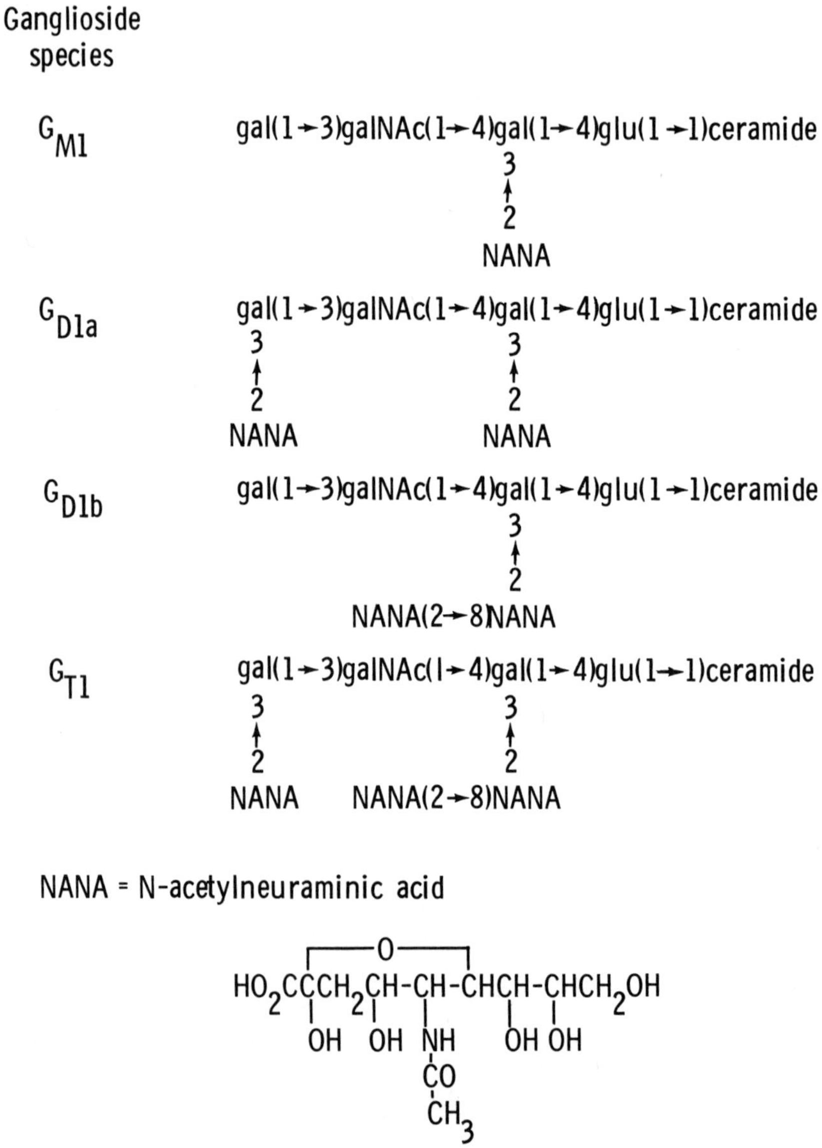

Ganglioside species

G_{M1} gal(1→3)galNAc(1→4)gal(1→4)glu(1→1)ceramide
                               3
                               ↑
                               2
                             NANA

G_{D1a} gal(1→3)galNAc(1→4)gal(1→4)glu(1→1)ceramide
               3   3
               ↑   ↑
               2   2
             NANA   NANA

G_{D1b} gal(1→3)galNAc(1→4)gal(1→4)glu(1→1)ceramide
                               3
                               ↑
                               2
                         NANA(2→8)NANA

G_{T1} gal(1→3)galNAc(1→4)gal(1→4)glu(1→1)ceramide
               3   3
               ↑   ↑
               2   2
             NANA   NANA(2→8)NANA

NANA = N-acetylneuraminic acid

$$HO_2CCCH_2CH-CH-CHCH-CHCH_2OH$$
with O bridge, OH, OH, NH, OH, OH substituents; NH-CO-CH_3

Figure 4.7 Structure of principal brain gangliosides and NANA. Nonenclature is that of Svennerholm.[9]

aqueous media and separate into the aqueous phase when partitioned between chloroform, methanol and water mixtures.

Gangliosides are membrane components and are found only in subcellular fractions that contain membranes. Their name arises from the discovery of their accumulation in ganglion cells in Tay-Sachs disease, but they are present throughout the nervous system. Gangliosides are also found in most other tissues, though in lower amounts and of different molecular structures. The concentration of gangliosides in nervous tissue tends to increase as one ascends the phylogenetic scale. In the brain, gangliosides are more concentrated in gray matter than in white, and microdissection techniques suggest that they are predominantly neuronal rather than glial. Subcellular fractionation procedures show gangliosides to be present in mitochondrial, microsomal and synaptosomal fractions.[30] The greatest amount is in the microsomal fraction, but the greatest concentration is in the synaptosomal fraction. The microsomal fraction in brain is ill-defined and contains plasma membranes of both neuronal and glial origin as well as endoplasmic reticulum and the Golgi apparatus. It contains most of the postsynaptic membrane that is not attached to synaptosomes. When bulk fractionation procedures are used to separate neurons from glia, the concentration of gangliosides is higher in the glial fraction. However, the neuronal fractions consist principally of neuronal perikarya, whereas the glial-enriched fractions normally contain many neuronal processes, especially dendrites, so that this result is not inconsistent with the location of gangliosides in neuronal processes. It is possible that gangliosides are concentrated at synapses (Chapter 5).

Gangliosides are thought to have their lipid moieties buried in the membrane with the carbohydrate tail protruding. Thus the sialic acid residue is probably on the surface of the membrane (extracellularly in plasma membranes). Approximately two-thirds of the sialic acid of the brain is in gangliosides, the remainder being in glycoprotein. Glycoprotein sialic acid is also on the membrane surface. Sialic acid residues play an important role in membrane excitability. Slices of cerebral cortex that have been stored in the cold for several hours lose their metabolic excitability to electrical stimuli and also lose their sialic acid. Excitability may be restored by the addition of purified gangliosides, but not sialic acid, to the incubation medium.[31] The principal brain gangliosides are distinguished only by the number and position of their sialic acid residues, and the possibility exists that alterations in these sialic acids could alter the properties of excitable membranes. Gangliosides (and sialoglycoproteins) bind Ca^{2+} at their hydrophilic ends and thus control the concentration of this ion, which is involved in membrane depolarization and neurotransmitter release.

Gangliosides are synthesized from ceramide. The first reaction is glycosylation, but the sugar added is glucose rather than the galactose used for galactocerebroside synthesis. Further glycosylation reactions, also involving uridine diphosphate derivatives, add on three more sugars. It has been suggested that multiglycosyltransferase complexes perform this sequence of reactions.

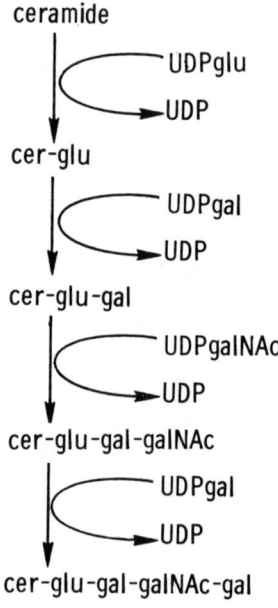

Sialic acid is transferred to the sugars via a cytidine nucleotide derivative, CMP-sialic acid (CMP-NANA). The first sialic acid group is transferred to the first galactose molecule and this addition probably precedes the addition of the last two sugars. Sialic acid is synthesized by condensation of N-acetylmannosamine-6-phosphate with phosphoenol pyruvate and subsequent dephosphorylation of the product.

$$\text{N-acetylmannosamine-6-phosphate} + \text{phosphoenol pyruvate}$$
$$\downarrow P_i$$
$$\text{N-acetylneuraminic acid-9-phosphate}$$
$$\downarrow P_i$$
$$\text{N-acetylneuraminic acid}$$

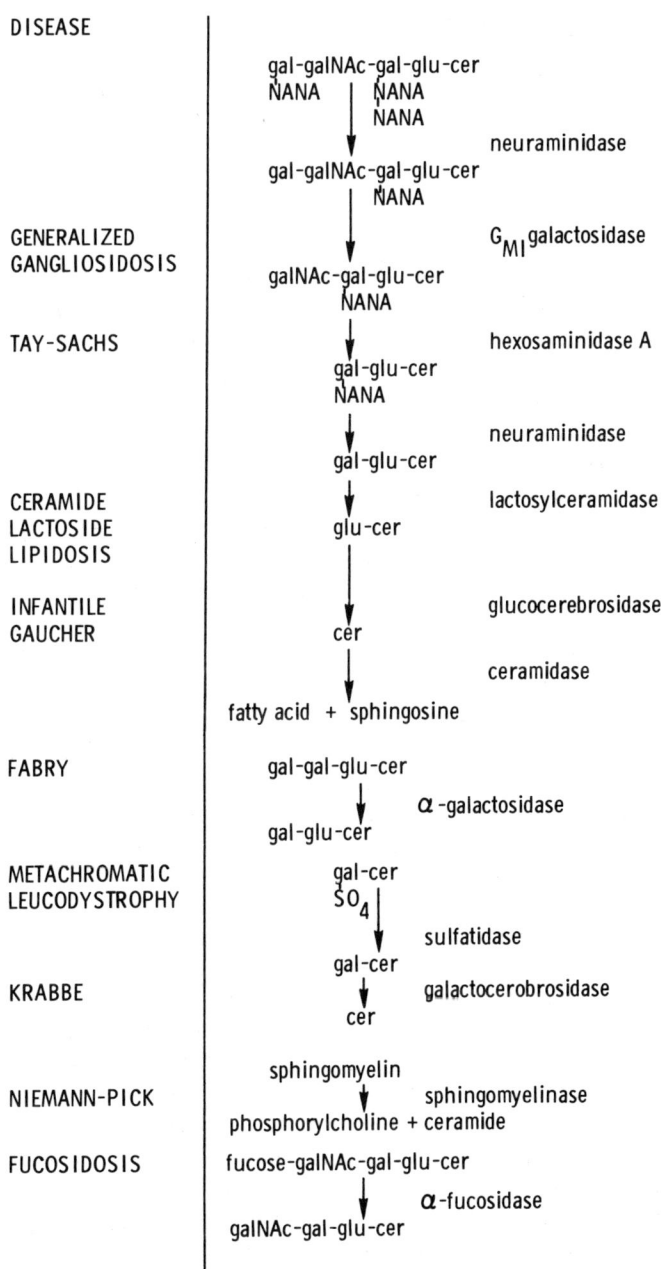

Figure 4.8 Known genetic diseases of lipid metabolism.

CMP-NANA is formed directly from CTP and sialic acid:

$$CTP + NANA \rightarrow CMP\text{-}NANA + PP_i$$

At least three sialyl transferases are used for brain ganglioside synthesis.

Kinetic data suggest that mitochondrial and synaptosomal gangliosides are synthesized from separate pools. Glycosyl and sialyl transferases are localized microsomally and perhaps also synaptosomally. This suggests that gangliosides may be synthesized locally at synapses, but recently axoplasmic transport of gangliosides from the nerve cell body to the synaptic terminal has been demonstrated in the optic nerve.[18] These transported gangliosides may be associated with mitochondria and other membranous organelles.

Ganglioside catabolism involves the initial removal of two NANA residues by sialidases (neuraminidases). The two terminal sugars are then removed by separate glycosidases (Figure 4.8). Further degradation is then similar to that of the other sphingolipids (Figure 4.6).

Several hereditary disorders are associated with impaired ganglioside breakdown.[10] Deficiencies of enzymes in this pathway may lead to the accumulation of specific intermediates. Many of these sphingolipidoses are characterized by the inability to cleave the carbohydrate chain. Figure 4.8 shows the known enzyme defects that cause the accumulation of the lipid preceding the block. Abnormal increases in total gangliosides also occur commonly in many neurological disorders not associated with a known specific enzyme defect. A deficiency of ganglioside sialic acid content has been found in Creutzfeldt-Jacob disease, which is characterized by neuronal destruction and astroglial proliferation. There is a relationship between the severity of neuron loss and the decrease of sialic acid. This may reflect the largely neuronal location of gangliosides.

v) Cholesterol

Cholesterol is the single most concentrated constituent of brain, comprising about 10 percent of the dry weight. In white matter the concentration is even higher (13 percent of the dry weight). Most of this cholesterol is in the free form; esters represent much less than one percent of total cholesterol, except early in myelination when the ester concentration is as high as 20 percent. Radioactively labeled cholesterol injected into the bloodstream is very poorly take up by the brain, which synthesizes most of its own cholesterol. A highly active cerebral synthesis has been demonstrated from precursors such as glucose or acetate. The biosynthetic pathway involves the initial condensation of three acetyl CoA molecules to form β-hydroxy-β-methylglutaryl CoA. A reduction with NADPH produces the key intermediate,

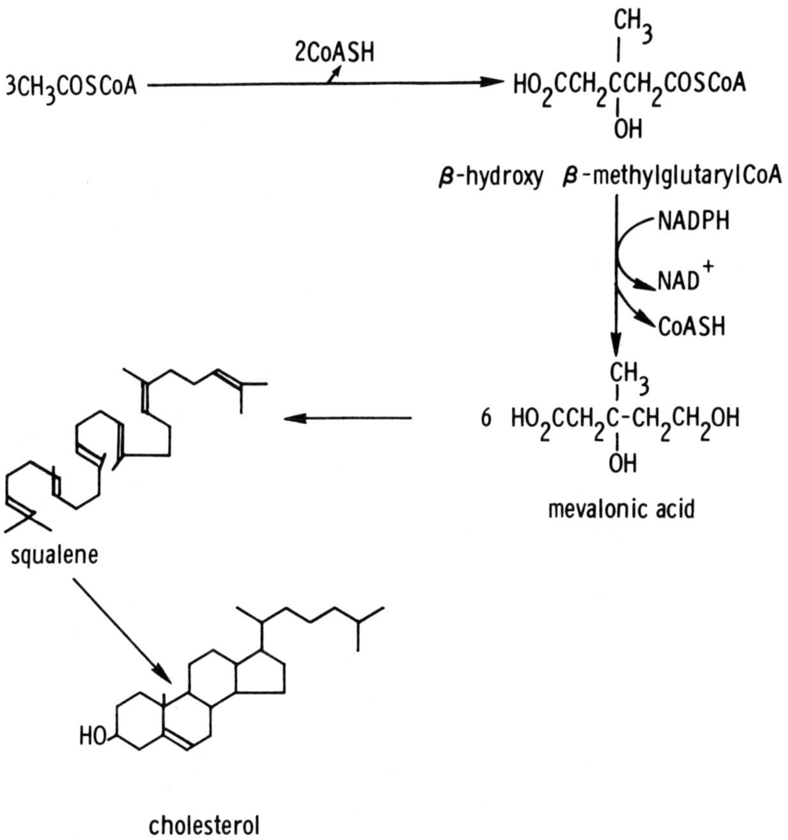

$$3CH_3COSCoA \xrightarrow{2CoASH} HO_2CCH_2\underset{OH}{\overset{CH_3}{\underset{|}{\overset{|}{C}}}}CH_2COSCoA$$

β-hydroxy β-methylglutarylCoA

$$\downarrow \begin{array}{l} \nearrow NADPH \\ \searrow NAD^+ \\ \searrow CoASH \end{array}$$

$$6\ HO_2CCH_2\underset{OH}{\overset{CH_3}{\underset{|}{\overset{|}{C}}}}-CH_2CH_2OH$$

mevalonic acid

squalene

cholesterol

Figure 4.9 Synthesis of cholesterol.

mevalonic acid. Six molecules of mevalonic acid pyrophosphate are then linked together by appropriate condensation reactions to form squalene. A series of further reactions then performs the four ring closures necessary to form cholesterol (Figure 4.9).

Cholesterol is not further metabolized appreciably in brain, though in other tissues it may serve as a precursor to steroids. Cerebral cholesterol catabolism, resulting from disease or injury, occurs by esterification and excretion.

vi) Glycoproteins

Glycoproteins are found in all tissues and consist of proteins to which chains of carbohydrate residues are covalently bound. Much of total cerebral protein is present as glycoprotein and some of these complexes are unique to the nervous system. In cerebral glycoproteins the protein and carbohydrate chains are generally connected by an O-glycosidic linkage between the hydroxyl group of a serine or threonine residue and a hydroxyl group of a hexosamine (D-glucosamine or D-galactosamine). The carbohydrate chain largely consists of 1 – 4 or 1 – 3 linked glucose, galactose or mannose residues, which are often present as the amine derivatives. The amino groups of hexomanines are frequently acetylated. Because of the many available linkages, a large degree of variation is possible in relatively short oligosaccharide chains with rather few constituent sugars.

Cerebral sialic acid is divided approximately 1:2 between glycoprotein and gangliosides. In sialoproteins the sialic acid residues are commonly found lateral to the main hexose chain, attached to the 3- or 6-carbon of galactose or N-acetylgalactosamine. The free carboxyl residue of sialic acid confers an acidic character to the carbohydrate chains of glycoproteins and gangliosides.

The sugar L-fucose (6-deoxy-L-galactose) has the form of a methylated pentose and is often found at the terminal of the carbohydrate chain, linked to the 2-carbon of a hexose or hexose derivative. The arrangement of the constituents in a hypothetical glycoprotein is:

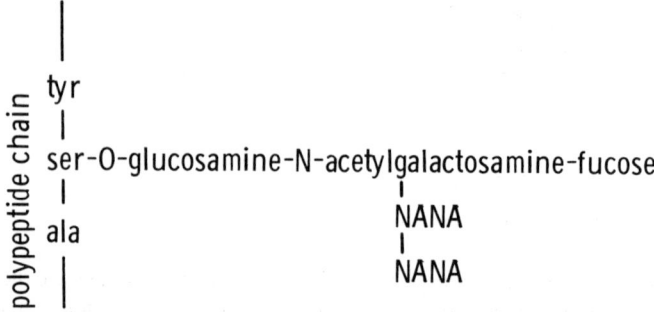

The protein part of glycoproteins is synthesized first by ribosomes, and the carbohydrates are subsequently added. This addition is performed by a series of transfer reactions involving nucleotide-sugar derivatives. The derivative is first synthesized from the sugar-phosphate and the nucleoside triphosphate. Then the sugar is transferred to the protein receptor releasing the nucleoside diphosphate. Thus in the case of glucosamine the sequence of reactions is:

glucosamine + ATP → glucosamine-6-phosphate + ADP

glucosamine-6-phosphate + UTP → UDPglucosamine + PP$_i$

UDPglucosamine + acceptor protein → protein-glucosamine + UDP

This sequence requires the hydrolysis of two energy-rich phosphate bonds and is reminiscent of the cytidine nucleotide dependent processes used in phospholipid synthesis. Additional sugars may be transferred from their nucleotide derivatives to the preceding sugar, forming carbohydrate chains.

Not all sugars are transferred by uridine derivatives, and there is a specificity of the nucleotide for a particular sugar. Thus fucose and mannose form guanosine diphosphate (GDP) derivatives, while sialic acid forms a cytidine *mono*phosphate derivative (CMP-NANA). However, uridine is by far the most common nucleoside involved, and is used in the transfer of glucose, glucosamine, galactose, galactosamine, glucuronic acid and the N-acetylated hexosamines. Uridine nucleotide sugars account for one-third to one-half of the soluble uridine nucleotides in brain. These same derivatives are used in the synthesis of the glycolipids and polysaccharides.

The hydrophilic carbohydrate parts of membrane glycoproteins, like the glycolipids, protrude into the aqueous surround.[29] In plasma membranes, the carbohydrates are exclusively on the outer surface. They may, therefore, play a role in cell surface recognition and transport phenomena. Considerable cell specificity may exist for glycoproteins, as they have a great variety of carbohydrate groups and many possible conformations.

E. THE MYELIN SHEATH

The axon is often enclosed by a lipoprotein sheath formed by the surrounding glial cells. This sheath, known as myelin, allows the nerve fiber to conduct impulses more rapidly, and also insulates the axon from the surrounding tissue. The myelin sheath originates from the membrane of a satellite cell that repeatedly wraps itself around the axon. Satellite cells of the central nervous system are oligodendroglia, while the corresponding cells of the peripheral nervous system are Schwann cells. The formation of the sheath has best been observed in peripheral nerve. During myelination, the Schwann cell slowly rotates around the axon to form the spiral sheath. In tissue culture a complete rotation takes approximately forty-four hours.

The axon is left bare at the junctions between Schwann cells. It is only at these gaps (the nodes of Ranvier) that the excitable membrane is exposed. The action potential can only move along the axon by depolarizing adjacent nodes. This "saltatory" condition from node to node greatly increases the velocity of nerve conduction, which can be as high as 120 meters per second. Myelinated fibers even of small diameter have high conduction velocities. The mechanism of the formation of CNS myelin sheath is unknown. Since oligodendroglia may myelinate more than one axon, the processes rather than the cell body must enfold the axons.

Myelin has been isolated in a relatively pure form, using density gradient centrifugation.[11] The preparation exploits the characteristic density of myelin which is distinctly lower (1.08 gm/ml) than other membrane fractions. When brain tissue is homogenized in 0.32M (isotonic) sucrose and layered over 0.8M sucrose, myelin alone remains at the surface of the 0.8M sucrose following centrifugation. Other insoluble fractions such as synaptosomes or mitochondria are denser, and sediment throughthe 0.8M sucrose. Cesium chloride gradients have also been used to purify myelin. Myelin prepared by these flotation techniques can be further purified by repeated resuspension in distilled water. This procedure osmotically lyses any vesicles within the myelin that may contain encapsulated soluble axoplasmic material, and pure myelin may then be centrifuged down.[12] Myelin purified in this way contains about 70 to 80 percent lipid and 20 to 30 percent protein (see table, p. 80). Such purification carries the risk that selective loss of myelin components may occur with repeated washing. It is also very likely that the axonal membrane itself (axolemma) is retained in these preparations. Axolemmal contamination of purified myelin may account for the ganglioside content which is specifically enriched in a monosialoganglioside, G_{M1}. This ganglioside may readily be converted to the disialo- and trisialogangliosides which predominate in the neuronal membrane. The addition of sialic acid groups may occur in unmyelinated regions where gangliosides may play a role in excitability (p. 91).

The major lipid components of myelin (cholesterol, phospholipids, cerebrosides and sulfatides) are very stable.[13] A relationship between the stability of myelin lipids and the length of their fatty acid constituents has been suggested on the basis of the rates of disappearance of radioactivity from myelin lipids labeled in their fatty acid substituents. Certain myelin components such as gangliosides and phosphoinositides seem to be more metabolically active. The stability of these compounds in myelin preparations differs from that of the same compounds in nerve cells. The half-life of rat brain myelin phosphoinositides is about forty days, while non-myelin neuronal phosphoinositides have a half-life of two days. Minor contamination of myelin by non-myelin fractions would drastically affect the calculated half-life of such compounds in myelin, which may thus be longer than forty days.

Myelin proteins have been less well characterized than myelin lipids.[14] This is in part due to their insolubility, which has made them difficult to manipulate. Three major protein groups have been isolated from CNS myelin: the proteolipid protein, the basic protein and the Wolfgram proteins. These groups are probably not homogeneous. A part of myelin protein is soluble in chloroform-methanol (2:1, v/v), and in a two-phase chloroform-methanol-water system this protein remains in the organic, chloroform-rich phase together with the lipids. This is the proteolipid protein first described by Folch-Pi *et al.*, which accounts for 35 to 50 percent of myelin proteins.[32] Its solubility in chloroform is due to the unusually high content (50 percent) of nonpolar amino acids. The polypeptide component has a molecular weight of 25,000.

Extraction of myelin with weak acid solutions solubilizes the basic protein fraction. The protein is lysine- and arginine-rich, and has an isoelectric point above pH 10. This protein, as purified from bovine brain, has a molecular weight of 18,000 and appears to be highly unfolded with little tertiary structure. The myelin basic protein is distinguished from the basic histones by its content of tryptophan, which is absent from histones. The basic proteins of several species (human, ox, rabbit, guinea pig) run identically on polyacrylamide gel electrophoresis as one band. The amino acid sequences of several of these have been determined. However, in the rat and mouse two bands appear: one of higher molecular weight corresponding closely in electrophoretic mobility, amino acid composition and encephalitogenic character with that of other species, the other appearing to be related to the first by a deletion of about forty amino acids.

The third class of myelin proteins, the Wolfgram proteins, includes those of high molecular weight and is probably heterogeneous. It is characterized by a high content of dicarboxylic acids. The Wolfgram proteins are proteolipid proteins and account for about 20 percent of myelin proteins. They are soluble in *acidified* chloroform-methanol.

The proteins of PNS myelin appear to be different from those of CNS myelin, although the basic protein is also present. Myelin proteins are all very stable and are infrequently replaced in the adult.[14] The rates of turnover of the proteolipid protein and basic protein are identical, but that of the

Wolfgram protein is different. One enzyme activity is always found in association with, and is largely confined to, CNS myelin: 2',3' cyclic AMP phosphodiesterase. Though its natural substrate and function are unknown, and it is also found in the erythrocyte membrane, this enzyme is a useful marker for the presence of myelin.

Injection of the basic protein of CNS myelin initiates an immunological process resulting in extensive demyelination and the specific destruction of central nervous tissue, which causes paralysis and encephalomyelitis. The process is known as experimental allergic encephalomyelitis (EAE).[15] A small (9-amino acid) peptide capable of causing EAE in the guinea pig has been isolated from partial hydrolysates of the myelin basic protein, though other portions of the molecule are effective in other species. Injection of myelin extracted from peripheral nerve can cause autoimmune destruction of peripheral myelin (experimental allergic neuritis). Thus peripheral and central myelin are antigenically as well as chemically distinct. Further evidence that the myelin types are distinct is that in many diseases there is a preferential attack on either central or peripheral myelin, but not on both.

The induced immune response is at the cellular level rather than mediated by circulating antibody. Lymphocytic attack on myelin sheaths has been observed during EAE. In the normal animal, autoimmune responses to myelin do not occur, probably because the myelin is separated from the vascular system by the blood-brain barrier, and the lymphatic system is very poorly developed in the nervous system. Myelin develops largely after the formation of the blood-brain barrier and thus in isolation from the immune system. This may account for the peculiar vulnerability of myelin to autoimmune attack when immunocompetent lymphocytes gain access to it. They may not be able to recognize the myelin proteins as "self."

Experimental allergic encephalomyelitis has several features in common with the human disease multiple sclerosis, and has been used as an experimental model for it. Both conditions are characterized by extensive demyelination, apparently by immunological attack, and elevated γ-globulin levels in the cerebrospinal fluid. However, it is possible that a virus plays a role in this disease, perhaps by disturbing the barriers that normally prevent the immune system from gaining access to nervous tissue.

There is much evidence that myelin exists as a highly compact bilayer. This may be due to the high cholesterol content which enhances lipid compaction. The sphingolipids, in which myelin is rich, are long enough to extend through the protein layer and to interdigitate with similar molecules of the adjoining myelin layer. This structure may provide the stability and density required for myelin's largely static and insulatory role.

The development of myelin occurs after the formation of axons. In the human this commences before birth and continues for several years postnatally, but animals such as rabbits, cats and dogs are born with very little myelin. During development, glial proliferation and myelin deposition coincide with increased coordination of movement and the appearance of the mature electroencephalogram. Optimal myelination is dependent upon the presence of several hormones and an adequate nutritional state during development. A deficiency of thyroid hormone leads to, amongst other things, a reduced rate of myelination.[16] Steroids such as cortisol are also needed for the myelination process. Administration of cortisol to very young animals can cause premature myelination, and thus the rise of steroid levels during development may be the factor initiating myelination. Precocious myelin development may impair completion of the phase of cerebral maturation involving glial proliferation and nerve cell body growth, resulting in an abnormally small brain.

Inadequate food intake has a less severe effect on the growth and size of the brain than of many other organs. However, cerebral deficits resulting from malnutrition are known. These include reduced brain size and decreased amounts of cerebral DNA, RNA, protein and lipids.[17] In the human, malnutrition during early childhood causes a reduction in mental abilities that appears to be largely irreversible. The immature, actively myelinating brain is much more vulnerable to dietary deficiencies than the mature brain. Dietary factors may affect the brain either directly or indirectly via systemic hormones.

Myelin metabolism may also be affected by a variety of toxic agents of the organophosphate type such as triorthocresylphosphate.[33] After administration of these compounds, there is typically a delay before the appearance of neurotoxic symptoms such as the ataxia indicative of peripheral demyelination. Central demyelination occurs to a lesser extent. As the Schwann cells are capable of a greater degree of axonal remyelination than the oligodendroglia, peripheral toxic symptoms may be reversible. The organophosphorus compounds that cause disturbances of myelin metabolism may exert their effect directly on myelin-forming cells, or demyelination may be a secondary response to a disturbance of neuronal metabolism.

The Jackson Laboratories at Bar Harbor, Maine, have developed a large collection of neurological mutants of the mouse. Several of these have genetic defects that result in disordered synthesis of myelin.[34] Since the immature animal does not require myelin for survival, defects of myelination are not immediately apparent. These mutants are autosomal recessives or X-linked. The homozygote is often not able to survive much beyond the time at which myelinogenesis normally occurs. Although their molecular basis is not known, these genetic defects are characterized by very low quantities of myelin, often of an abnormal type. While many such mutants contain low concentrations of synthetic enzymes, especially those concerned with cerebroside or sulfatide synthesis, it is not clear whether this is a primary defect or a reflection of the failure of the oligodendroglia to differentiate normally. A more recent view is that the primary defect may involve one of the myelin proteins — possibly the proteolipid protein, which is almost absent before the onset of myelination. Other genetic disorders of myelin such as metachromatic leucodystrophy may involve an insufficient level of a catabolic enzyme.

F. AXOPLASMIC TRANSPORT

The axon connects the cell body with the synaptic effector areas that impinge on other cells. The cell body contains the genetic material within the nucleus and much of the machinery of the cell for the synthesis of RNA, protein and carbohydrate. In contrast, the synapse has a very limited capacity for the synthesis of macromolecules. While small molecules may be taken up locally by the synapse, macromolecules are not extensively exchanged between cells. In addition to its ability to transmit action potentials, the axon can transport materials between the perikaryon and the synapses. The synapse thus depends for its supply of macromolecules on axonal transport from the cell body. Conversely, the cell body receives material from the synapses that may control the supply of material to the synapse. Effective intracellular communication within the neuron may lay the foundation for the sophisticated intercellular communication that characterizes nervous tissue.

The passage of materials along the axon was first suggested by Weiss, who showed that the ligation of an axon resulted in an accumulation of materials on the perikaryal (proximal) side of the block.[35] Later work showed that mitochondria and catecholamine-containing vesicles were among the accumulated materials.[36] A lesser accumulation of particles appeared on the synaptic (distal) side of the ligature, indicating that axonal transport could take place in both directions. Direct microscopic observation of living axons also suggested that particles migrated both toward and away from the perikaryon.

These observations were extended by the administration of radioactive compounds in the region of the nerve cell body. In this way radioactive atoms can be incorporated into intracellular materials and their movement within the axon can be followed. Movement can be detected by radioactive analysis following dissection and chemical fractionation, but may be better followed by radioautography. The use of radioautography to determine the precise location of labeled molecules, in combination with biochemical techniques to determine their nature, has established that many classes of compounds migrate within the axon toward the synaptic termini.[18]

Axoplasmic transport assures the axon and the nerve terminals of a constant supply of structural and enzymic proteins needed for the maintenance of both morphological integrity and the capacity for neurotransmission.

i) Molecules transported

Neurotransmitters

The location of catecholamine neurotransmitters can be determined by fluorescence microscopy. The accumulation of catecholamines on the proximal side of a ligatured nerve has been visualized by this means. Such studies are readily carried out in peripheral nerve bundles such as the sciatic nerve, where the axon is relatively accessible and of considerable length.

Reserpine treatment results in a depletion of neuronal catecholamines. This is followed by a compensatory increased rate of synthesis of neuronal catecholamines (p. 181). Following reserpine treatment this increase in the amount of catecholamine can be detected by fluorescence microscopy. The catecholamines first appear in the nerve cell bodies, then gradually spread distally along the axons.

There is also evidence for a proximodistal migration of acetylcholine and GABA. However, since much local synthesis occurs presynaptically, the bulk of neurotransmitters may not be synthesized in the perikarya and transported axoplasmically to the synapses.

Proteins

A flow of proteins along the axon has been demonstrated in many systems, largely with the use of radioisotopic tracers. One useful experimental model is the visual system. Isotopes injected into the vitreous humor of the eye may be incorporated into macromolecules in the retinal ganglion cell bodies, which lie at the innermost margin of the retina. Radioactive macromolecules may be transported to the nerve termini of the ganglion cells, which lie within the primary visual areas of the brain. In the case of non-mammalian vertebrates these termini consist of the optic lobes, which are readily accessible and each of which is innervated by a single eye (Figure 4.10). In such animals the optic nerve is totally crossed over at the chiasm, so that there is only direct cellular communication with the contralateral optic lobe. Both optic lobes may accumulate radioactivity by diffusion or by way of the vascular system, but only the contralateral lobe may receive it directly by transmission within cells. Any excess radioactivity found in the contralateral lobe over the ipsilateral lobe is presumably due to axoplasmic flow. Using this system, it has been found that the major part of axonal protein migrates at a rate of 2 mm to 10 mm per day. This slow axoplasmic transport of protein commences at an early stage of cerebral differentiation, when the axons are growing out from the perikaryon. At this time the rate of movement of axonal protein is several times the rate of axonal outgrowth. A considerable amount of the total protein synthesized within the perikaryon of the retinal ganglion cell is transported along the axon. The migrating proteins are both soluble and particulate, and the microtubular protein, tubulin, also migrates at this slow rate. Water molecules within the axon are not freely diffusible, and it may be that the entire content of the axon migrates as a whole. Within this moving column, migration of specific components may occur at a faster rate. A small proportion of proteins migrate extremely

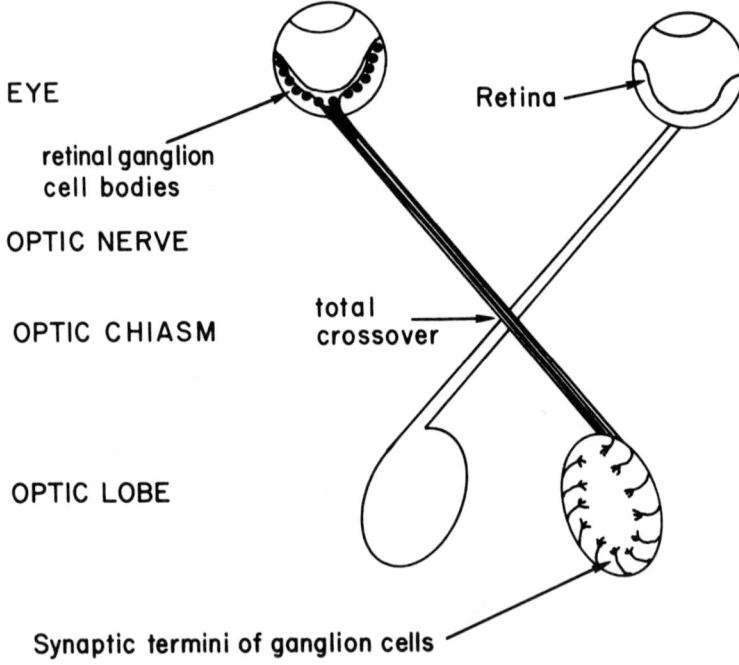

Figure 4.10 The avian visual system.

rapidly at around 200 mm per day.[19] In the chick embryo this rapid transport process develops only after the completion of axonal outgrowth, at the period of maximal synaptogenesis.[37] This is several days prior to the onset of myelination and coordinated electrical activity. Analysis of the fastest and slowest flow rates is performed more easily than for intermediate rates. It may be that a spectrum of flow rates exists within the axon.

Barondes has examined the overall axoplasmic migration of proteins within the central nervous system by studying the labeling of the protein of the synaptosome fraction after intracerebral injection of radioactive amino acids.[38] There is a delay in the labeling of this fraction relative to that of other subcellular fractions which may reflect the time taken for protein synthesized perikaryally to migrate to the synapse. These experiments enable the estimation of the average axonal length in various cerebral areas.

Ligation experiments, similar to those described in the section on neurotransmitters, have suggested the transport of several enzymes, demonstrating their accumulation at the points of ligation. The enzymes include specific neuronal enzymes such as choline acetylase and acetylcholinesterase.

Axoplasmic transport is used in the translocation of the neurohypophyseal peptide hormones from their hypothalamic sites of synthesis to the sites within the posterior pituitary gland where they are released (Chapter 6). Using the technique of injecting a single nerve cell body with radioactive amino acids, Gainer has identified a specific neurosecretory neuron in the land snail, which synthesizes a distinct class of polypeptides.[39] These peptides are transported along the axon in granules prior to liberation at the synaptic terminus. Their synthesis and migration are regulated by physiological conditions. The hypothalamic neurosecretory mechanisms of higher organisms, while more complex, may essentially operate in a similar manner.

Glycoproteins, glycolipids and phospholipids

Glycoproteins are exported to a great extent from the perikaryon of the retinal ganglion cells. Over half the glycoprotein labeled by radioactive fucose in the cell body migrates to the synapse at a rate more than 100 times faster than the bulk of migrating protein. These glycoproteins are rather stable upon reaching the synaptic junction and thus rapid transport of such molecules is probably quantitatively minor relative to the total axoplasmic transport process. The role of these molecules at the synaptic junction is unknown but they may have a relation to the specialized features of the synaptic cleft, which is rich in carbohydrate-staining material.

The main carbohydrate chains of glycoproteins contain galactose, mannose and fucose, generally attached to protein by glycosidic linkages to the hydroxyl residues of serine or threonine. This process occurs in the nerve cell body, probably within the Golgi apparatus. Recent studies suggest that galactosyl transferase and similar enzymes are not present in pure synaptic preparations. However, neuraminic acid, which is always lateral to the main carbohydrate chain of glycoproteins and gangliosides, may be attached at the synapse rather than at the nerve cell body since sialyl transferases do appear in synaptosomal fractions. Neuraminic acid appears to reduce the intracellular mobility of compounds to which it is added. It may be that such addition occurs upon the conversion of transported glycoproteins and gangliosides to constituents of the synaptic or axonal plasma membrane.[40] Sulfated glycoproteins have also been shown to migrate along the axon; the addition of the sulfate residue to these molecules takes place in the nerve cell body rather than at the synapse.

A rapid migration of perikaryally synthesized gangliosides and phospholipids toward the synapse also occurs. As with glycoproteins, the neuraminic acid component of gangliosides may be added at the synaptic junction. Like glycoproteins, transported gangliosides are relatively stable and persist for a long time at the synapse.

RNA

Though ribosomes are generally not seen in electron microscope sections of the axon, small amounts of RNA have been reported within axoplasm and RNA appears to migrate toward the synaptic terminus from the nerve cell body. This process occurs at a rather slow rate (approximately 12 mm per day in the chick), and less than 5 percent of the RNA synthesized in the cell body passes into the axon and appears at the synaptic junction.[40] Migrating RNA is largely ribosomal but may contain other types of RNA. Transported RNA may permit the synthesis of proteins to occur at the synapse. This synthesis could be immediately responsive to changes in synaptic activity. The extent of autonomous synaptic protein synthesis is uncertain. While synaptosomes can incorporate labeled amino acids into protein, it is difficult to be sure that these preparations are free of postsynaptic or glial elements that may contain ribosomes (p. 148). A migration of RNA from the nerve cell body in a distal direction along dendrites has been clearly demonstrated by autoradiography (p. 60).

ii) Mechanism

Several mechanisms have been proposed to account for axoplasmic transport. Though the basis of this process is unknown, several possibilities can be ruled out.[19]

1. The transport is not due to diffusion, since proteins could not diffuse as

rapidly as observed flow rates. In addition, axoplasmic transport is an energy-requiring process. Ochs has shown that fast axoplasmic transport is very temperature-dependent and abolished by inhibitors of oxidative phosphorylation such as dinitrophenol.

2. The mechanism of axoplasmic transport cannot be peristalsis of the axonal membrane, because axoplasmic flow is highly selective and may take place simultaneously in two directions within a single nerve fiber (see below).

3. Axoplasmic flow is not a consequence of the outflow of perikaryally produced material. Following axonal section, transport continues in the distal segment of the axon for a considerable time and is thus a local axonal phenomenon. Axoplasmic transport requires the local generation of ATP and can be prevented by anoxia or metabolic inhibitors acting on an axonal segment. Transport is not possible in an axonal region that has been frozen and thawed.

4. Protein synthesis is not essential for axoplasmic transport, as transport continues even after inhibition of perikaryal protein synthesis by acetoxycycloheximide.

5. Axoplasmic transport does not depend upon the presence of a myelin sheath, as transport also occurs within non-myelinated axons.

6. Axoplasmic transport is not dependent upon the electrical excitability of the axonal membrane, since flow is not inhibited by tetrodotoxin which abolishes the action potential. The effect of functional activity on axoplasmic transport has been examined in several laboratories. The most elegant of such studies is that of Kreutzberg and his colleagues who have been able to insert a multibarreled electrode into the cell body of an individual spinal motoneuron.[41] Radioactive amino acids can then be iontophoretically introduced into the neuron through one barrel, while another barrel may serve to stimulate the neuron. The axoplasmic flow of protein is then determined by radioautography. In this way it has been found that although activation may lead to an increase of the amount of axoplasmic flow, the velocity of the process appears to be unaffected.

Electron microscopy of axons reveals a very distinct pattern of longitudinally arranged tubules and filaments (Figure 1.7). The protein constituents of these axonal structures can be dissociated into subunits of molecular weight 45,000 to 60,000 which are arranged in helical or linear aggregates longitudinally within the axon. Neurotubules closely resemble the microtubules found in mitotic cells and within cilia.[20] The similarity between microtubules and neurotubules extends to the biochemical level. Both structures bind the mitotic inhibitor colchicine and are rather specifically precipitated by vinblastin. The concentration of vinblastin-precipitable protein is higher in the nervous system than in any other tissue. Since mature nervous tissue has a very low mitotic index, the bulk of this precipitated protein is probably derived from neurotubules. Microtubules in mitosing cells appear to be related to the intracellular transport of materials preceding cell division. There is evidence that neurotubules may function in a similar manner in intracellular transport along the axon since vinblastin or colchicine inhibit axonal transport, especially the rapid component. Cytochalasin B, which disrupts the polygonal patterns of neurofilaments, has a much lesser effect on axoplasmic transport but severely inhibits axonal outgrowth. Electron microscope radioautography has shown protein to move distally along the axon largely in areas adjacent to microtubules. Colchicine-binding protein from brain (tubulin) has features that resemble muscle actin (p. 119). When mixed with muscle myosin, the resulting solution undergoes viscosity changes analogous to those occurring in actomyosin. The precise relationship between axoplasmic flow and neurotubules is unclear, but it is possible that contractile tubular elements working in succession can progressively shunt other substances forward by reversibly binding to them.

Tubulin is one of the most abundant brain proteins and has a half-life of approximately 4 days in the mouse. It constitutes 15 percent of total soluble protein in the adult brain and over 40 percent of soluble protein in embryonic brain. A considerable fraction of the total protein synthetic machinery of the brain must be directed toward tubulin synthesis. There is evidence that neurotubular protein may be reversibly phosphorylated. This could transiently affect the conformation of the protein and thus its sequestering abilities. Alternation of phosphorylation and dephosphorylation cycles in successive subunits of the tubules, may be a means of moving materials in either direction along the nerve.

Colchicine inhibits many cellular secretory mechanisms thought to involve exocytosis, such as neurotransmitter release or liberation of thyroid hormones from thyroid slices stimulated with thyrotropin. Thus tubulin-like proteins may also be involved in the export of materials from a variety of cells.

iii) Transneuronal and Retrograde Transport

Radioautographic studies suggest that a small amount of protein reaching the synaptic termini may cross the synapse and enter the postsynaptic cell in an intact form.[42] The possibility of large molecules moving between nerve cells suggests a means by which complex information could be exchanged.

In this way, neurons could reciprocally regulate their metabolism, and the information transfer could also account for the neurotrophic control of innervated cells. However, in a study in which protein synthesis in the ciliary ganglion of the chick was inhibited by puromycin, Droz concluded that the transneuronal transport of amino acids which were subsequently incorporated into protein, accounted for most if not all of the radioactive protein observed postsynaptically.[43] He could find no evidence for the transfer of intact proteins. Therefore, very little (if any) transneuronal transport of axoplasmically transported proteins occurs in this system.

The rapid changes in the histology of the perikaryon following nerve section indicates that the nerve cell body is responsive to the periphery (Chapter 3). This chromatolytic response occurs more rapidly when axotomy is close to the cell body, and the ascending signal appears to move at about 5 mm per day. The response could be caused by the cessation of retrograde migration of specific factors following nerve section or injury. The absence of this material may result in the derepression of genes, leading to the synthesis of new proteins. Alternatively, a positive chemical signal may be transported axoplasmically.

If horseradish peroxidase or albumin-tagged Evans blue dye (which forms a fluorescent complex) is injected into CNS regions containing nerve endings, these proteins can later be histochemically demonstrated within the corresponding nerve cell bodies. Thus entire protein molecules can be taken up at the synapse. Such uptake and retrograde transport may be increased during neural activity. Peroxidase can also be taken up in an intact form by nerve cell bodies and transported distally along axons and dendrites. By these means, pathways within the CNS can be traced.[44]

After ligature of a peripheral nerve bundle such as the sciatic, a gradual accumulation of certain enzymes (e.g. acetylcholinesterase, choline acetylase) occurs in both the proximal and distal nerve sections directly adjacent to the ligation. This also suggests a bidirectional movement of materials along the axon. It has recently been possible to directly observe the migration of particles within the living axons of peripheral nerve, using time-lapse cinematography in conjunction with optical diffraction techniques. Intra-axonal particles move "purposefully" in either direction in a saltatory manner. There appear to be channels for passage in a specific direction.

While proximodistal flow of material may enable the cell body to modify synaptic events, a flow of materials in the reverse direction could permit a reciprocal modulation of activity within the perikaryon by distal areas within the nerve.

CHAPTER 4 REFERENCES

Reviews and General References

1. Johnson, P. V., and Roots, B. I. *Nerve Membranes,* Pergamon Press, New York, 1972.
2. Katz, B. *Nerve, Muscle and Synapse,* McGraw-Hill, New York, 1966.
3. Cohen, L. B. Changes in neuron structure during action potential propagation and synaptic transmission. *Physiol. Rev.* 53:373–418, 1973.
4. Hawthorne, J. N., and Kai, M. Metabolism of phosphoinositides. In *Handbook of Neurochemistry,* Vol. 3 (Ed. A. Lajtha), Plenum Press, 1970, pp. 491–508.
5. Swanson, P. D., and Stahl, W. L. Ion transport. In *Basic Neurochemistry* (Ed. R. W. Albers, G. J. Siegel, R. Katzman, and B. W. Agranoff), Little, Brown, Boston, 1972, pp. 21–40.
6. Tower, D. B. *Neurochemistry of Epilepsy,* Thomas Press, Springfield, Ill., 1960.
7. Davson, H., and Danielli, J. F. *The Permeability of Natural Membranes,* Cambridge University Press, London, 1952.
8. Morell, P., and Braun, P. Biosynthesis and metabolic degradation of sphingolipids not containing sialic acid. *J. Lipid Res.* 13:293–310, 1972.
9. Svennerholm, L. Gangliosides. In *Handbook of Neurochemistry,* Vol. 3 (Ed. A. Lajtha), Plenum Press, New York, 1970, 425–52.
10. Brady, R. O. Inborn errors of lipid metabolism. *Advances in Enzymology,* 38:293–315, 1973.
11. Spohn, M., and Davison, A. N. Separation of myelin fragments from central nervous system. In *Research Methods in Neurochemistry,* Vol. 1 (Ed N. Marks and R. Rodnight), Plenum Press, New York, 1972, pp. 33–43.
12. Norton, W. T. Myelin. In *Basic Neurochemistry* (Ed. R. W. Albers, G. J. Siegel, R. Katzman, and B. W. Agranoff), Little, Brown, Boston, 1972, pp. 365–86.
13. LeBaron, F. N. Metabolism of myelin constituents. In *Handbook of Neurochemistry,* Vol. 3 (Ed. A. Lajtha), Plenum Press, New York, 1970, pp. 561–73.
14. Eylar, E. H. Myelin-specific proteins. In *Proteins of the Nervous System* (Ed. D. J. Schneider), Raven Press, New York, 1973, pp. 27–44.
15. Einstein, E. R. Basic protein of myelin and its role in experimental allergic encephalomyelitis and multiple sclerosis. In *Handbook of Neurochemistry,* Vol. 7 (Ed. A. Lajtha), Plenum Press, New York, 1972, pp. 107–29.
16. Balázs, R. Biochemical effects of thyroid hormones in the developing brain. In *Cellular Aspects of Growth and Differentiation* (Ed. D. C. Pease), University of California Press, Los Angeles 1971, pp. 273–320.
17. Dobbing, J. Undernutrition and the developing brain. In *Handbook of Neurochemistry,* Vol. 6 (Ed. A. Lajtha), Plenum Press, New York, 1971, pp. 255–66.
18. Bondy, S. C. Axoplasmic transport. In *Research Methods in Neurochemistry,* Vol. 4 (Ed. N. Marks and R. Rodnight), Plenum Press, New York, in press.
19. Ochs, J. Axoplasmic flow — the fast transport system in mammalian nerve fibers. In *Macromolecules and Behavior,* 2nd ed. (Ed. J. Gaito), Meredith Corp., New York, 1972, pp. 147–66.
20. Shelanski, M. L. Microtubules. In *Proteins of the Nervous System* (Ed. D. J. Schneider), Raven Press, New York, 1973, pp. 227–41.

Literature Cited

21. DeVries, G. H., Norton, W. T., and Raine, S. Axons: Isolation from mammalian central nervous system. *Science* 175:1370–72, 1972.
22. Clark, H. R., and Strickholm, A. Evidence for a conformational change in nerve membrane with depolarization. *Nature* 234:470–71, 1971.
23. Nachmansohn, D. Proteins in bioelectricity: the control of ion movements across excitable membranes. *Proc. Nat. Acad. Sci., U.S.A.* 61:1034–41, 1968.
24. McIlwain, H. Tetrodotoxin and the cation content, excitability and metabolism of isolated mammalian cerebral tissues. *Biochem. Pharmacol.* 16:1389–96, 1967.
25. Post, R. L., Kume, S., Tobin, T., Orcutt, B., and Sen, A. K. Flexibility of an active center in sodium-plus-potassium adenosine triphosphatase. *J. Gen. Physiol.* 54:306S – 26S, 1969.
26. Wheeler, K. P., and Whittam, R. The involvement of phosphatidylserine in adenosine triphosphatase activity of the sodium pump. *J. Physiol.* 207:303–28, 1970.
27. Whittam, R. The dependence of the respiration of brain cortex on active cation transport. *Biochem. J.* 82:205–12, 1962.
28. Singer, S. J., and Nicolson, G. L. The fluid mosaic model of the structure of cell membranes. *Science* 175:720–31, 1972.
29. Nicolson, G. L., and Singer, S. J. The distribution and asymmetry of mammalian cell surface saccharides utilizing ferritin-conjugated plant agglutinins as specific saccharide stains. *J. Cell Biol.* 60:236–48, 1974.
30. Avrova, N. F., Chenykaeva, E. Yu., Obukhova, E. L. Ganglioside composition and content of rat-brain subcellular fractions. *J. Neurochem.* 20:997–1004, 1973.
31. McIlwain, H. *Chemical Exploration of the Brain: a study of cerebral excitability and ion movement,* Elsevier Press, Amsterdam, 1963, pp. 16–20.
32. Folch, J., Ascoli, I., Lees, M., Meath, J. A., and LeBaron, F. N. Preparation of lipide extracts from brain tissue. *J. Biol. Chem.* 191:833–41, 1951.
33. Johnson, M. K. A phosphorylation site in brain and the delayed neurotoxic effect of some organophosphorus compounds. *Biochem. J.* 111:487–95, 1969.
34. Neskovic, N. M., Sarlieve, L. L., and Mandel, P. Biosynthesis of glycolipids in myelin deficient mutants: brain glycosyl transferases in Jimpy and Quaking mice. *Brain Research* 42:147–57, 1972.
35. Weiss, P. Endoneural edema in constricted nerve. *Anat. Rec.* 86:491–522, 1943.
36. Dahlström, A., and Häggendahl, J. Recovery of noradrenaline in adrenergic axons of rat sciatic nerves after reserpine treatment. *J. Pharm. Pharmac.* 21:633–38, 1969.
37. Bondy, S. C., and Madsen, C. J. Development of rapid axonal flow in the chick embryo. *J. Neurobiol.* 2.279–86, 1971
38. Barondes, S. H. Further studies of the transport of protein to nerve endings. *J. Neurochem.* 15:343–50, 1968.
39. Gainer, H. Effects of experimentally-induced diapause on the electrophysiology and protein synthesis patterns of identified molluscan neurons. *Brain Research* 39:387–402, 1972.
40. Bondy, S. C., and Madsen, C. J. The extent of axonal transport during development, determined by migration of various radioactively-labeled materials. *J. Neurochem.* 23: 1974.
41. Lux, H. D., Schubert, P., Kreutzberg, G. W. and Globus, A. Excitation and axonal flow:

autoradiographic study on motoneurons intracellularly injected with a ^{3}H-amino acid. *Exptl. Brain Res.* 10:197–204, 1970.
42. Specht, S. and Grafstein, B. Accumulation of radioactive protein in mouse cerebral cortex after injection of ^{3}H-fucose into the eye. *Exptl. Neurol.* 41:705–22, 1973.
43. Droz, B., Koenig, H. J. and Di Giamberardino, L. Axonal migration of protein and glycoprotein to nerve endings. I. Radioautographic analysis of the renewal of protein in nerve endings of chicken ciliary ganglion after intracerebral injection of [^{3}H]lysine. *Brain Research* 60:93–127, 1973.
44. LaVail, J. H. and LaVail, M. M. Retrograde axonal transport in the central nervous system. *Science* 176:1416–17, 1972.

V. The Synapse

A. CHEMICAL NEUROTRANSMISSION

A synapse is a specialized junction between two neurons. It occurs most often between an axon and a dendrite or the cell soma, but axo-axonal, dendro-dendritic, somato-dendritic and somato-somatic synapses also exist. There are two principal types of synapses: *chemical synapses* and *electrical synapses*.* Electrical synapses have been observed mainly in invertebrate systems, but recently they have been observed in the central nervous system of mammals and may be more prevalent than hitherto thought.

*Chemical and electrical synapses may be distinguished electrophysiologically by the presence or absence, respectively, of a significant time delay (*synaptic delay*) as an impulse is transmitted across the junction. They may be distinguished morphologically by the presence of a space 100 Å to 200 Å wide called the *synaptic cleft* between the neuronal plasma membranes at chemical synapses, whereas at electrical synapses there may be a small 20 Å gap (gap junctions) or the membranes may be fused (tight junctions). Electrical synapses are also devoid of the special morphological features of chemical synapses (described below), are unaffected by drugs that affect chemical synapses, do not require calcium for activity and may often, but not always, conduct impulses in both directions.

This chapter is concerned only with chemical synapses and chemical neurotransmission.

The most striking feature of chemical synapses is their asymmetry. This is evident at both the functional and morphological levels. An impulse may only be transmitted in one direction at a single synapse (always from an axon). The synapse thus acts as an electrical rectifying device analogous to an electronic diode. In electron micrographs, synapses may be distinguished by a pronounced thickening (the *synaptic thickening*) of the plasma membranes of both neurons over their area of contact (Figures 1.8, 5.1). In many synapses this thickening is asymmetrical, the presynaptic membrane being thinner than the postsynaptic one which may exceed 100 Å. Studies of the specificity of histological stains suggest that, especially in the postsynaptic region, the thickening itself is composed of protein.[1] The synaptic cleft is not empty but filled with carbohydrate material. This is probably the carbohydrate moieties of glycoproteins of the membranes, though it may also include glycolipids and mucopolysaccharides.[1]

The presynaptic region is characterized by the presence of vesicles (Figure 1.8). These vesicles are variable in size, shape and appearance, and it is thought that most of them contain neurotransmitter material stored ready for release. There is currently some speculation that the appearance of the vesicles (round, flat, smooth, coated, or dense-cored) or the intensity of staining may indicate the particular neurotransmitter stored.[1] Synaptic vesicles are not seen in the postsynaptic region which does, however, contain ribosomes, which are not seen presynaptically. Occasionally the ribosomes are particularly concentrated close to the synapse on the postsynaptic side, but this is not normal. Mitochondria often congregate presynaptically, and lysosomes may be present. These features of synapses are summarized diagrammatically in Figure 5.1.

Neurotransmission is thought to function in the following way: An electrical impulse travels down the axon to the presynaptic region, where the terminal membrane is depolarized. The depolarization results in the secretion or release into the synaptic cleft of molecules of chemical neurotransmitter that diffuse across the cleft and interact with specific receptors on the postsynaptic membrane. This interaction results in a postsynaptic potential (PSP) on the dendrite or soma of the receiving neuron. The PSP may be either excitatory (EPSP), resulting in a depolarization, or inhibitory (IPSP), resulting in a hyperpolarization, depending on the particular synapse, and in general is characteristic for a given neurotransmitter. (But see p. 125.) The neurotransmitter in the synaptic cleft is rapidly inactivated, either by catabolic enzymes or by being actively taken up into neuronal and possibly glial cells. In either case some recycling of the neurotransmitter may occur.

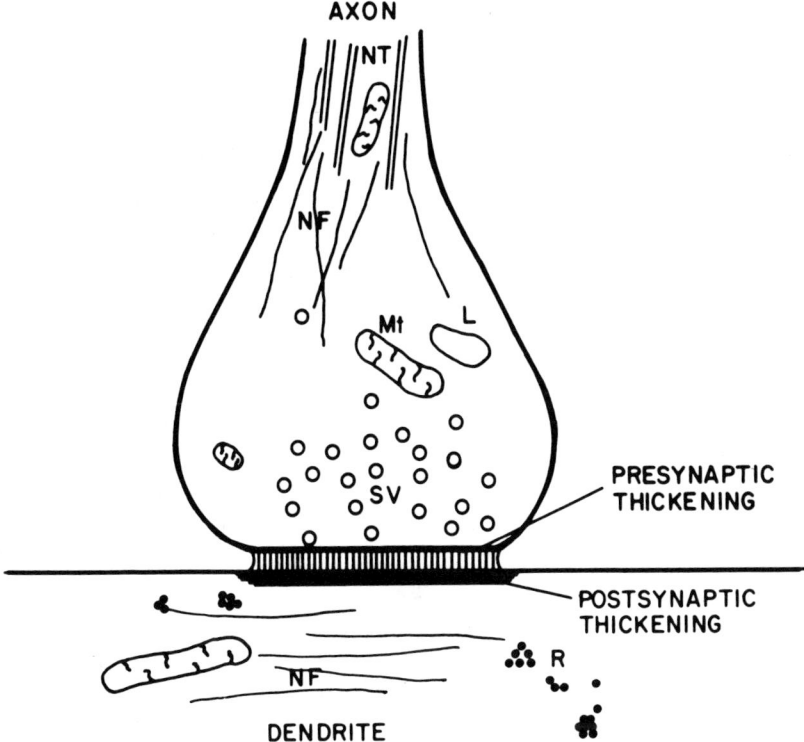

Figure 5.1 A schematicized synapse, showing synaptic vesicles (SV), mitochondria (Mt), lysosomes (L), neurotubules (NT), neurofilaments (NF) and ribosomes (R).

There is presently some discussion over the immediate source of neurotransmitter and the mechanism of its release. Two decades ago, Fatt and Katz observed in a frog neuromuscular preparation that there were spontaneous (i.e., unstimulated) small depolarizations of the muscle membrane (sarcolemma). These were called *miniature endplate potentials* (MEPP's) and were found to be quantal in nature; that is to say, the magnitude of successive MEPP's seemed to be low-number multiples of single quanta. Fatt and Katz speculated that this corresponded to the release of small variable numbers of uniformly sized "packets" of chemical neurotransmitter (in this case acetylcholine).[2] When the motor neuron was stimulated electrically, large numbers of quanta were released producing comparatively large depolarizations of the sarcolemma, and the quantal effect was buried. Subsequently, attempts were made to link this quantal phenomenon with the presynaptic vesicles. The amount of acetylcholine released on stimulation was related to the depolarization produced, and it was estimated that one vesicle contained just enough acetylcholine to correspond to one quantum of the MEPP. These estimates were based upon consideration of molecular size and packing, and also on the chemical assay of acetylcholine and counting of purified synaptic vesicles, and were necessarily very approximate.

The idea that the neurotransmitter for release was contained in vesicles immediately suggested a possible mechanism, namely *exocytosis* (Figure 5.2).

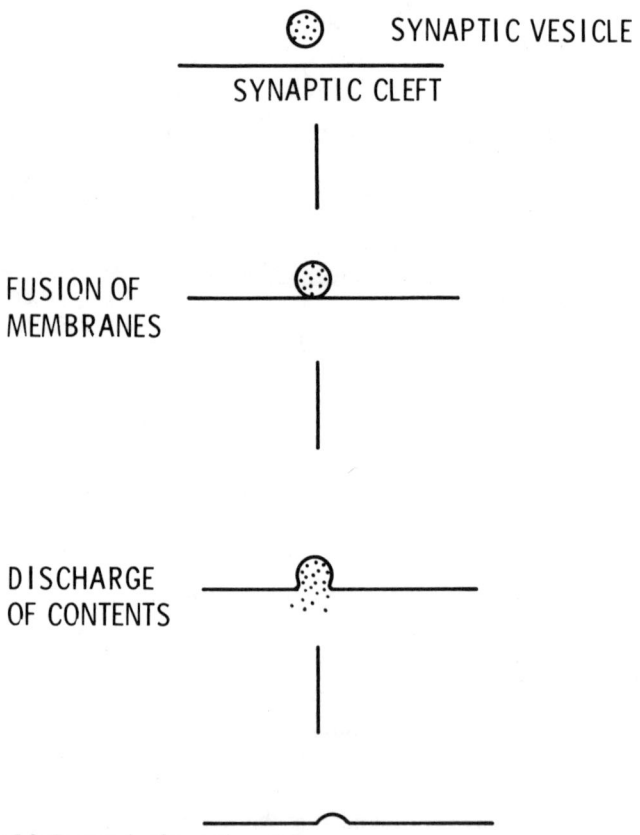

Figure 5.2 Exocytosis of synaptic vesicles.

The vesicle would move very close to the presynaptic membrane; the presynaptic and vesicle membranes would fuse and then split, leaving the vesicle as a small invagination in the presynaptic membrane. The vesicle contents would be discharged into the synaptic cleft and the invagination flat-

tened so that the vesicle membrane would now become part of the presynaptic membrane. Several predictions follow from this hypothetical mechanism:
1. The number of presynaptic vesicles should be depleted by stimulation.
2. The total contents of the vesicle should be secreted extracellularly, thus the secreted material should correspond exactly to the former contents of the vesicle.
3. The plasma membrane should increase in area corresponding to the addition of vesicle membrane.
4. A mechanism must exist for taking up excess presynaptic membrane, possibly using it to make new vesicles.
5. The components of the vesicle membrane should all be present in the presynaptic membrane.

Attempts to show a depletion of synaptic vesicles with prolonged stimulation have generally been unsuccessful. This has been ascribed to the large number of vesicles or a high rate of resynthesis, or both. However, results with black widow spider venom have shown such depletion. The venom applied to the frog sartorius muscle preparation has been shown to result in a dramatic stimulation of the muscle which subsides only after ten to fifteen minutes.[11] At this time the muscle may no longer be stimulated by electrical stimulation of the neuron. During this period of stimulation a large proportion of the acetylcholine was released from the neurons. Electron microscopic examination of the nerve terminals showed almost total depletion of synaptic vesicles when activity had ceased. While the depletion of vesicles *per se* is good evidence that the store of acetylcholine is vesicular, it does not argue for any particular release mechanism. However, the electron micrographs also showed a large increase in the amount of presynaptic membrane, which appeared to correlate with the extent and the amount of vesicle depletion. More recently, vesicle depletion has been shown in the same preparation using physiological stimulation (see p. 119).[12] These observations provide strong support for an exocytotic mechanism of acetylcholine release at the neuromuscular junction.

Further evidence for an exocytosis mechanism arises from observations of the adrenal medulla. Epinephrine is stored in the adrenal medulla in large, densely staining vesicles known as *chromaffin granules* which also contain ATP, chromogranins (soluble proteins) and an enzyme involved in the synthesis of epinephrine, dopamine-β-hydroxylase (DBH). When the medulla is stimulated neurally, epinephrine is released and the number of chromaffin granules decreases. ATP, chromogranins and DBH are also released, and the ratios of epinephrine to ATP and chromogranins released are the same as observed in purified preparations of chromaffin granules. This strongly suggests that exocytosis of the granules has occurred and electron micrographs have shown apparent exocytosis in the adrenal medulla. Synaptic vesicles (about half the size of chromaffin granules) containing the neurotransmitter norepinephrine have been isolated from the sympathetic nervous system, and these also contain DBH, chromogranin A (the principal adrenal chromogranin) and ATP in approximately the same proportions as in the chromaffin granules. Using the hypogastric nerve–vas deferens system, Axelrod has shown that electrical stimulation *in vitro* results in the release of norepinephrine and soluble DBH in proportions similar to those found in the tissue itself. Thus exocytosis seems likely in this system. Plasma contains detectable amounts of DBH even in adrenalectomized animals. 6-hydroxydopamine, a drug which causes the degeneration of catecholamine-containing nerve terminals but does not affect the adrenals, depresses plasma DBH activity. Thus the circulating DBH cannot originate solely in the adrenal medulla and may originate in the sympathetic nervous system. This is indirect evidence for an analogy between norepinephrine release from sympathetic neurons and epinephrine release from the adrenal medulla, and supports the vesicle exocytosis hypothesis.

Conflicting data have been reported from studies where the *specific radioactivity* of neurotransmitter released is compared with that stored in the tissue. The specific radioactivity is a measure of the amount of radioactivity in the chemical compound and is defined as the number of disintegrations per minute (dpm) per unit of compound (grams or moles). In the case of acetylcholine, the specific radioactivity can be measured after administration of either radioactive choline or acetate. The specific radioactivity of acetylcholine released on stimulation is very much higher than that remaining in the tissue. Similar results have also been obtained for the catecholamines. This may indicate that a certain fraction of the acetylcholine (for example, that in particular neurons or at particular synapses) is synthesized and degraded (turned over) very rapidly, while the bulk of the tissue acetylcholine is more stable. However, measurements of the specific radioactivity of the acetylcholine from the tissue show that whereas the specific radioactivity of the vesicle-bound acetylcholine is low, that of the free acetylcholine is high, comparable to that released. Though the origin of free acetylcholine is not known, it is probably a mixture of newly synthesized acetylcholine, acetylcholine released by rupture of vesicles during tissue preparation, and other sources. The results have been interpreted to mean that it is the free, not the vesicular acetylcholine that is released upon nervous stimulation, and that the vesicles are merely a stable store. However, another possibility is that there are two types of vesicles, and that those that are about to release neurotransmitter are fragile and do not survive homogenization procedures. This type of vesicle, which may be derived from the other more stable type, may turn over very rapidly, thus explaining the specific radioactivity data.

There has also been some interest in the possible recycling of the vesicle membrane. Recently, Heuser and Reese have rather convincingly demonstrated that recycling of the synaptic vesicle membrane does occur at neuromuscular junctions of the frog.[12] When the motor nerve was stimulated for short periods, the number of synaptic vesicles was decreased, there was an increase in the number of coated vesicles, and cisternae appeared. When the stimulation was prolonged, the number of synaptic vesicles was further depleted and the amount of cisternae greatly increased. Calculations suggested that the membrane from the synaptic vesicles could be approximately accounted for in the coated vesicles and cisternae. Electron micrographs are consistent with the view that the cisternae may be formed by the coalescence of coated vesicles. When the unstimulated muscle is bathed in a solution of horseradish peroxidase (for which there is a specific histochemical stain), the peroxidase does not penetrate undamaged synaptic terminals. However, when the nerve is stimulated, peroxidase is found in coated vesicles and later in cisternae. With prolonged stimulation the peroxidase also appears in the synaptic vesicles where it is not found after short periods of stimulation. A series of kinetic experiments were entirely consistent with the idea that the presynaptic membrane undergoes pinocytosis* to form coated vesicles. The coated vesicles then coalesce to form the cisternae from which the synaptic vesicles are subsequently formed. This elegant series of experiments provides very good evidence for the series of processes depicted in Figure 5.3.

The biochemical data show that the proteins and glycoproteins of the synaptic vesicle membranes are all present in the synaptic plasma membranes.[13] The phospholipids and the ratio of cholesterol to phospholipids are also similar for synaptic vesicles and synaptic plasma membranes.[14] However, gangliosides, which are especially concentrated in synaptic plasma membranes, are not found in synaptic vesicles. Moreover, there are proteins in the synaptic plasma membrane that are not found in synaptic vesicles. Therefore, if recycling does occur, there must be some molecular selection when the presynaptic membrane is pinocytosed to form coated vesicles.

Little is known concerning the molecular mechanism of exocytosis. It is known that cytochalasin B, colchicine and vinblastin inhibit the release of norepinephrine from sympathetic nerve terminals, and that colchicine and vinblastin also inhibit the secretion of epinephrine from the adrenal medulla. Recently an interesting mechanism for the release process has been postulated by Berl and his co-workers.[15] Brain contains an actomyosin-like protein, neurostenin, which is concentrated in the synaptosomal fraction (8 to

*Pinocytosis is the reverse of exocytosis. The presynaptic membrane invaginates and buds off, forming a vesicle (see Figure 5.2).

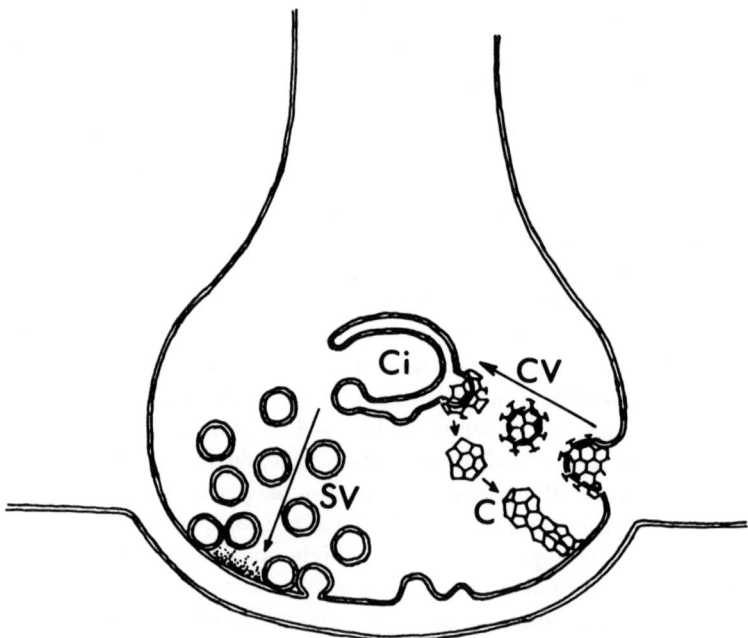

Figure 5.3 The recycling of synaptic vesicle membrane. Synaptic vesicles (SV) exocytose and their membrane becomes part of the presynaptic membrane. Coated vesicles are formed by pinocytosis of the synaptic plasma membrane. These coated vesicles are fused to form cisternae (Ci) from which new synaptic vesicles are made. The coats (C) must return to the synaptic plasma membrane. (Adapted from Heuser and Reese[12].)

10 percent of synaptosomal protein is neurostenin). The actin-like neurin interacts with muscle myosin and brain stenin in a similar manner, and myosin and stenin are molecularly similar. Berl has recently shown that synaptosomal plasma membranes are enriched in neurin, whereas synaptic vesicle membranes are enriched in stenin. Thus he has suggested that during exocytosis a muscle-like contraction may occur between the stenin of the vesicles and the neurin of the presynaptic membrane. Ca^{2+}, which is essential for neurotransmitter release, could be the trigger for this interaction just as it is in muscle. Furthermore, neurotubular protein will interact with myosin in an actin-like manner (muscle actin is also precipitated by vinblastin). Thus molecular interaction of the neurotubules with vesicular stenin could provide a mechanism for axoplasmic transport similar to that which Schmitt has proposed.[16] At present it is far from clear how these mechanisms could be compatible with the occurrence of recycling of vesicular membrane. One possibility is that the rough coat on coated vesicles is stenin being returned for incorporation into synaptic vesicles.

B. SYNAPTOSOMES

A most important impetus has been given to the understanding of chemical neurotransmission from the use of synaptosomes. In the late 1950's Whittaker and de Robertis independently fractionated homogenates of brain in isotonic sucrose by differential and sucrose gradient centrifugation (Figure 5.4). In this way fractions were produced that were enriched in particles which, under the electron microscope, closely resembled nerve terminals of brain sections (see Figures 1.8, 5.5).[17] These same fractions contained most of the acetylcholine of the homogenate. The particles were called synapto-

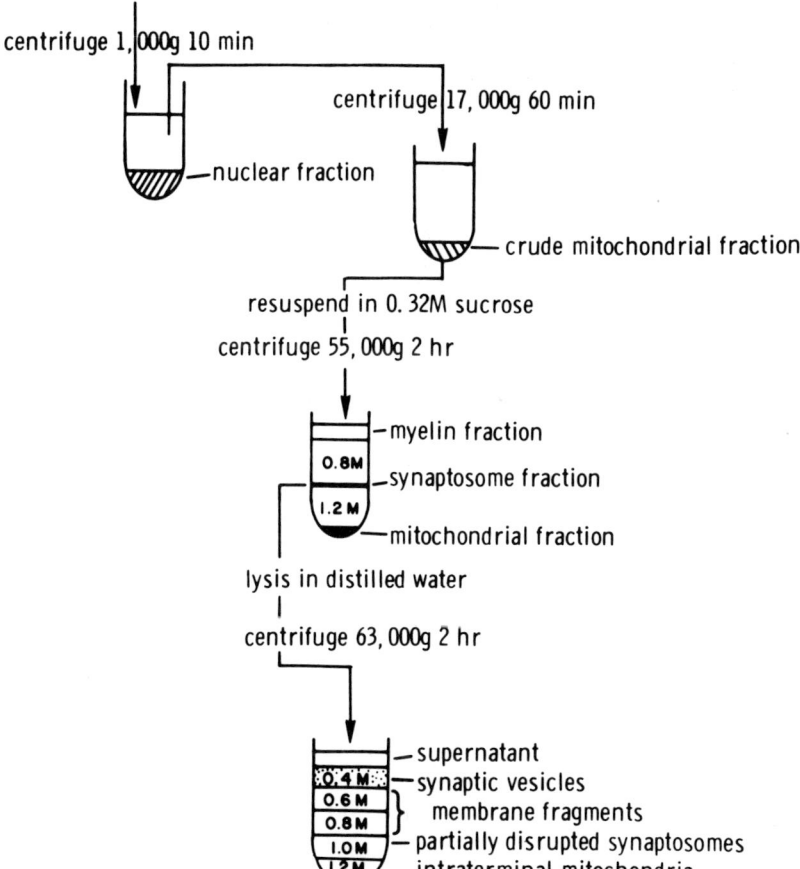

Figure 5.4 The preparation of synaptosomes and synaptosomal subfractions. (Adapted from Whittaker and Barker[18].)

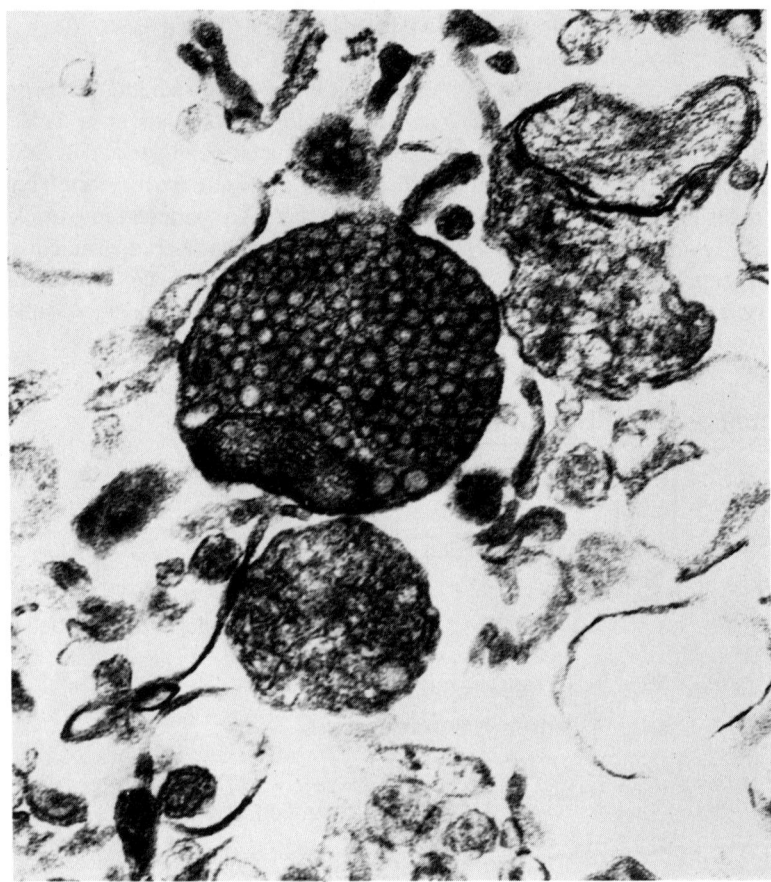

Figure 5.5 Electronmicrograph of synaptosomes prepared from Ficoll gradients. Note the synaptic vesicles and mitochondrion. (Synaptosomes Dr. A. Dunn, electron microscopy Mrs. M. Bernstein).

somes and much work over the past fifteen years strongly supports the idea that they are isolated nerve terminals. Apparently during the process of homogenization the terminals are pinched off and the membrane reseals to give a completely enclosed particle. The synaptosomes, as normally isolated, may have postsynaptic attachments ranging from postsynaptic thickenings to resealed postsynaptic terminals. Morphologically, they correspond very closely to terminals seen in microscope sections. Synaptosomes contain vesicles, mitochondria and lysosomes, and exhibit presynaptic thickenings (Figure 5.5). The synaptosomes are autonomous and synthesize ATP if adequately oxygenated, and can maintain K^+ and Na^+ gradients across their membranes corresponding to those observed in intact cells. They actively accumulate compounds other than ions, including glucose, amino acids and various neurotransmitters and precursors. A drawback is that even with improved techniques using sucrose-Ficoll gradients,[18] synaptosomes have not been isolated uncontaminated by other subcellular components, notably membranes and their inclusions. It is also not known whether synaptosomes are a representative collection of nerve terminals or a biased sample. Nevertheless, much of our understanding of synaptic mechanisms stems from experiments involving their use.

When crude synaptosome preparations are centrifuged on continuous sucrose gradients, a kind of chemical fractionation may be achieved. Synaptosomes containing different neurotransmitters appear in different regions of the gradient. Thus GABA-containing synaptosomes separate from norepinephrine-containing ones.[19] This separation can be detected either by chemical assay or by observing the uptake of radioactive neurotransmitters or appropriate precursors *in vivo* and *in vitro*. It appears that only terminals that utilize a particular neurotransmitter take up significant amounts of it. By autoradiography of synaptosomes previously incubated with radioactive neurotransmitters or precursors, the neurotransmitter specificity of isolated synaptosomes may be determined. These studies have indicated differences in morphology (especially of the synaptic vesicles) corresponding to different neurotransmitters. Such studies suggest that GABA and glycine account for about 50 percent of the synaptic terminals in spinal cord, and that catecholamines account for only 5 percent of the terminals in cerebral cortex.[20]

Synaptosomes may be lysed osmotically and, under suitable conditions, subsynaptosomal fractions may be purified using sucrose gradients (Figure 5.4). Particularly important have been the preparations of synaptic vesicles and synaptic plasma membranes. Detergents disrupt these membranes and release neurotransmitters from synaptic vesicles. Plasma membranes may also be isolated using density gradients, especially with zonal centrifuge rotors. In this way, using non-ionic detergents such as Triton under carefully controlled conditions, junctional complexes consisting of the contacting pre- and postsynaptic membranes (i.e., in the area of the synaptic thickening) have been isolated in relatively pure form by Cotman and others.[21]

C. NEUROTRANSMITTERS

Several different neurotransmitters have now been identified in various systems, and probably many more remain to be discovered. The known neurotransmitters are all small molecules and all amines. Though a neuron may receive inputs from more than one type of neurotransmitter, as far as is known a given neuron synthesizes and secretes only one chemical neurotransmitter, which is thus characteristic for the cell (Dale's law). For example, excitatory neurons to lobster leg muscles appear to use glutamate; inhibitory neurons use GABA. The enzyme for the synthesis of GABA is present only in the inhibitory neurons and not in the excitatory neurons, which would not need it. Thus in one type of cell, because of the need for GABA, a considerable proportion of the Krebs cycle metabolism is channeled through the GABA shunt (p. 30).

The overall processes of storage, secretion and reception are rather similar for all known neurotransmitters. The bulk of neurotransmitter synthesis probably occurs in the presynaptic terminal; that which arrives by axonal transport is probably insignificant in terms of total metabolism. The mechanism of storage into vesicles is not understood. In the case of norepinephrine, the last synthetic step is completed by an enzyme, dopamine-β-hydroxylase, which is present in the vesicle. This is not the case for acetylcholine, serotonin or GABA.

The release of neurotransmitter requires the presence of calcium ions and may be blocked by calcium ion binding agents such as ethylene diamine tetraacetic acid (EDTA) or better, ethyleneglycol bis(aminoethylether) tetraacetic acid (EGTA) which is a more powerful binding agent. Neurotransmitter secretion can also be blocked by high concentrations (50 mM) of Mg^{2+}, which presumably competes for the Ca^{2+} effector sites.

Following secretion, the neurotransmitters bind to specific receptors on the postsynaptic membrane and subsequently produce their postsynaptic effects. They are inactivated in the synaptic cleft either by enzymic reactions or by being taken up into cells. In the case of acetylcholine a catabolite, choline, may also be taken up by the neuron and resynthesized into active neurotransmitter.

What is the advantage of chemical over electrical synaptic transmission? It is not the ability to conduct unidirectionally, since many electrical synapses can do this. An important advantage of the chemical synapse is the ability to inhibit as well as to excite postsynaptic membranes. The biological significance of this is indicated by the predominance of inhibitory over excitatory synapses in the brain. One may also ask why, if the overall effects of neurotransmissions are so similar, are different neurotransmitters used? There are several possible answers. Initially it was thought that chemical coding existed so that when a neurotransmitter was released, only neurons receptive to that particular neurotransmitter would be activated. But since neurotransmitters are very rapidly inactivated in the synaptic cleft, it is unlikely that significant amounts of neurotransmitter find their way to other postsynaptic membranes. However, it is possible that this type of coding may be important in the initial establishment of synapses. Thus a particular cell may be predisposed as to the chemical types of innervation that it will accept (see Chapter 6). In this way the formation of certain pathways could be genetically predetermined.

A second possibility is that the nature of the postsynaptic effect may be specific for each particular neurotransmitter. We know that, in general, certain neurotransmitters such as GABA, glycine and norepinephrine tend to be inhibitory, whereas others such as glutamate and acetylcholine tend to be excitatory. This generalization is misleading, however, since in almost every case there are exceptions. An extreme case is that of acetylcholine in *Aplysia,* where, depending on the rate of stimulation, acetylcholine may be both inhibitory and excitatory for a particular synapse in the abdominal ganglion. Two different types of receptor with different affinities for acetylcholine are thought to be involved in this case.[22] However, the function of a neurotransmitter may be more complicated than just the production of excitatory or inhibitory postsynaptic potentials. Postsynaptic reception may initiate processes other than postsynaptic potential changes. These processes, which are not presently understood, may feed back presynaptically or otherwise to influence the subsequent behavior of the synapse. They may thus form the basis of plasticity. These secondary properties might be characteristic for a particular neurotransmitter.

The third and perhaps most important reason for the multiplicity of neurotransmitters is a chemical coding of functional pathways. If these pathways were specific in the neurotransmitter used, then it would be possible to regulate them by gross control throughout the nervous system of the metabolism of the particular neurotransmitter involved. There is evidence that functional pathways may be to some extent chemically coded. For example, in the hypothalamus the pathways for eating apparently use norepinephrine, whereas those for drinking use acetylcholine. It is remarkable that nearly all the known psychoactive substances affect the metabolism of one or more neurotransmitters. Such drugs often have relatively specific behavioral effects. The biological significance of these observations may be that behavior is physiologically controlled to some degree by controlling the metabolism of particular neurotransmitters. We know that circulating norepinephrine and epinephrine potentiate the activity of the sympathetic nervous system which uses catecholamines as neurotransmitters. Thus secretion of epinephrine from the adrenal medulla can hormonally regulate the sympathetic nervous system.

In the central nervous system, Parkinson's disease is characterized by a loss of neurons which originate in the substantia nigra and innervate the neostriatum. These neurons use dopamine as their neurotransmitter (the biproducts of dopamine metabolism include melanin, which gives the substantia nigra its characteristic color). Administration of L-DOPA, the precursor of dopamine, potentiates the activity of the nigrostriatal neurons and in many cases alleviates some of the symptoms of Parkinsonism (the rigidity and facial akinesia, but generally not the tremor). Another example of peripheral control of CNS transmitters is the reflection of dietary state in brain serotonin concentrations, mediated via the plasma concentrations of the serotonin precursor, tryptophan (p. 138). It is likely that this neurotransmitter coding may be the mechanism the body uses to regulate the relative activities of nervous system pathways. The body may even manufacture its own neurotransmitter-active drugs (perhaps the prostaglandins). This system could form the molecular basis of mood (see Chapter 8). The possibility of controlling neurotransmitter-coded pathways also adds a new dimension to electronic models of the brain. The synapse may be considered the analogue of the semiconductor. The activity of the synapse may be regulated hormonally in the same way that the electrical bias may control the activity of the semiconductor. In the brain, however, the hormone has the ability to selectively control the activities of all the synapses of a particular kind.

Criteria for the establishment of a chemical substance as a neurotransmitter at a particular junction

Because of the problems of unequivocally identifying a substance as a neurotransmitter and of identifying the neurotransmitter at a given junction, a series of criteria have been established for practical use:

1. The suspected neurotransmitter must be present in the presynaptic cell.
2. A mechanism for the synthesis of the suspected neurotransmitter or for its assimilation must exist in the presynaptic cell.
3. The suspected neurotransmitter must be released (into the extracellular fluid) by presynaptic stimulation of the particular cells without activation of adjacent cells.
4. A mechanism must exist for inactivating the suspected neurotransmitter in the synapse. This may be a catabolic enzyme and/or an active system for the uptake of the neurotransmitter into the presynaptic cell (re-uptake), the postsynaptic cell or the surrounding glial cells.
5. The postsynaptic effect of exogenously administered suspected neurotransmitter must mimic presynaptic stimulation.
6. The effect of drugs on synaptic transmission should be the same for presynaptic electrical stimulation as it is following the application of exogenous transmitter.

While these criteria provide good general guidelines for the identification of a neurotransmitter, they are not definitive. Especially in the central nervous system there are many serious problems in localizing suspected neurotransmitters or their metabolic enzymes to particular cells. Released neurotransmitters may be very difficult to collect, there may be difficulty in selectively stimulating particular cells, and drugs may not readily penetrate the tissue. Particular anatomical distributions of substances and their enzymes are useful, but in practice there has been increasing reliance on the use of drugs with well-characterized activities. Thus known blocking agents should block the neurotransmission, whereas drugs that inhibit the inactivating systems should potentiate the transmission. As a greater variety of drugs with specific actions become available, the process of neurotransmitter identification will become both easier and more definitive.

i) Acetylcholine (ACh)[2,3]

Acetylcholine is synthesized by the enzyme choline O-acetyltransferase (choline acetylase) from choline and acetylCoA.

$$\text{choline} + \text{acetylCoA} \rightarrow \text{acetylcholine} + \text{CoASH}$$

The choline is produced from hydrolysis of phosphatidylcholine or acetylcholine itself (Figure 5.6); it cannot be produced by direct methylation of ethanolamine. It is uncertain whether or not choline can be synthesized in

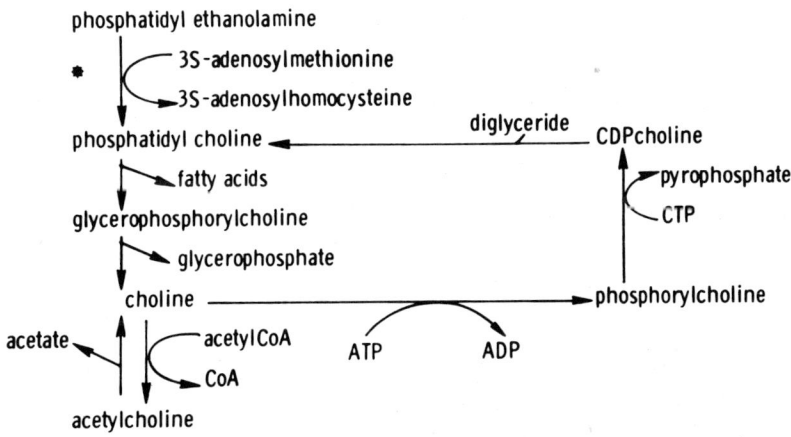

Figure 5.6 Synthesis and catabolism of acetylcholine. *This reaction has not been detected in brain.

the brain,[23] but physiologically considerable amounts of choline are taken up from the plasma by a mechanism sensitive to hemicholinium. Upon subcellular fractionation of brain tissue, the greatest concentration of choline acetylase is found in the synaptosome fraction. When the synaptosomes are osmotically lysed, the enzyme is associated with the vesicle fraction, but in the presence of physiological concentrations of salts it is soluble. Thus the attachment to vesicles is thought to be artifactual. Choline acetylase has a molecular weight of 65,000 and is sensitive to sulfhydryl reagents. The synthesis of ACh is most probably under direct feedback control since pharmacological treatments that block neurotransmission, or hydrolysis of ACh, fail to elevate its concentration more than twofold. The results of *in vitro* studies on isolated synaptosomes are also consistent with direct feedback control of ACh synthesis.

The studies of Whittaker and de Robertis showed that acetylcholine itself was concentrated in the synaptosome fraction and that the vesicles isolated after osmotic lysis of the synaptosomes were rich in ACh. Nevertheless a large amount (50 percent or more) of the acetylcholine in synaptosomes was not associated with vesicles. Attempts to incorporate either radioactive choline or acetylcholine into vesicles *in vitro* have been relatively unsuccessful, and very little is understood about the storage of ACh in vesicles. However, Whittaker and his co-workers have recently provided evidence that a specific protein, vesiculin, may be involved in packing the ACh into the vesicles along with ATP, as in the case of the catecholamines.[24]

Acetylcholine is inactivated by cholinesterase, which hydrolyzes it to choline and free acetate.

$$\text{acetylcholine} + H_2O \rightarrow \text{choline} + \text{acetate}$$

Cholinesterases are ubiquitous in the body and there are several of them. They are not specific for acetylcholine and have activity for other choline esters. They have been divided into two classes: acetylcholinesterases (also called specific cholinesterases or "true" cholinesterases) and butyrylcholinesterases (also called nonspecific or "pseudo" cholinesterases, or sometimes propionylcholinesterases). This classification is based on the best substrate for the hydrolysis reaction; acetylcholinesterases hydrolyze ACh faster than other esters, while butyrylcholinesterases work faster with butyrylcholine. The types of cholinesterase present are characteristic of the particular tissue, and generally neural tissue contains acetylcholinesterase, and nonneural tissue, butyrylcholinesterase. However, neural tissue (e.g., autonomic ganglia) may contain butyrylcholinesterase and nonneural tissue (e.g., red blood cells) may contain acetylcholinesterase. Glial cells contain butyrylcholinesterase; this may be important in inactivating the acetylcholine released at cholinergic synapses before it diffuses to other areas.

When mammalian brain is homogenized and subfractionated by differential centrifugation, acetylcholinesterase activity is principally associated with the mitochondrial and microsomal fractions, the latter being the more enriched. This suggests that the enzyme is associated with membranes of the endoplasmic reticulum. Histochemical studies have shown that cholinesterase activity is associated with all types of membrane, both endoplasmic reticular and plasma, neuronal and glial, and in the central and peripheral nervous systems. The enzyme has been isolated from the electric organ (electroplax) of the electric eel and crystallized; its molecular weight is 260,000. It has a turnover number of 64,000 molecules of ACh per second per molecule of enzyme, which is among the highest turnover rates known for any enzyme.

Acetylcholine receptors[4]

Pharmacologists have distinguished two types of cholinergic receptors, *nicotinic* and *muscarinic,* named after two compounds which exclusively mimic the respective acetylcholine activities. Cholinergic receptors on skeletal muscles or in autonomic ganglia are nicotinic. They may be stimulated by direct application of ACh or nicotine but not muscarine, and this activity is unaffected by atropine. Parasympathetic organs innervated by cholinergic fibers are muscarinic. They may be stimulated by ACh or muscarine but not nicotine, and this activity is antagonized by atropine which is a specific muscarinic blocker. Autonomic ganglia and also cortical and subcortical regions of brain (which was formerly thought to be exclusively nicotinic) are now known to contain small numbers of muscarinic receptors.

Acetylcholine receptors have been studied mainly in the electroplax of the electric eel or torpedo, since these are rich sources of exclusively cholinergic tissue. It has long been known that the acetylcholine-binding properties of the receptor were rather similar to those of acetylcholinesterase. Nevertheless, in the electroplax they are distinct, since proteases destroy cholinesterase activity but not ACh-binding activity, whereas the reverse is true for sulfhydryl reagents such as p-hydroxymercuribenzoate. These observations do not apply to mammalian ACh receptors, which may include cholinesterase.

Much progress has been made recently following the discovery of α-bungarotoxin, a component of the venom of the snake *Bungarus multicinctus.*[4] This toxin inhibits ACh-induced depolarization of vertebrate skeletal muscle and the electroplax. The inhibition is virtually irreversible, and is accompanied by a very high affinity binding of radioactively labeled toxin in the region of the receptors. Both the binding and the inhibition of depolarization may be prevented by agonists such as carbachol and by reversible antagonists such as d-tubocurarine which also block α-bungarotoxin binding in detergent-dispersed preparations. This evidence, plus a quantitative relationship between ACh receptor activity and α-bungarotoxin binding sites (for example, during denervation sensitization of muscle), strongly suggests that the toxin binds to the receptor at the ACh site. The use of radioactively labeled α-bungarotoxin has greatly expedited the biochemical purification of receptors. However, the present data on the nature and the activity of these isolated receptors are very conflicting.

Membrane effects

In addition to its role as a neurotransmitter, acetylcholine may have a direct effect on axonal membranes. It can depolarize nerve axons in the absence of specific receptors. It may also depolarize intestinal smooth muscle and hyperpolarize atrial muscle in the absence of neural activity. The significance of this effect of ACh is unknown but is also observed with glutamate, glutamine and aspartate. (See also Nachmansohn's theory, p. 75.)

Assay of acetylcholine

Acetylcholine may be assayed by quantifying its effects on various neuromuscular preparations, in particular the dorsal muscle of the leech and the guinea pig ileum. These assays are difficult and time-consuming, and this has seriously hampered work on acetylcholine. Gas chromatography is now being used and some enzymatic assays have recently been developed. In these, choline, liberated from acetylcholine by hydrolysis, is phosphorylated by choline kinase using $[\gamma\text{-}^{32}P]$ ATP so that the product choline phosphate is radioactive. The choline phosphate is then separated from the other reactants by ion-exchange chromatography and the radioactivity determined. ACh may be determined by comparison of the radioactivity with known standards. This method is sensitive to 1 picomole of ACh, which is slightly more sensitive than the bioassay procedure.

ii) Catecholamines[3,5,6,7,8]

Three known neurotransmitters are catecholamines: namely, dopamine, norepinephrine (noradrenaline) and epinephrine (adrenaline). Their structures are all based on 3,4-dihydroxyphenylethylamine and they are all synthesized from tyrosine (Figure 5.7).

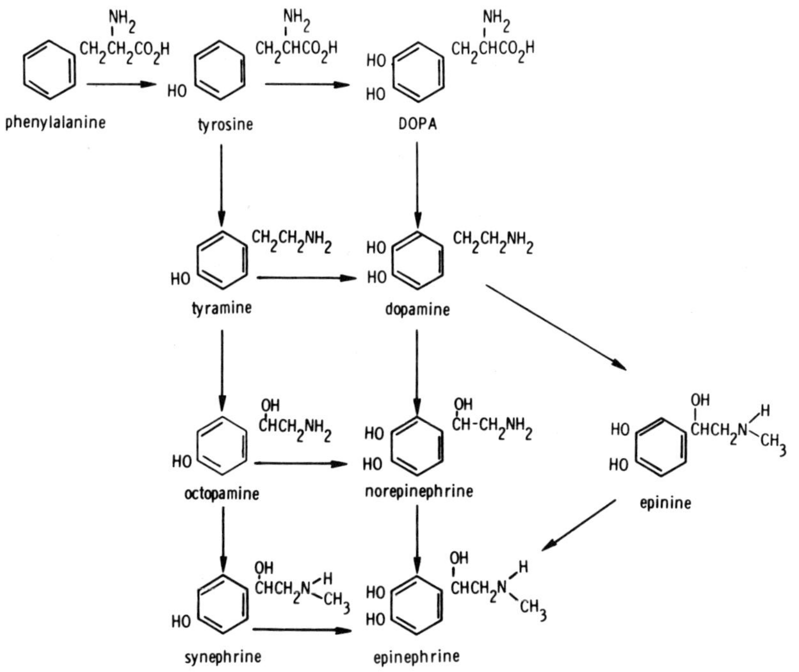

Figure 5.7 Synthesis of catecholamines.

Synthesis

Tyrosine may be synthesized in the body from phenylalanine by phenylalanine hydroxylase, but this enzyme is apparently absent from brain. The liver probably performs this function for the brain, supplementing dietary tyrosine (see p. 31).

In the synthesis of catecholamines, tyrosine is further hydroxylated to 3,4-dihydroxyphenylalanine (DOPA) by tyrosine hydroxylase (TH). This enzyme requires molecular oxygen, Fe^{2+} and a reduced pteridine as cofactors. The natural pteridine cofactor is thought to be dihydrobiopterin, but this has not been conclusively shown.

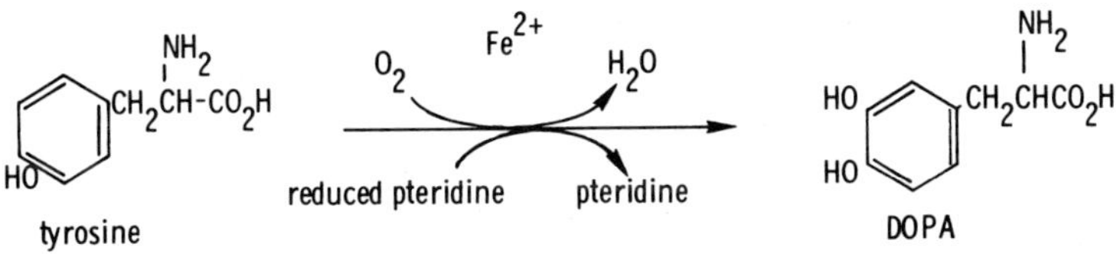

While tyrosine hydroxylase is very similar in activity and cofactor requirements to phenylalanine hydroxylase, the two enzymes are distinct and phenylalanine is a very poor substrate for tyrosine hydroxylase. This is also apparently true *in vivo*, since phenylketonuria sufferers are normal when provided with adequate tyrosine and reduced amounts of phenylalanine in the diet.

Tyrosine hydroxylase is a soluble enzyme and is located principally in the synaptosomal fraction. TH is probably rate-limiting for catecholamine biosynthesis and is inhibited by norepinephrine. This may be the mechanism for the feedback control of catecholamine synthesis. Other potent inhibitors of TH, both *in vivo* and *in vitro*, are α-methyl-p-tyrosine (αMpT) and iodinated derivatives of tyrosine.

DOPA is decarboxylated to form dopamine by DOPA decarboxylase.

$$\text{DOPA} \xrightarrow[\text{pyridoxal phosphate}]{-CO_2} \text{dopamine}$$

A non-specific L-aromatic amino acid decarboxylase may be used to decarboxylate DOPA, 5-hydroxytryptophan and histidine, but there is a specific histidine enzyme and there is some evidence that may indicate the existence of separate enzymes for DOPA and 5-hydroxytryptophan.[25] The enzyme requires pyridoxal phosphate (vitamin B_6) as a cofactor. It is a soluble enzyme found in all subcellular fractions that contain soluble cytoplasm. In brain, aromatic amino acid decarboxylase activity is 100 to 1,000 times higher than that of tyrosine hydroxylase, but the activities of the specific enzymes have not been reported.

Dopamine is converted to norepinephrine (NE) by the enzyme dopamine-β-hydroxylase (DBH). This enzyme is not specific for dopamine but will oxidize any β-phenylethylamine to the β-hydroxy derivative, e.g., tyramine to octopamine. It requires oxygen and ascorbic acid (vitamin C) as cofactors. The enzyme contains copper and is inhibited by copper chelating reagents. It is stimulated by fumarate and other dicarboxylic acids, but the mechanism and significance of this are unknown. The enzyme is particulate in the brain, adrenal medulla and sympathetic nervous system and is thought to be associated with the catecholamine storage granules, where a part of it is associated with the membrane. Its activity in brain is comparable to that of DOPA decarboxylase. The activities of both TH and DBH may be controlled by neural activity (see p. 181).

HO–C₆H₃(OH)–CH₂CH₂NH₂ (dopamine) →[O₂, reduced ascorbate / H₂O, ascorbate]→ HO–C₆H₃(OH)–CH(OH)CH₂NH₂ (norepinephrine)

Norepinephrine is methylated to epinephrine by phenylethanolamine-N-methyltransferase (PNMT). The enzyme from adrenal medulla has low substrate specificity and will methylate octopamine to synephrine, and epinephrine itself may be further methylated to N-methylepinephrine. It requires as a methyl donor S-adenosylmethionine (SAM), which it converts to S-adenosylhomocysteine (SAH). The enzyme is soluble and appears in cytoplasmic fractions from the adrenal medulla. Since DBH is contained in the chromaffin granules, this poses a problem for epinephrine synthesis. Apparently, either the NE is transferred to the cytoplasm after its synthesis and then returned to the vesicles, or the *in vivo* synthesis pathway is via epinine (Figure 5.7). PNMT is found in brain especially in areas concerned with olfaction, but only in low concentrations. The enzyme is distinct from the nonspecific N-methyl transferase found in several tissues, notably lung and recently also in brain.

norepinephrine →[SAM / SAH]→ epinephrine

Storage and release

Catecholamines are stored in vesicles analogous to acetylcholine vesicles. The mechanism of storage is unknown, but both in the adrenal medulla and in the sympathetic nervous system dopamine-β-hydroxylase is associated with the vesicles. Thus the final step of synthesis of norepinephrine and the penultimate step of epinephrine synthesis (unless it is synthesized from epinine, see above) may be completed inside them. In the adrenal medulla and splenic nerve the vesicles also contain ATP (1 molecule for each 4 molecules of catecholamine) and soluble proteins called chromogranins. There are at least eight chromogranins, but the principal one, chromogranin A, accounts for 40 percent of the total. The ATP and chromogranins apparently neutralize the positively charged amines to enable them to be packed into the vesicles. The vesicles also contain an Mg^{2+}- and Ca^{2+}-dependent ATPase. Since calcium is necessary for release of the catecholamines, this enzyme may have a role in the release mechanism and may be identical with stenin (p. 119). Ca^{2+} may well be the trigger for the exocytosis process.

When the catecholamines are released, the ATP and chromogranins are also released along with small amounts of DBH. The significance of this as evidence for exocytosis has been discussed above, but the reason for such an apparently wasteful process is obscure. New proteins (chromogranins and DBH) are required for storage of the amines, but the protein-synthetic capacity of presynaptic terminals is very low, if it exists at all (see p. 148). This means that new proteins must be supplied from the cell body by axoplasmic flow. While there is considerable axoplasmic flow of catecholamine vesicles, this is not adequate for the needs of the synapse, and protein may be transported in other forms. Alternatively, it is possible that mechanisms exist for the re-uptake of these proteins from the extracellular space, similar to those for the catecholamines themselves (see below). Nevertheless, DBH and chromogranins do circulate in the plasma.

Receptors

Very little is known about the receptors for catecholamines. As in the case of the cholinergic systems, in the peripheral nervous system there are two types of receptors: α-receptors and β-receptors. These receptors are defined pharmacologically by the ability of two classes of drugs to block receptor activity. The most commonly used α-blockers are phenoxybenzamine, the ergot alkaloids and phentolamine; the most commonly used β-blockers are dichloroisoproterenol and propanalol. Both types of receptor are stimulated by the catecholamines themselves and the sympathomimetics to differing extents, whereas the blocking agents generally affect one type of receptor exclusively. The receptors themselves are uncharacterized other than pharmacologically. The central nervous system receptors have different properties, and though they may have α- and β-like properties many pharmacologists dislike this classification. Reception in some systems, notably the Purkinje cells of the cerebellum (which have β-receptors) and pyramidal cells in the hippocampus, has been shown to activate the enzyme adenyl cyclase (see p. 186).

Catabolism

Catecholamines are degraded by two enzymes, monoamine oxidase (MAO) and catechol-O-methyltransferase (COMT), which may act sequentially in either order. Monoamine oxidase oxidizes the amine groups to an aldehyde. The aldehyde may then be further oxidized to the acid or reduced to the alcohol by a dehydrogenase or a reductase, respectively. MAO will also oxidize amines other than catechoamines, for example, tyramine, tryp-

V. The Synapse

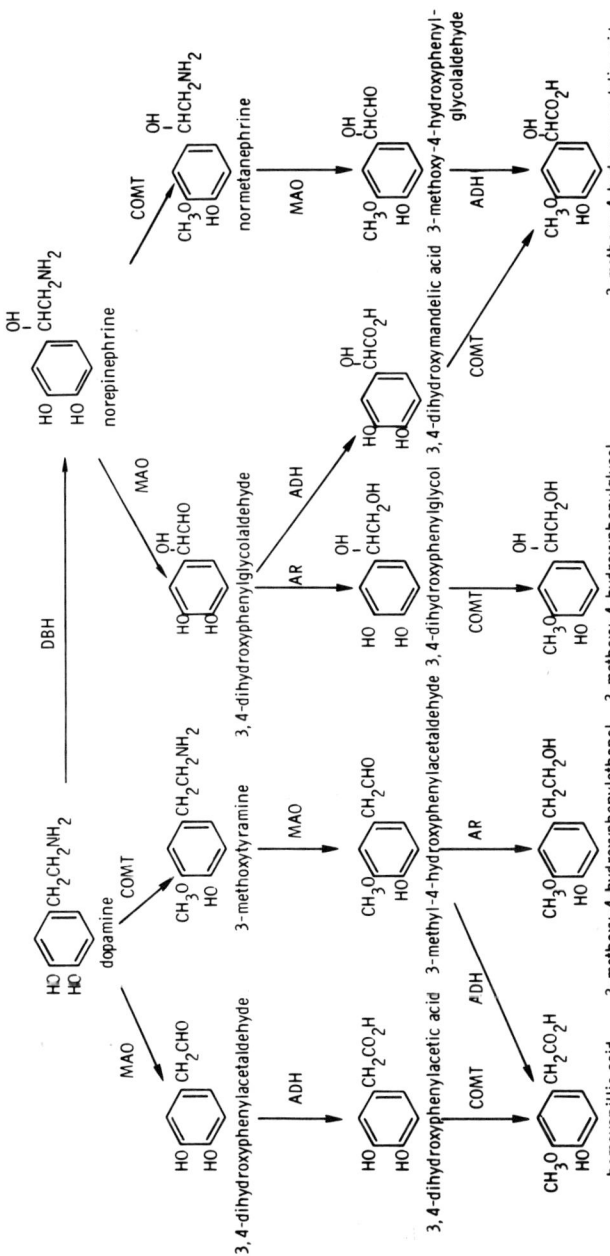

Figure 5.8 Catabolism of dopamine and norepinephrine. ADH, aldehyde dehydrogenase; AR, aldehyde reductase; DBH, dopamine-β-hydroxylase; COMT, catechol-O-methyl transferase; MAO, monoamine oxidase.

$$\text{dopamine (HO, HO, CH}_2\text{CH}_2\text{NH}_2) + O_2 + H_2O \longrightarrow \text{3,4-dihydroxyphenylacetaldehyde (HO, HO, CH}_2\text{CHO)} + H_2O_2 + NH_3$$

tamine and 5-hydroxytryptamine. It will also oxidize secondary amines but only if the substituted group is methyl, as in epinephrine. Monoamine oxidase is a particulate enzyme located in the outer membrane of mitochondria. However, at least in peripheral nerve, it is also found extraneuronally, since when a fiber is cut the MAO does not disappear when the terminals do. The enzyme has been solubilized from mitochondria with the use of detergents and at least four different forms (isozymes) exist in the brain with different substrate reactivities and inhibitor specificities. It is probably a flavoprotein. The mitochondrial location of MAO is surprising, but its location on the outer membrane would permit access to catecholamines without their transport into the mitochondria. Its importance as a catabolic enzyme is indicated by the excretion in the urine of large amounts of dihydroxyphenylacetic acid and homovanillic acid (see Figure 5.8). However, MAO apparently plays a minor role in the inactivation of catecholamine neurotransmitters, since inhibitors of the enzyme have little effect on sympathetic nervous system activity. The physiological effects of MAO-inhibitors are not correlated with their ability to inhibit MAO.

Catechol-O-methyltransferase methylates the 3-hydroxyl group of catecholamines. The methyl group is donated by S-adenosylmethionine, and Mg^{2+} is required for activity. COMT is a soluble cytoplasmic enzyme.

$$\text{dopamine} \xrightarrow{\text{SAM} \quad \text{SAH}} \text{3-methoxytyramine}$$

While it is not known whether it exists extraneuronally in the brain, it is present in other tissues, notably liver and kidney, where it is probably involved in the catabolism of drugs. COMT is inhibited by pyrogallol or tropolone derivatives. Inhibition of COMT activity has very little effect on sympathetic activity, though a slight prolongation of the response has been observed in some systems.

If neither MAO or COMT significantly affects sympathetic neurotransmission, what then is the mechanism of inactivation of the released neurotransmitter? When sympathetic nerves are stimulated, very little norepinephrine is released into the circulation. This suggests that the transmitter may be re-taken up into the nerves. Evidence that this occurs arises from studies using radioactive tracers. [^{3}H]norepinephrine injected intravenously is taken up very actively into the sympathetic nervous system and only about half of it is catabolized by MAO and COMT. The uptake is approximately proportional to the amount of sympathetic innervation; thus spleen and heart are the most active. Similar results are obtained when [^{3}H]norepinephrine is injected intraventricularly into the brain. The radioactivity is best taken up in regions that have high endogenous NE concentrations. Further evidence that the uptake is important comes from the use of the tricyclic antidepressants such as amitryptyline and imipramine. These drugs depress both central and peripheral nervous system concentrations of NE and also inhibit uptake of radioactive NE *in vivo*. Studies with isolated synaptosomes have shown that they possess very active energy-dependent uptake mechanisms for both dopamine and norepinephrine. Only the uptake of norepinephrine into noradrenergic neurons is inhibited by the tricyclic antidepressants. The evidence is thus consistent with very active presynaptic neuronal catecholamine uptake mechanisms, which probably constitute the major route of inactivation of catecholamine neurotransmitters in the synaptic cleft.

Assay of catecholamines

Very sensitive fluorometric assays exist for the catecholamines. Several different procedures exist with varying specificities. The assays are imperfect and not easy to perform, but are extensively used because of their sensitivity. Most important is the histological use of fluorescence techniques. Exposure of tissue sections (preferably freeze-dried ones) to warm, dry formaldehyde gas results in the formation of fluorescent derivatives of the biogenic amines. Different amines exhibit different excitation and emission spectra, and refinement of the technique has permitted DOPA, dopamine, norepinephrine, epinephrine, serotonin and histamine all to be distinguished from each other. This technique has been useful for the study of the location of these amines and especially for the determination of neuronal pathways in the brain by tracing the fluorescent axons. It has thus been important in neuroanatomical studies, besides revealing chemical information.

A new and very sensitive assay uses COMT to methylate the catecholamines with [^{3}H]methyl groups from [Me-^{3}H]S-adenosylmethionine.[26]

Two drugs which affect catecholamines deserve special mention: L-DOPA and 6-hydroxydopamine. The natural metabolite L-DOPA is particularly effective in alleviating symptoms of Parkinson's disease (p. 125–6).

Injection of 6-hydroxydopamine into the body causes the death of catecholamine-containing neurons, thus performing a chemical sympathectomy on systems to which it is exposed. The drug does not cross the blood-brain barrier, but by injecting into precise sites in the brain catecholamine-containing neurons in that area alone can be selectively destroyed. In the brain this effect is irreversible. The technique has been used to study behavioral involvement of catecholaminergic pathways. It is possible to adjust the treatment to deplete either norepinephrine or dopamine-containing neurons selectively, but some damage may well be done to both systems. The mechanism of action of 6-hydroxydopamine is unknown. It is probably toxic to all cells but is only taken up by catecholaminergic ones, presumably by the specific mechanisms for the re-uptake of released catecholamines.

iii) Serotonin (5-hydroxytryptamine, 5HT)

Serotonin was first discovered as the factor from serum that stimulated smooth muscle, hence its name. It occurs widely in nature. In man its greatest concentration is in the pineal gland but most 5HT in the body is in the gastrointestinal tract, with only a small percent in the brain.

Serotonin is synthesized from tryptophan by hydroxylation and decarboxylation (Figure 5.9). Tryptophan hydroxylase is present in very low concentrations in the brain. The oxidation requires molecular oxygen and reduced pteridine cofactors and *in vitro* requires a sulfhydryl compound for stability. It is probably a soluble cytoplasmic enzyme. It is potently inhibited by p-chlorophenylalanine (pCPA), a drug widely used to determine the behavioral significance of serotonin pathways. The decarboxylation is performed by an aromatic amino acid decarboxylase which may be the same enzyme as used for catecholamine biosynthesis or may be specific.[25]

Tryptophan hydroxylation is the rate-limiting step in serotonin biosynthesis. The decarboxylase is much more active than the tryptophan hydroxylase and has a lower Michaelis constant. However, the hydroxylation itself seems to be limited mainly by the availability of substrates. Elevation of tryptophan or oxygen results in elevated 5HT concentrations if the other substrate is not limiting. Feedback control from 5-hydroxytryptophan (5HTP) or 5HT appears to be minimal, and brain concentrations of 5HT can be elevated several-fold by breathing pure oxygen or administering tryptophan. The diurnal rhythm of brain 5HT is apparently a reflection of the rhythm of brain tryptophan, which is itself a reflection of fluctuations in plasma tryptophan caused by dietary intake (see Chapter 2). This is a good example of a case in which the brain is not isolated from the metabolism of the rest of the body, and may have special significance for appetitive mechanisms.

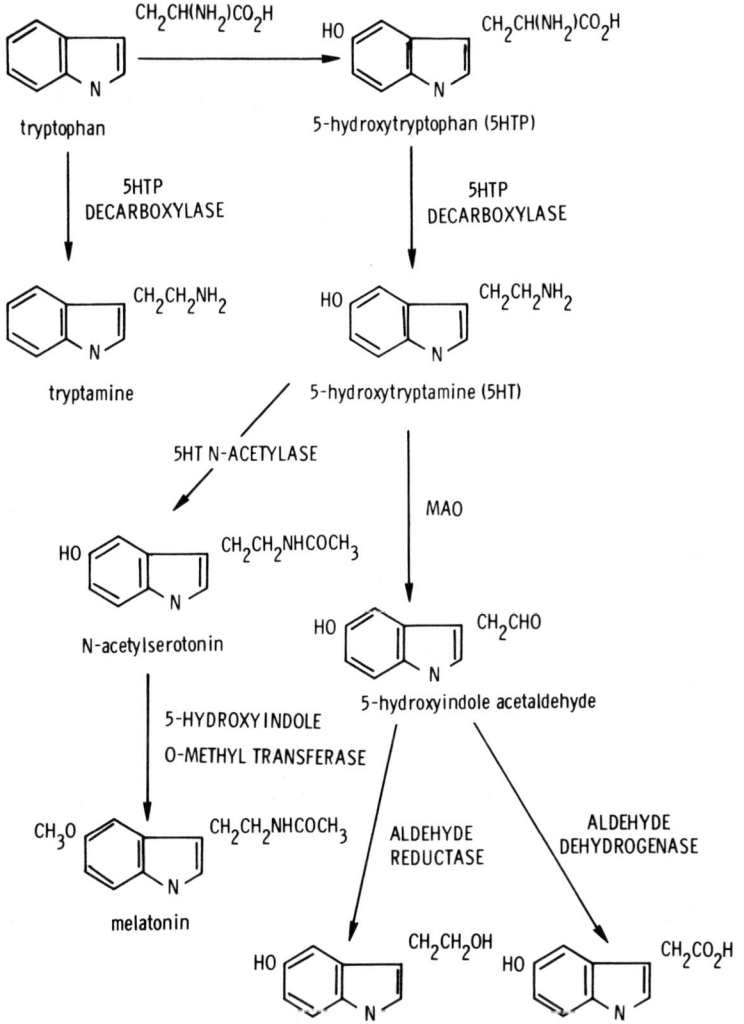

Figure 5.9 Synthesis and catabolism of serotonin (5HT).

Serotonin appears to be stored in vesicles within nerve terminals analogous to the acetylcholine- and catecholamine-containing vesicles. The storage process is disrupted by reserpine, which also disrupts catecholamine storage in vesicles.

Treatment of smooth muscle preparations with neuraminidase destroyed their ability to be stimulated by 5HT. Activity could be restored by addition of purified gangliosides to the preparations.[27] It has thus been suggested that gangliosides are involved in the receptor site. Nevertheless, there is little reason to suppose that gangliosides need be the receptor itself, or even part of the receptor site. The hallucinogenic drug lysergic acid diethylamide (LSD) is a 5HT analogue and interferes with 5HT metabolism in the peripheral nervous system, possibly by competing for receptor sites. It is possible that LSD blocks serotonin receptors in the brain, but the data are equivocal and cannot be distinguished from other possible effects on 5HT metabolism such as LSD mimicking 5HT. It seems unlikely that receptor-blocking activity alone could account for the behavioral effects of LSD, since 2-bromoLSD, which is also a serotonin blocker in the peripheral nervous system, does not have similar behavioral effects in the brain. It may be that the behavioral effects of LSD are concerned with substance P metabolism (p. 41), since LSD inhibits the degradation of this peptide but 2-bromoLSD does not.

The principal route of serotonin degradation is oxidation by monoamine oxidase to the aldehyde. After further oxidation to 5-hydroxyindoleacetic acid (5HIAA) or reduction to the alcohol, it is excreted in the urine. Uptake of serotonin by nervous tissue is not as active as in the case of the catecholamines. Nevertheless, radioactive serotonin is taken up into the nerve endings after intraventricular injection and also into isolated synaptosomes. This process is inhibited by the tricyclic antidepressants, notably amitryptyline, which inhibits 5HT uptake more effectively than it does norepinephrine uptake.

The pineal is a very small gland located dorsal to the thalamus. It is innervated only from the superior cervical ganglion. In the pineal, serotonin is further converted by acetylation and methyl transfer to melatonin (Figure 5.9). Acetylation is performed by the enzyme 5HT-N-acetyltransferase which uses acetyl coenzyme A. The methyl transfer occurs from S-adenosylmethionine using the enzyme 5-hydroxyindole O-methyltransferase. Both these enzymes are found only in the pineal. The O-methylation is rate-limiting for melatonin biosynthesis.[28]

The activity of melatonin synthesis seems to be controlled by the activity of the sympathetic nervous system and the light-dark cycle. Increased activity or light increases concentrations of 5HT but decreases those of melatonin. In mammals, these two factors are not independent; denervation suppresses the light sensitivity and the effect of light is mediated through the eyes, since blinded animals show no diurnal rhythm. In amphibians, reptiles and birds, the effect of light on the pineal is direct. Apparently there are photoreceptors in the pineal, and light penetrates the thin skull to activate these receptors. The activities of both the acetylating and methylating enzymes are increased by darkness and rapidly decreased by light, the former enzyme being decreased with a half-life of three minutes. Cyclic AMP stimulates the overall rate of 5HT and melatonin synthesis. Norepinephrine has a similar effect and it is thought that adenyl cyclase in the pineal is activated by a norepinephrine input from the superior cervical ganglion. In this way neural activity in the superior cervical ganglion may control the synthesis of melatonin in the pineal. In animals such as frogs and toads, whose skin contains melanophores, melatonin induces lightening of the skin by causing aggregation of the pigmented granules in the melanocytes. Skin color is thus controlled by a balance between the pituitary melanocyte stimulating hormone (MSH) and melatonin. In other animals, melatonin is apparently important in sexual development, as it suppresses formation of the female gonads and the size of seminal vesicles.[29]

Assay of serotonin

Serotonin can be assayed by fluorometric assays which are sensitive to 1 nanogram or less. As in the case of the catecholamines, fluorescence techniques have been adapted to histological use. This technique has revealed that most serotonin containing neurons are in the pons and brain stem in nuclei known as the Raphé nuclei. Serotonin may also be assayed *in vitro* by the transfer of [³H]methyl groups from [Me-³H]S-adenosylmethionine by 5-hydroxyindole-O-methyltransferase, following acetylation by 5HT-N-acetyltransferase.[30]

iv) Glutamic Acid[3,9]

Glutamate is almost certainly the excitatory neurotransmitter in lobster motor neurons and probably performs a similar function in the central nervous system of mammals. Application of glutamate may be excitatory, and it is released by stimulation, but to date the specificity necessary for unequivocal definition as a CNS neurotransmitter has not been established. Nevertheless, glutamate is the probable neurotransmitter in the dentatothalamic and rubrothalamic tracts. It does not display a characteristic regional distribution like other neurotransmitters, and its high concentration throughout the brain is puzzling. A possible explanation is that glutamate has the role of a general excitatory substance. In common with acetylcholine and aspartic acid, glutamic acid shares the property of being excitatory to axons. Low concentrations of these compounds in the physiological range (except possibly acetylcholine) applied extracellularly significantly depolarize axonal membranes. The threshold for the firing of cortical neurons is 0.14 mM for glutamate, whereas the net tissue concentration is 10 mM. The depolarization effects are caused by an increased sodium conductance (up to five-fold). A postulated mechanism is that glutamate, aspartate and acetylcholine are analogues of the polar head groups of membrane phospholipids (see p. 76). In the case of glutamate and aspartate, the α-carboxyl group may effect the Na^+ transport. This general excitation-inhibition effect is discussed below (pp. 143, 179).

Glutamate metabolism is discussed in Chapter 2 (p. 34). Recently two derivatives have proved important for analyzing its neurotransmitter activity. Glutamic acid diethyl ester apparently blocks synaptic transmission at glutamate synapses, probably by competition for the postsynaptic receptor.[31] In contrast, glutamic acid dimethyl ester blocks the uptake of glutamate and potentiates synaptic transmission.[31] This is good evidence for a re-uptake mechanism of synaptic inactivation for glutamate.

v) Gamma-aminobutyric Acid (GABA)[3,9]

Gamma-aminobutyric acid is found in animals almost exclusively in the brain and to a very limited extent in the kidneys. GABA is produced by α-decarboxylation of glutamic acid by glutamic acid decarboxylase (GAD) (p. 36). Glutamic acid decarboxylase is found in the synaptosome fraction. Work on the nerves that innervate the walking leg muscles of lobsters suggests that only neurons that produce and use GABA as a neurotransmitter contain GAD. In the mammalian brain, the distribution of GAD closely parallels that of GABA itself. Glutamic acid decarboxylase from the lobster is inhibited by GABA providing a simple feedback control mechanism for GABA synthesis. The mouse brain enzyme, however, is not affected by GABA, so that here the control mechanism is unknown.

GABA is catabolized by transamination with α-ketoglutarate by a specific transaminase (GABA-T) to succinic semialdehyde. Succinic semialdehyde may then be oxidized to succinate and reincorporated into the tricarboxylic acid cycle. This pathway, which forms the GABA shunt, is discussed in Chapter 2 (p. 30 and Figure 2.4). GABA transaminase occurs in the mitochondrial fraction but is not enriched in mitochondria of synaptosomal origin. GABA-T is found in both excitatory and inhibitory motor neurons in the lobster but the activity is higher in the latter. Both the decarboxylase and transaminase require pyridoxal phosphate (vitamin B_6) as a cofactor. In vitamin B_6 deficiency GABA levels are depressed. This is probably because GAD has a lower affinity for pyridoxal phosphate than does GABA-T, so that it is less active than the transaminase. Both hydroxylamine and aminooxyacetic acid are potent inhibitors of GAD and GABA-T *in vitro*, but *in vivo* GABA-T is inhibited much more than GAD. These two inhibitors may elevate the brain content of GABA up to five-fold.

GABA has been well established as an inhibitory neurotransmitter in several invertebrate systems and probably has this role in the brain and spinal cord, though in the central nervous system of the lobster it may be excitatory. The concentration of GABA in the brain increases in a rostral to caudal direction, which may reflect the larger number of inhibitory pathways found caudally, especially in the cerebellum. Little is known of the storage and secretion of GABA, though it is rapidly taken up by some synaptosomes. Its postsynaptic effect is inhibited by picrotoxin and also by bicuculline, which probably competes for the receptor.

In addition to its role as a neurotransmitter, GABA may perform a general inhibitory function. GABA has a hyperpolarizing effect on nerve axons. In this respect it opposes the effect of glutamate, and it has been suggested that the balance of these two compounds may control the general excitation-inhibition state of the brain (see p. 179). The effects of glutamate and GABA on axons suggests that they may have been primordial neurotransmitters, active before specific receptors evolved. It is highly significant in this regard that glutamate, the excitatory neurotransmitter, is the direct precursor of GABA, the inhibitory one.

Huntington's chorea is an autosomal dominant genetic disease characterized by continuous extensive involuntary movement. Patients with this disease have abnormally low concentrations of GABA in the substantia nigra, putamen-globus pallidus and caudate nucleus. This is associated with deficiency of GAD and may reflect a degeneration of the GABA-containing cells in these tracts.[32]

vi) Glycine[3,9]

The work of Aprison has indicated that glycine is the neurotransmitter in the inhibitory interneurons of the spinal cord.[33] While GABA may also be an inhibitory transmitter in the cord, the distribution of glycine in the cord, especially after anoxia, suggests strongly that it is the transmitter for the interneurons. It is likely that glycine is also an inhibitory neurotransmitter in the brain but the evidence for this is not yet conclusive.

In addition to its availability in the diet, glycine may be synthesized from serine by serine hydroxymethyltransferase:

serine + tetrahydrofolate ↔ glycine + 5,10-methylenetetrahydrofolate

It may also be produced by transamination of glyoxylate:

$$HCOCO_2H + HO_2CCH_2CH_2CH(NH_2)CO_2H \leftrightarrow$$
glyoxal glutamate
$$HCH(NH_2)CO_2H + HO_2CCH_2CH_2COCO_2H$$
glycine α-ketoglutarate

Some 25 percent of the synaptosomes from spinal cord have a very active sodium-dependent mechanism for glycine uptake. Thus re-uptake is probably the mechanism of synaptic inactivation for glycine. Because it is such a ubiquitous metabolite, very little has been worked out concerning its special neurotransmitter metabolism. However, the action of strychnine in blocking the postsynaptic inhibitory effect of glycine in spinal cord may be specific.

vii) Histamine

The possible role of histamine as a neurotransmitter is uncertain, though it undoubtedly occurs in significant concentrations in the brain and in other nerve tracts. It is produced from histidine by decarboxylation (Figure 5.10) and recently a specific histidine decarboxylase has been isolated from cat brain. Histamine is N-methylated in mammalian nervous systems, and this may be the major route of histamine catabolism (Figure 5.10).

viii) Other Neurotransmitters

Undoubtedly many other neurotransmitter substances remain to be discovered. Aspartate and several other amino acids are suspected to be neurotransmitters.[9] In Chapter 2 the possibility that substance P is a neurotransmitter was referred to, and the same may be true for other peptides. We have discussed here only those compounds which we are reasonably certain are neurotransmitters.

The foregoing discussion of individual neurotransmitters suggests that the predominant site of synthesis of neurotransmitters is the presynaptic nerve terminals. In most cases the synthetic enzymes are concentrated there and the specific uptake mechanisms are found there. Also, the systems for vesicular storage seem to operate in the presynaptic nerve terminal. Nevertheless, experiments studying axoplasmic flow by ligation of nerves have suggested that vesicles containing catecholamines and acetylcholine are transported axonally from the perikaryon. What is the significance of this transport? One possibility is that the axonally transported vesicles are a

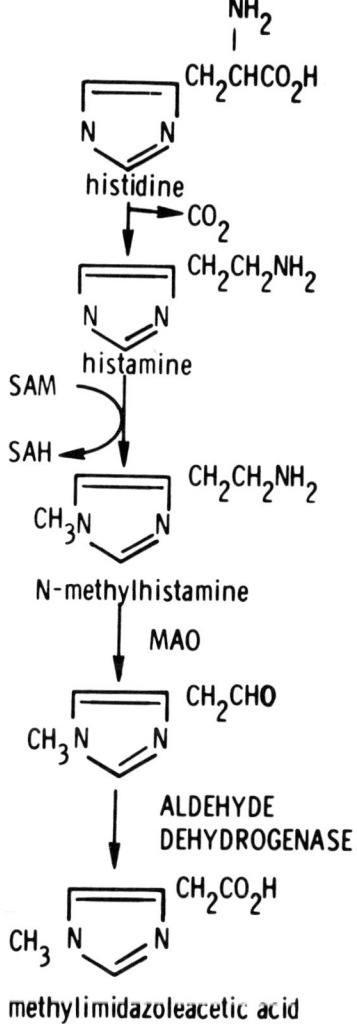

Figure 5.10 Synthesis and catabolism of histamine.

means of providing a fresh supply of vesicle membrane and other components lost by the wear and tear of repeated use. These materials may be conveniently packaged in the perikaryon and transported as intact vesicles. This possibility is particularly pertinent in the case of norepinephrine, where, as pointed out above, important proteins are lost following secretion.

ix) Turnover of Neurotransmitters

An important characteristic of a neurotransmitter is the rate of its secretion and how this is influenced by cerebral processes. In practice, all that can be measured is the rate of turnover. The measurement of turnover has been approached in several ways, none of which is free of artifact:

1. Blocking the synthesis of neurotransmitter and observing the decrease in its concentration. This method has the disadvantages that side effects of the necessary drugs may affect the turnover rate, that the secretion rate may depend to some extent upon the available store, and that any decrease in activity due to depleted stores may feed back into the system and decrease secretion rates.

2. Observing the rate of catabolism of labeled neurotransmitter, either injected or synthesized by the brain from a suitable precursor. This method has the disadvantages that the rate of labeling must be assumed to be uniform in all neurons, and that, if labeled neurotransmitter itself is administered, this neurotransmitter is incorporated only into cells that actively secrete it. A variation of this method is to examine the rate of synthesis of the neurotransmitter from a suitable precursor. Because the concentration of precursor may affect the rate of synthesis, tracer techniques using precursors of high specific radioactivity must be used. For this method the rate of uptake by the tissue is an important factor that must be taken into consideration.

Neither of these methods can resolve the problem that different neurons containing the same neurotransmitter may have different turnover rates. Also, these methods measure the *net* turnover rate; re-uptake and recycling processes will decrease the observed rates. These processes may be blocked pharmacologically but not without disturbance of normal metabolism.

3. A more indirect method that has been used is the study of the secretion of neurotransmitter metabolites in CSF, plasma or urine. While this method is important since it can be used clinically, it is difficult to get unequivocal data because of variable re-uptake, the many alternate catabolic pathways and, clinically, the inability to determine endogenous concentrations.

For norepinephrine, turnover has been estimated by using α-methyl-p-tyrosine to inhibit synthesis, or radioactive norepinephrine, tyrosine or DOPA as precursors. A problem is that dopaminergic neurons may take up radioactive norepinephrine though they do not secrete it. The results obtained with these diverse methods do not disagree widely. MAO inhibitors such as pargyline have been found to reduce the turnover rate of radioactive norepinephrine by about 50 percent, whereas electroconvulsive shock treatment increases turnover by about the same amount. During the rebound of REM sleep that follows its chronic deprivation, norepinephrine turnover nearly doubles.

In contrast, serotonin turnover rates vary greatly according to the method of measurement. The rate of decay of radioactive 5HT injected intracerebrally corresponds to a half-life of about four to five hours. However, turnover estimated by inhibiting MAO and observing the subsequent elevation of 5HT concentration gives much faster rates. This discrepancy may be due to selective uptake of 5HT into more stable storage systems, since when radioactive tryptophan is used as a precursor the faster turnover rates are obtained.

D. SYNAPTIC COMPONENTS OTHER THAN NEUROTRANSMITTERS

i) Gangliosides

The structures of the gangliosides are shown in Figure 4.7. The essential features are a lipid part, ceramide, and a carbohydrate part consisting of an oligosaccharide chain to which variable amounts of sialic acid are attached. Ganglioside synthesis and metabolism are considered in Chapter 4 (p. 89). They are membrane components, probably of neurons, and their greatest concentration is in the synaptosomal fraction. This suggests that they may play some role in synaptic transmission; their role in electrical excitability in the cortex (p. 91) reinforces such a theory. Gangliosides may also be involved in the serotonin receptor (p. 140). Isolated gangliosides interact with tetanus toxin[34] and cholera toxin,[35] and may thus form the site of the blocking activity of these toxins.

Since gangliosides are believed to have their lipid parts buried in the membrane with the carbohydrate tails protruding, the sialic acid moieties may be exposed to the extracellular space.* This would permit the extracellular transfer of sialyl groups to change the species of ganglioside. Such chemical modification could alter the properties of the excitable membrane or the synapse. In agreement with these ideas, sialyl transferases are found in the synaptosome fraction. Since Ca^{2+} is bound to the hydrophilic sialic acid, it is possible that gangliosides control the calcium essential for neurotransmitter release.

*Some recent data suggest that the sialic acid of gangliosides in synaptosomal and microsomal membranes is not accessible to sialidase.[36]

ii) Proteins

Proteins exist at the synapse both as components of the membranes (structural proteins) and as soluble proteins, presumably enzymes. The bulk of these proteins are probably supplied by axoplasmic flow, but there may also be some local synaptic protein synthesis. Isolated synaptosomes have been shown to contain small amounts of RNA and to actively incorporate amino acids into proteinaceous material, but ribosomes have never been seen in electronmicrographs of presynaptic nerve terminals, either in tissue sections or in synaptosome preparations. At least a part of synaptosomal protein synthesis is due to mitochondria enclosed within the synaptosomes. Since mitochondria contain ribosomes of the prokaryotic (70S) type, protein synthesis in mitochondria is inhibited by the drug chloramphenicol. Some 30 percent of the amino acid incorporation of synaptosome preparations is inhibited by chloramphenicol, which suggests that this fraction is accounted for by mitochondria. The remainder is sensitive to cycloheximide, which inhibits protein synthesis by ribosomes of the eukaryotic (80S) type. However, synaptosome preparations are not pure nerve terminals. Electron microscopy has shown that they are contaminated with small packets of ribosomes completely enclosed in membrane. Radioautographic studies have shown that about half the incorporation of radioactive amino acids is into these ribosomal packets. Since these packets represent only about 5 percent of the total processes, they are of very high specific radioactivity.[37,38] The remainder of the incorporation is into synaptosomes and about 20 percent of this is chloramphenicol sensitive. The chloramphenicol-insensitive grains in the synaptosomes appear to be associated with the limiting membranes.

Previously, synaptosomal plasma membranes purified by density gradient centrifugation had been shown to incorporate many different amino acids into protein *in vitro*.[39] Recently, highly purified synaptosomal plasma membranes have been shown to incorporate amino acids into three specific protein bands. All three of these components are Triton-insoluble and may thus be within the synaptic membrane itself (see p. 123).[40] In this case the amino acid incorporation was inhibited by chloramphenicol, which conflicts with earlier data.[39] For the present we may only conclude that if protein synthesis does occur in presynaptic regions other than in mitochondria, then it is severely limited and probably specifically associated with the neuronal membrane.

iii) Glycoprotein

Biochemical analysis suggests that a large number of the proteins isolated from synaptosomes are perchloric-acid-Schiff (PAS) positive, and so probably contain carbohydrate. Histological staining of brain tissue, in particular with ruthenium red, suggests that carbohydrate is attached to the neuronal plasma membrane and that the synaptic cleft is filled with carbohydrate.[1] This is probably attributable to glycoproteins that form part of the membrane structure, though glycolipids (especially gangliosides) may also be involved. The synaptic cleft is wider than the expected length of the carbohydrate portion of glycoproteins of the membrane, so that glycoproteins, polysaccharides and mucopolysaccharides that are not part of the membrane may exist in the cleft.

Our understanding of the synthesis of glycoproteins in the brain is limited. Probably most, if not all, of the polypeptide is synthesized on ribosomes in the cell body. The carbohydrates may be added either during synthesis or subsequently. In the liver the carbohydrates are added principally in the Golgi apparatus, but the situation in the brain is less clear. Roseman and his co-workers showed that the enzymes for the transfer of galactose, N-acetylglucosamine and N-acetylneuraminic acid from their respective nucleotide derivates (UDPgal, UDP-N-acetylglucosamine, CMP-NANA) to proteins and lipids were concentrated in the synaptosome fraction.[41] However, other workers have found little UDPgalactose-galactosyltransferase activity in this fraction, the bulk being in the microsome fraction.[13] Nor do synaptosomes have any detectable capacity for the incorporation of fucose.[42]

The radioisotope tracer data are also confusing. Barondes has shown that whereas there was a delay in the appearance of radioactivity from $[^{14}C]$leucine in the proteins of the synaptosome fraction, there was no such delay in the incorporation of $[1\text{-}^{14}C]$glucosamine into glycoprotein.[43] Furthermore, the protein synthesis inhibitor acetoxycycloheximide did not immediately inhibit the glucosamine incorporation. Kinetic studies suggested that the glucosamine incorporation was only affected later, when the supply of proteins transported axoplasmically from the cell body was depressed. The interpretation was that the polypeptide acceptors were synthesized perikaryally and transported to the terminals, where the carbohydrate (glucosamine, galactosamine, glucuronic acid) was added. This was consistent with the extensive *in vitro* incorporation of glucosamine into glycoprotein of isolated synaptosomes. However, when $[^3H]$fucose was used as a precursor of glycoprotein, radioactivity did not immediately appear in the synaptosome fraction, but there was a delay consistent with a very rapid axoplasmic transport of fucosyl glycoproteins.[43] This rapid axoplasmic transport of glycoproteins has been confirmed in a number of systems using fucose, glucosamine or N-acetylmannosamine as precursors. A possible explanation is that Barondes did not observe some of the transported glucosamine-labeled glycoprotein because he did not anticipate the velocity of the transport. Yet the data are also consistent with the possibility that glucosamine or one or more of its carbohydrate metabolites may be added locally at the nerve terminal.

Recently, it has become possible to prepare pre- and postsynaptic membranes as junctional complexes recognizable in the electron microscope by their staining with phosphotungstic acid.[21] These complexes contain protein, glycoprotein, phospholipid and sialic acid. Most of the sialic acid is in glycoproteins rather than gangliosides. Enzymes normally associated with synaptic plasma membranes, such as acetylcholinesterase, 5'-nucleotidase and alkaline phosphatase, are almost completely removed by the Triton treatment used to prepare the complexes.

Like gangliosides, the glycoproteins in the synapse probably play some role in neurotransmission, but the nature of this is as yet unknown. By analogy with the immunological and other roles of cell-surface carbohydrates, glycoproteins are thought to be involved in cell-cell interaction, and possibly in the recognition involved in synapse formation (Chapter 6).

E. SYNAPTIC MODIFICATION[44]

One of the ways in which communication between neurons could be altered is by synaptic modification. This would result in an altered probability of the occurrence of a postsynaptic potential or a change in its magnitude. Several possibilities exist for such modifications:

1. a change in the amount of transmitter released;
2. a change in the width or composition of the synaptic cleft such that the rate of diffusion of the neurotransmitter across the cleft is altered;
3. a change in the activity of the enzymes or the uptake mechanisms that inactivate the neurotransmitter;
4. a change in the affinity of the postsynaptic receptor sites for the neurotansmitter;
5. a change in the response of the postsynaptic membrane to neurotransmitter-receptor interaction.

These changes could all be readily adaptable but longer-term possibilities would include major structural reorganization of the entire synapse. The feasibility of some of the above mechanisms has already been demonstrated pharmacologically. Interference with neurotransmitter inactivation mechanisms by inhibition of the catabolic enzymes or of the re-uptake is known to potentiate neurotransmitter action. Similarly, blockage of receptors will block neurotransmitter action. A decrease in the amount of neurotransmitter released could occur if the presynaptic stores become depleted. This has been postulated to be the mechanism of habituation. (After repeated presynaptic stimulation, the magnitude of the postsynaptic potential is temporarily reduced.) Many other mechanisms are possible. Certain data suggest that the presynaptic terminal may have receptors for the neurotransmitter that have the ability to modulate the amount of transmitter released. Thus the magnitude of the release may be regulated by the synaptic efficacy of the released neurotransmitter.[20] There may also be feedback from the postsynaptic cell to the presynaptic one. Such feedback might occur by the secretion of a diffusible substance (e.g., cyclic AMP) from the postsynaptic cell subsequent to neurotransmitter reception. There has also been some discussion, but little convincing evidence, concerning the possible transynaptic transfer of macromolecules, especially proteins (see p. 108). Given what is now known concerning the uptake of macromolecules by cells, this is at least feasible. The synapse is an important control point in interneuronal communication and thus in information transfer. This and the many possibilities for rapid modulation have led many neuroscientists to view the synapse as the most important structure in the brain.

CHAPTER 5 REFERENCES

Reviews and General References

1. *Structure and Function of Synapses* (Ed. G. D. Pappas and D. P. Purpura), Raven Press, New York, 1972.
2. Hubbard, J. I. Microphysiology of vertebrate neuromuscular transmission. *Physiol. Rev.* 53:674–723, 1973. An excellent review of acetylcholine.
3. Krnjević, K. Chemical nature of synaptic transmission in verebrates. *Physiol. Rev.* 54: 418–540, 1974.
4. *Neurochemistry of Cholinergic Receptors* (Ed. E. de Robertis and J. Schacht), Raven Press, New York, 1973.
5. Molinoff, P. B., and Axelrod, J. Biochemistry of catecholamines. *Ann. Rev. Biochem.* 40:465–500, 1971.
6. *Neurotransmitters and metabolic regulation.* (Ed. R. M. S. Smellie), *Biochemical Society Symposia #36*, The Biochemical Society, London, 1972.
7. Catecholamines (Ed. L. L. Iversen), *Brit. Med. Bull.* 29:#2, 1973.
8. Molinoff, P. B. The regulation of the noradrenergic neuron. In *Catecholamines and Their Enzymes in the Neuropathology of Schizophrenia* (Ed. S. S. Kety and S. W. Matthyse), Pergamon Press, London, 1974.

9. Snyder, S. H., Young, A. B., Bennett, J. P., and Mulder, A. H. Synaptic biochemistry of amino acids. *Fed. Proc.* 32:2039–47, 1973.
10. *New Concepts in Neurotransmitter Regulation* (Ed. A. J. Mandell), Plenum Press, New York, 1973.

Literature Cited

11. Clark, A. W., Hurlbut, W. P., and Mauro, A. Changes in the fine structure of the neuromuscular junction of the frog caused by black widow spider venom. *J. Cell Biol.* 52:1–14, 1972.
12. Heuser, J. E., and Reese, T. S. Evidence for recycling of synaptic vesicle membrane during transmitter release at the frog neuromuscular junction. *J. Cell Biol.* 57:315–44, 1973.
13. Morgan, I. G., Breckenridge, W. C., Vincendon, G., and Gombos, G. The proteins of nerve-ending membranes. In *Proteins of the Nervous System* (Ed. D. Schneider), Raven Press, New York, 1973, pp. 171–92.
14. Morgan, I. G., Zanetta, J.-P., Breckenridge, W. C., Vincendon, G., and Gombos, G. The chemical structure of synaptic membranes. *Brain Research* 62:405–11, 1973.
15. Berl, S., Puszkin, S., and Nicklas, W. J. Actomyosin-like protein in brain. *Science* 179:441–46, 1973.
16. Schmitt, F. O. Fibrous proteins—neuronal organelles. *Proc. Nat. Acad. Sci., U.S.A.* 60:1092–1101, 1968.
17. Whittaker, V. P. The synaptosome. In *Handbook of Neurochemistry*. Vol. 2 (Ed. A. Lajtha), Plenum Press, New York, 1969, pp. 327–64.
18. Whittaker, V. P., and Barker, L. A. The subcellular fractionation of brain tissue with special reference to the preparation of synaptosomes and their component organelles. In *Methods of Neurochemistry*, Vol. 2 (Ed. R. Fried), Marcel Dekker, New York, 1972, pp. 1–52.
19. Iversen, L. L., and Snyder, S. H. Synaptosomes: different populations storing catecholamines and gamma-aminobutyric acid in homogenates of rat brain. *Nature* 220:796–98, 1968.
20. Iversen, L. L. Biochemical aspects of synaptic modulation. In *The Neurosciences, Third Study Program* (Ed. F. O. Schmitt and F. G. Worden), M.I.T. Press, Cambridge, Mass., 1974, pp. 905–15.
21. Cotman, C. W., and Taylor, D. Isolation and structural studies on synaptic complexes from rat brain. *J. Cell Biol.* 55:696–711, 1972.
22. Gardner, D., and Kandel, E. Diphasic postsynaptic potential: a chemical synapse capable of mediating conjoint excitation and inhibition. *Science* 176:675–78, 1972.
23. Dross, K., and Kewitz, H. Concentration and origin of choline in the rat brain. *Naunyn-Schmiederbergs Arch. Exp. Path. Pharmak.* 274:91–106, 1972.
24. Whittaker, V. P., Dowdall, M. J., and Boyne, A. F. The storage and release of acetylcholine by cholinergic nerve terminals: recent results with non-mammalian preparations. *Biochem. Soc. Symp.* 36:49–68, 1972.
25. Sims, K. L., and Bloom, F. E. Rat brain L-3,4-dihydroxyphenylalanine and L-5-hydroxytryptophan decarboxylase activities: differential effect of 6-hydroxydopamine. *Brain Research* 49:165–75, 1973.
26. Coyle, J. T., and Henry, D. Catecholamines in fetal and newborn rats. *J. Neurochem.* 21:61–67, 1973.

27. Woolley, D. W., and Gommi, B. W. Serotonin receptors, VII. Activities of various pure gangliosides as the receptors. *Proc. Nat. Acad. Sci., U.S.* 54:959–63, 1965.
28. Wurtman, R., Axelrod, J., and Kelly, D. E. *The Pineal*, Academic Press, New York, 1968.
29. Axelrod, J. The pineal gland: a neurochemical transducer. *Science* 184:1341–48, 1974.
30. Saavedra, J. M., Brownstein, M., and Axelrod, J. A specific and sensitive enzymatic-isotopic microassay for serotonin in tissues. *J. Pharmacol. Exp. Therap.* 186:508–15, 1973.
31. McLennan, H., and Haldeman, S. The actions of the dimethyl and diethyl esters of glutamic acid on glutamate uptake by brain tissue. *J. Neurochem.* 20:629–31, 1973.
32. Perry, T. L., Hansen, S., and Kloster, M. Huntington's chorea: deficiency of γ-aminobutyric acid in brain. *N.E.J. Med.* 288:337–42, 1973.
33. Aprison, M. H., Davidoff, R. A., and Werman, R. Glycine: its metabolic and possible transmitter roles. In *Handbook of Neurochemistry*, Vol. 3 (Ed. A. Lajtha), Pergamon Press, New York, 1970, pp. 382–97.
34. Van Heyningen, W. E., and Mellanby, J. Tetanus toxin. In *Microbial Toxins*, Vol. 2 (Ed. S. J. Ajl), Academic Press, New York, 1971, pp. 69–108.
35. Cuatrecasas, P. Interaction of *Vibrio Cholerae* enterotoxin with cell membranes. *Biochemistry* 12:3547–58, 1973.
36. Dicesare, J. L., and Rapport, M. M. Availability to neuraminidase of gangliosides and sialoglycoproteins of neuronal membranes. *J. Neurochem.* 20:1781–83, 1973.
37. Cotman, C. W., and Taylor, D. A. Autoradiographic analysis of protein synthesis in synaptosomal fractions. *Brain Research* 29:366–72, 1971.
38. Gambetti, P., Autilio-Gambetti, L., Gonatas, N. K., and Shafer, B. Protein synthesis in synaptosomal fractions, ultrastructural radioautographic study. *J. Cell Biol.* 52:526–35, 1972.
39. Appel, S. H. Macromolecular synthesis in synapses. In *Macromolecules and Behavior*, 2nd ed. (Ed. J. Gaito), Appleton-Century-Crofts, New York, 1972, pp. 185–203.
40. Ramirez, G., Levitan, I. B., and Mushynski, W. E. Highly purified synaptosomal membranes from rat brain. Incorporation of amino acids into membrane proteins *in vitro*. *J. Biol. Chem.* 247:5382–90, 1972.
41. Roseman, S. The synthesis of complex carbohydrates by multiglycosyltransferase systems and their potential function in intercellular adhesion. *Chem. Phys. Lipids* 5:270–97, 1970.
42. Zatz, M., and Barondes, S. H. Particulate and solubilized fucosyl transferases from mouse brain. *J. Neurochem.* 18:1625–37, 1971.
43. Zatz, M., and Barondes, S. H. Rapid transport of fucosyl glycoproteins to nerve endings in mouse brain. *J. Neurochem.* 18:1125–33, 1971.
44. Bloom, F. E. Dynamics of synaptic modulation: perspectives for the future. In *The Neurosciences, Third Study Program* (Ed. F. O. Schmitt and F. G. Worden), M.I.T. Press, Cambridge, Mass., 1974, pp. 989–99.

VI. Cell – Cell Interaction

In complex organisms the existence of discrete tissues is maintained by specific interactions among cells. Both in living organisms and in explants or cell dispersions, cells aggregate into clumps of distinctive morphology. For the competent functioning of a complex organism, cells must be cognizant of one another and their interrelationships must be coordinated. These interrelationships are important in the development of the organism and are later maintained by surface contact between adjacent cells and by hormones in noncontacting cells. A failure of these mechanisms occurs in malignant tissue where cells behave in a primitive manner, growing and dividing without regard for the position and nature of nearby cells. Unregulated cell proliferation is not found in normal cells.

Within the nervous system several types of interaction occur among neurons and between neurons and other cells. These can conveniently be classified into (1) developmental processes preceding functional maturation, (2) the maintenance of structural differentiation by trophic effects of neurons on other cells, (3) interactions between cells and tissues that they do not directly innervate and (4) neuronal interactions relating to the passage of the action potential.

A. THE DEVELOPMENT OF NERVE CONNECTIONS—NEUROTROPISM[1,2]

The primary afferent and efferent pathways of the nervous system are connected according to a genetically predetermined plan. The formation of these connections precedes modifications that may occur through use or disuse. The development of such connections have been extensively studied in the visual system of reptiles, amphibians and birds, where the major primary visual area of the brain is the optic tectum. During embryogenesis, fibers from the retinal ganglion cells of the eye grow toward the contralateral optic tectum and ultimately innervate it. There is a map of the retina on the surface of the tectum with a correspondence between the relative positions of points on the retina and their representation in the tectum. Lower vertebrates have a considerable capacity for axonal regeneration following section of the optic nerve. Thus the way in which these outgrowing axons reach their appropriate destinations may be examined by surgery of the visual pathway of these animals. In a classical study, Sperry removed the eye of a newt, rotated it through 180 degrees and reimplanted it in the orbit.[11] After regeneration of the optic nerve from the retinal ganglion cells, there was inversion of the normal behavior of the animal in response to visual stimuli in that eye. Thus the animal struck to the left when presented with a lure placed high in right side of its field of vision, and struck downward at a lure placed high in the visual field. Detailed electrophysiological mapping showed that there had been a highly selective reconnection of nerve fibers to their original termini. It appeared as though the axon from each ganglion cell were destined for a precise locus in the optic tectum.

These observations raised two related questions: (1) How do the retinal ganglion fibers find their way to the contralateral optic tectum? (2) Once in the tectum, how do they identify the appropriate tectal neuron to make the specific connections? A suggested answer to the first question is that the afferent fibers grow toward the source of a particular attractant in the manner of salmon migrating from the ocean up the rivers to their original home stream. The homing salmon apparently achieve their goal using an acute olfactory sense which detects chemical substances in the water. The existence of a chemical gradient of the attractant would ensure continuous growth in the correct direction. No attractant substance for growing nerve fibers has yet been isolated.

A possible explanation for the point-to-point specificity between retina and tectum is that each tectal neuron is specific and is recognized by one and only one retinal ganglion cell fiber. Sperry considered this to be unlikely and postulated the existence of gradients of receptor substances across the tectal surface. Gradients of two or more substances would be needed to achieve the necessary specificity. Thus fibers could distinguish the relative proportions of the receptor substances in order to determine their destination. Jacobson has pointed out that the behavioral and electrophysiological data do not justify the claim of precise point-to-point specificity, but that there is only specificity in the *relative* positions of the innervating fibers. This agrees well with the idea of a gradient of attractant substances.

Remarkable specificity of innervation has been demonstrated in another sensory system. Jacobson transplanted pieces of skin of frog tadpoles from the back to the belly and vice versa.[12] After metamorphosis, the transplant was integrated into its new location and had been reinnervated, but its coloration corresponded to its site of origin. Yet when the transplanted skin was stimulated, the frog behaved as though the skin were in its *original* location in the body. Presumably, either the sensory nerves that had previously innervated the piece of skin had traveled across the body to reinnervate it, or the transplanted skin had been innervated nonspecifically and had signaled the central nervous system of its previous location. Jacobson felt the latter possibility was more likely and that substances from the transplanted skin transmitted the "false" information to the CNS. Whichever mechanism is correct, substances from the skin are clearly able to influence the growth of nerve fibers in a sophisticated way.

That cellular affinity between specific neurons may exist has recently been shown by Roth.[13] A trypsinized suspension of radioactively labeled cells was made from dorsal and ventral halves of chick embryo retinae. When incubated with a section of the optic tectum, the retinal cells selectively and preferentially adhered to that region of the optic tectum that they normally innervated. This *in vitro* system presents unprecedented opportunities for biochemical studies of this specificity.

The problem of how the fibers decide which cells to innervate is still unresolved. It is not known whether the fiber grows out touching all cells in its path until it finds one that will trigger synapse formation, or whether the fiber grows only toward cells with which it can form synapses. No definitive evidence exists to distinguish between the specificity being a property of the surface of the cells or a property of trophic attractants released by the recipient cells.

The nature of none of the substances that confer specificity is known. Any trophic attractant would have to combine a high degree of chemical specificity with a molecular weight low enough to allow adequate diffusion. The class of compounds that may best fulfill these criteria is peptides, though nothing definitive is known in this respect. There has been much speculation that carbohydrates on the cell surface could provide the specificity for the innervation. This is because the changes in cellular interactions that occur during neoplasia are accompanied by loss of carbohydrates from the cell surface. Non-neoplastic cells restrict each other's growth by a process termed *contact inhibition*. The characteristic of neoplastic cells is the lack of this contact inhibition, exhibited in their unrestricted growth. It is also known that the immunological specificity of antisera from foreign cells resides in the nature and pattern of carbohydrates on the cell surface.

Cell-surface carbohydrates may occur in glycoproteins and glycolipids, both of which are common components of neuronal plasma membranes. The wide variety of carbohydrate sequences and patterns in glycoproteins (p. 96) might contain specificity to the extent required by the observation on the development of the nervous system.

The reeler is a mouse mutant in which neurological impairment can at least in part be accounted for by the inability of the nerve cells to align themselves correctly with respect to one another. The reeler carries a non-lethal recessive mutation which results in cerebral malformation and a consequent impairment of balance. Dissociated cerebellar cortical cells from an eighteen-day-old normal mouse embryo will reassociate to form a symmetrical structure in which neurons are aligned with an outer molecular layer of nerve cell bodies and an inner zone consisting largely of nerve fibers. A similar suspension of cerebellar cortical cells from the embryo of the reeler mutant will not reaggregate to form such an ordered structure but appears to coalesce in random clumps.[3]

Cyclic AMP has been shown to mediate the rearrangement of isolated thyroid cells which, when exposed to TSH (thyroid-stimulating hormone), form follicle-like structures.[14] Thus cyclic AMP may play a role in regulating the alignment of cells to each other, in addition to its important intracellular functions.[4]

B. EFFECTS OF NEURONS ON INNERVATED TISSUES—NEUROTROPHISM

When outgrowing axons have come into contact with their target cells, the formation of synapses occurs. The two cells connected in this manner are capable of profoundly influencing each other. Within the nervous system, neurons are vulnerable to changes in both the neurons upon which they synapse (retrograde effects) and neurons which synapse upon them (transneuronal effects). When an efferent neuron is cut, there may be degenerative changes in both the ganglion or nucleus from which the cell emerged and in the nervous structure innervated.

The visual system has been of use in following the course of the elaboration of neuronal circuitry. If the embryonic eye of lower vertebrates is removed, the contralateral optic tectum does not receive its major source of afferentation. Cowan has shown that when this enucleation was carried out in the early chick embryo (at three days of incubation), there was no discernible effect on the development of the optic tectum for the next ten days of incubation.[5] Cell proliferation and differentiation within the tectum continues normally in the absence of outgrowing axons from retinal ganglion cells. However, after this period a progressive hypoplasia becomes apparent in the optic tectum, followed by cell loss in certain lower tectal layers. This failure may perhaps be due to the absence of normal synaptogenesis. These events precede the development of the electrical maturity of the optic nerve. Thus the development of postsynaptic cells in the tectum may depend on chemical factors secreted by the nerve terminals of retinal ganglion cells, and not on the occurrence of action potentials. On the other hand, it should be borne in mind that all living cells have a charged surface and that nonnervous electrical coupling can result in coordinated activity which may be mechanical (as in the movements of early embryos) and possibly also chemical. Enucleation of chicks at hatch results in severe retardation of the development of the denervated optic lobe.[6] Growth of the lobe is largely arrested and there is a retarded appearance of neurotransmitters and enzymes associated with their metabolism. These include acetylcholine, choline acetylase and acetylcholinesterase. The normal increase in concentration of myelin-specific lipids is also severely impaired. This failure of myelination may be secondary to the impaired differentiation of the postsynaptic neuron. Thus, the differentiation of the glia depends on the integrity of the neuron. The means by which signals are exchanged between the nuclear genetic material and peripheral areas of the neuron which are in contact with neighboring cells may be the migration of materials in both directions along the axon. Cells which are appropriately located can act as mutual inducers, each being essential for the maturation of the other. Thus a defect in one cell species can cause a widespread retardation of development.

As cerebral differentiation proceeds, the axon becomes capable of electrical conduction. At this point, not only is further development of the central nervous system dependent on the genetic program, but the nature of the sensory environment becomes increasingly important. The visual system is also useful as a tool to determine the role of afferent input in cerebral development, since modification of visual information from the eye to visual areas can be achieved in many ways (Chapter 7). Reduction of visual stimuli by maintaining an animal in darkness or by closure of the eyelid results in imperfect development of the optic centers. Thus eyelid suture in rats results in a loss of spines from the apical dendrites, the postsynaptic elements of the visual cortical pyramidal cells.[15] Additionally, there is a reduction of the size of neurons and the number of synapses within the lateral geniculate nucleus. Defects caused by sensory deprivation are often more severe during development than in the adult animals. There appears to be a critical period during maturation when susceptibility to sensory deprivation is maximal, and if deprivation is prolonged these defects become irreversible. This time may be when synaptogenesis is maximal. In man, abnormal visual input due to astigmatism has been shown to permanently modify cerebral connectivity.[16]

Knowledge of the way in which the brain interprets visual information gives clues as to how neurons become interconnected in a meaningful manner. When there is a change of the illumination falling on retinal photoreceptor cells, they may activate the retinal ganglion cells by way of interneurons. The ganglion cells relay initially to the primary visual centers, and from there pathways lead to associative cerebral areas. As one moves from neurons closely related to the sensory receptors to neurons that are more indirectly related to the initial sensory stimulus, the responses of nerve cells to light become increasingly complex. Hubel and Wiesel have found neurons in the cat and monkey visual cortex that have narrow, band-shaped receptive fields of precise width, length and retinal position.[17] The appropriate pattern of light within this restricted retinal area results in the neuron firing. Other higher-order neurons fire only when such bands are moving in a certain direction within a rather large area of retina. Such cells then are able to generalize stimulus position and respond to a specific pattern that may be initially detected by photoreceptors located in many retinal positions. This work has led to new ideas concerning the way in which visual information is processed by the brain. The brain does not interpret a photograph-like image transmitted from the eye. Rather, the eye acts essentially by detecting the edges of areas of differing light intensity. These patterns effect the firing of adjacent retinal ganglion cells in a certain order. The angle and velocity of these edges are reported to neurons with inputs from many ganglion cells. Such cerebral neurons integrate information from their many inputs and fire only to a specific stimulus pattern. Information then passes to higher-order cells that respond only to more specific stimuli. It may be this arrangement of orders of complexity that makes it possible to rapidly recognize a familiar face from several angles and at various distances even though very different images may be cast on the retina.

Reduced neural use may result in subtle transneuronal changes. Events within a single neuron have a spatial and temporal relationship to events in neighboring neurons. Neurons can interact and influence the output of each other. In the case of the visual system, the particular firing pattern in the afferents is ultimately reflected in secondary visual and associative cerebral areas. The development of the organization of the higher centers may be profoundly influenced by synaptic events in closely related areas occurring at very nearly the same time. There is evidence that neighboring retinal ganglion cells must fire simultaneously for them both to have inputs to the same neuron in the lateral geniculate nucleus.[18]

Blakemore has found that the nature of early visual experience may modify the distribution of visual receptive fields in the cortex.[19] This was demonstrated by maintaining kittens, from the time before their eyes opened, in an environment consisting entirely of either vertical or horizontal black and white bars. This difference in early visual experience resulted in the receptor fields of the kitten becoming specialized so that they responded maximally only to the visual input to which they had previously been exposed. Neurons in the visual cortex of kittens reared in the presence of vertical bars responded very poorly to horizontal bars and vice versa. These deficits indicate the need for effective functional activity during the specification of nerve connections.

Interactions between nerve cells and other cells are not merely essential for the normal development of cerebral structures, but are equally vital for the maintenance of the differentiated state of most innervated cells. Considerable knowledge about the trophic effects of nerve on the periphery has come from studies of the influences of innervation on striated muscle.

i) Effects of Nerve on Muscle

Section of the nerve to a muscle leads to degenerative changes within the muscle. Tissue differentiation cannot be reestablished by electrical stimulation of the muscle or by the topical application of acetylcholine (the neurotransmitter at the neuromuscular junction). As long as muscle has an intact nerve supply, it will remain differentiated, even if it is immobilized and inactive.

In the innervated muscle, sensitivity to acetylcholine is confined to the region of the motor endplate. Soon after the muscle is denervated, the acetylcholine sensitivity increases and spreads across the surface of the muscle membrane (sarcolemma). This phenomenon is known as *denervation supersensitivity*. Study of the acetylcholine receptors has been made easier by the use of the snake-venom toxin, α-bungarotoxin.[20] This compound binds very strongly and specifically to the receptors (p. 129). Radioactively labeled α-bungarotoxin has been used to determine the number and location of ACh receptors on the sarcolemma. Following denervation, the number of receptors increases more than a hundredfold and they spread from their usual location at the motor endplates to a more uniform distribution over the membrane. Denervation supersensitivity can be blocked by cycloheximide and thus appears to involve the synthesis of new proteins, perhaps the receptor molecules themselves.

The disease myasthenia gravis is characterized by severe muscle weakness and this has been attributed to the low content of acetylcholine receptors in the affected muscle, as assayed by its α-bungarotoxin binding capacity. Vinblastin and colchicine interfere with axoplasmic flow by neurotubule disruption (p. 107) but do not interfere with the passage of the action potential. When these compounds are applied to a motor neuron, neither the electrical properties of the nerve nor the contractility of the muscle are impaired.[21] However, the muscle membrane undergoes denervation-like changes including partial depolarization and spreading of the sensitivity to acetylcholine.

These data suggest the existence of neurogenic factors that are essential for the maintenance of normal muscle. Other evidence for the existence of such factors arises from experiments in which the innervation of slow and fast muscles is surgically interchanged.[22] Following such an operation there are histological, physiological and biochemical changes such that the originally fast muscle comes to more closely resemble slow muslce, and the slow muscle comes to resemble fast muscle. These changes may be due to neurotrophic factors, but they may also be caused by the altered firing pattern of the new nerve supply.

It is possible that many diseases of muscle tissue may be due to a failure of the secretion by the nerve of chemicals that are essential for muscle maintenance. Duchenne muscular dystrophy is associated with a substantial loss of muscle motor endplates at an early stage in the disease.[23] Mouse strains are known that have a genetic defect resulting in a disorder resembling human muscular dystrophy. When minced muscle from normal mice is transplanted into this dystrophic strain, it fails to develop.[24] Conversely, minced muscle from dystrophic mice can be grafted into normal mice and will subsequently revert to apparently normal muscle. Thus the primary deficit associated with this disorder may be not within the muscle tissue but rather in the environment in which the tissue must develop.

Further experiments suggesting the existence of neurotrophic factors essential for muscle differentiation have been carried out in organ culture of whole muscle. A diffusible heat-labile factor derived from nerve homogenates is capable of inducing a rise in the level of acetylcholinesterase in the muscle.[25] Other heat-labile factors have been extracted from nerve tissue that are able to enhance the rate of protein synthesis in the denervated muscle by as much as 40 percent. Thus a considerable proportion of the biosynthetic activity of muscle may be directed by neurotrophic factors. It may be significant that the fall in rates of protein synthesis and cell division that follow denervation of regenerating newt limb muscle are preceded by a fall in the rate of RNA synthesis in muscle tissue

The diffusability and heat-labile nature of these factors suggest that they may be peptides. Loewenstein has found that the junctional membranes formed between cells are permeable to molecules of a molecular weight of over 10,000.[26] Thus macromolecules could be exchanged between adjacent cells and information about each other communicated. Tumor cells do not exhibit such permeability and the lack of communication with neighboring cells could account for their unregulated proliferation and dedifferentiated nature. In addition, they frequently do not possess the electrical coupling found between normal cells.

The ability to regenerate limbs after their amputation is found in many but not all anurans (tailless amphibians such as toads and frogs). A strong correlation exists across many amphibian species between the regenerative capacity and the amount of axoplasm available at the cut surface (a function of the number and diameter of nerves present), which suggests the paramount importance of neural factors in such regeneration.[7] Sensory organs are also dependent on their nerve connections: section of the afferent nerve fibers from the taste buds of the tongue causes a rapid loss of their structure. As the sensory nerve regenerates, the taste bud morphology is restored.

Just as innervated cells may be influenced by their nerve supply, so neurons are frequently affected by postsynaptic events. Thus the diameter of the axons of motor neurons may increase following overload of innervated muscles. Loss of neuromuscular contact by nerve section has been shown to lead to a retraction of the dendrites of motor neurons of adult rats. Regeneration of the distal nerve segment results in a restoration of the neuromuscular junction and this is followed by a reexpansion of the dendritic tree. In such experiments it is difficult to distinguish possible trophic influences of peripheral tissue from functional changes resulting from altered neuronal activity. However, using a mouse cell culture system, it has recently been reported that the choline acetyltransferase activity of mouse spinal cord neurons is increased more than tenfold when neuromuscular junctions are formed with simultaneously incubated muscle cells.[27] Thus muscle apparently has a marked and highly specific trophic effect on the cholinergic neurons that innervate it. Information, probably of a chemical nature, may travel up the axon in a retrograde direction (p. 109). The chromatolytic response of the nerve cell body to axonal injury (p. 62) indicates the existence of such a mechanism, and also that the perikaryon is rapidly informed of peripheral events.

There has been no adequate direct biochemical demonstration of the passage of neurotrophic substances from neurons to the innervated tissue. Korr and co-workers showed that following the injection of [^{14}C]amino acids into the hypoglossal nucleus of the rabbit, radioactivity traveled down the nerve and appeared in the muscles of the tongue.[28] More recently, several workers have demonstrated the transfer of radioactive proteins (synthesized from amino acids in the retina) from the optic nerve to the optic tectum and in one case to the striate cortex. The problem with all of these experiments is that the radioactive proteins may be degraded in the nerve terminals to their constituent amino acids, which may then pass into the postsynaptic neuron and be reincorporated into proteins (see p. 108).

C. EFFECTS BETWEEN NEURONS AND CELLS THAT THEY DO NOT INNERVATE

Nerve cells may affect and be responsive to cells that are not innervated. Such cells may be directly in contact with neurons (e.g., glia) or may be at a distance from nerve cells, mutual influences being mediated via the vascular system.

i) Neuronal-Glial Interaction

There is a very intimate relationship between neurons and glial cells in the central nervous system. Nerve cells are in direct contact with other nerve cells only at synapses; the rest of the neuron is surrounded by glial cells. Malfunctions of glial cell metabolism can rapidly lead to failure of effective neuronal transmission. This is apparent in a variety of human genetic demyelinating diseases in which a key enzyme of myelin metabolism is missing or present in insufficient amounts. Glial cells in turn are responsive to neuronal damage and may proliferate in response to cerebral injury. As discussed above, the denervation of the developing avian optic tectum prevents its normal myelination. Damaged nerve cells may be selectively phagocytosed by microglia. Diseases involving axonal destruction (e.g., amyotrophic lateral sclerosis) frequently lead to a secondary degeneration of the myelin sheath (Wallerian degeneration).

The concept of a neuronal-glial unit in which the metabolism of these cells is closely linked has frequently been suggested. In support of this, Hydén has demonstrated reciprocal relationships in the neuronal and glial content of certain chemicals.[29] Stimulation of the vestibular nuclei (by rotation of the animal) increases the content of RNA and the activity of certain respiratory enzymes (cytochrome oxidase and succinic dehydrogenase) in the large Dieter's nerve cells, while their concentrations were diminished in the surrounding oligodendroglia. Hydén suggested that large molecules are exchanged between cells and that, since glial cells entirely surround neurons, they are able to regulate the supply of energy to the neuron, perhaps by alterations in their own metabolic rate.

Glial cell metabolism may also be influenced by neuronal activity. Recently, Perkins has demonstrated that treatment of astrocytoma cells grown in culture with low concentrations of norepinephrine or dopamine causes a large increase in their cyclic AMP content.[30] Elevated cyclic AMP concentrations have frequently been associated with genetic depression of tissues by hormones (p. 171). Thus glial cell metabolism may be regulated by the amount of free neurotransmitter liberated by nearby neurons through variations of the intracellular content of cyclic AMP. In this way the electrical activity in the neuron could be paralleled by changes in the rate of glial cell metabolism. It is interesting that there appears to be a correlation between the amount of cyclic AMP excreted in the urine and the extent of cerebral excitation in manic depressives.

Other tissue culture studies suggest that glial cells synthesize the glial-specific S-100 protein only when they are in contact with other glial cells and not proliferating. Contact inhibition of cell division may initiate the expression of the specialized genes.

Nonelectrical interactions between neurons may also occur. Experiments with sensory nerves suggest that substances regulating growth are transported along the axon and secreted at the nerve terminals. These substances suppress sprout formation. When the nerve from a skin receptor is cut, there is degeneration of the distal segment in the innervated area of the skin. Sprouts from nerves innervating adjacent areas of skin then invade and subsequently innervate the deafferented area. The application of colchicine to the fiber results in similar sprouting of adjacent nerves.

ii) Neurosecretion[8, 9]

Nerve cells are able to influence tissues that they do not contact by means of chemicals liberated into the circulatory system. This process is known as neurosecretion. Specialized regions exist in the brain (e.g., the neurohypophysis) and in the periphery (e.g., the adrenal medulla) that are neurosecretory. The neurosecretory cell is capable of propagating action potentials, but it does not synapse on other cells. Rather, its axon terminates at blood spaces into which chemicals, especially polypeptides, are released.

The hypophysis (pituitary) consists of two adjacent parts (Figure 6.1). The posterior part (neurohypophysis) is truly neural, but the anterior part (adenohypophysis) is formed from ectodermal tissue from the roof of the mouth. Though both anterior and posterior parts secrete hormones into the circulation, there are important differences.

The neurohypophysis consists of the axonal terminals of neurons whose cell bodies lie in the hypothalamus. The peptide hormones, oxytocin and vasopressin (antidiuretic hormone), are synthesized in these cell bodies and transported down the axons to the neurohypophysis. They are released from the neurohypophysis in response to action potentials caused by stimulation in the hypothalamus.

The adenohypophysis does not contain neurons but consists largely of cells which synthesize trophic peptide hormones: growth hormone (GH), adrenocorticotrophic hormone (ACTH), thyrotropin (TSH), follicle-stimulating hormone (FSH), luteinizing hormone (LH) and prolactin. Neurons in the hypothalamus (hypophysiotropic neurons) also synthesize a series of releasing hormones (releasing factors), one for each adenohypophyseal hormone.[9] These releasing factors are secreted at the median eminence into a local hypophyseal vascular system (the portal circulation), whence they are transported to the adenohypophysis. The neurohypophyseal release factors can stimulate the release of the corresponding adenohypophyseal hormone into the general circulation. Prolactin and growth hormone are exceptions to this, being under inhibitory control; the prolactin and growth hormone release-inhibiting hormones (PRIH and GHRIH) secreted in the median eminence respectively inhibit the release of prolactin and growth hormone from the

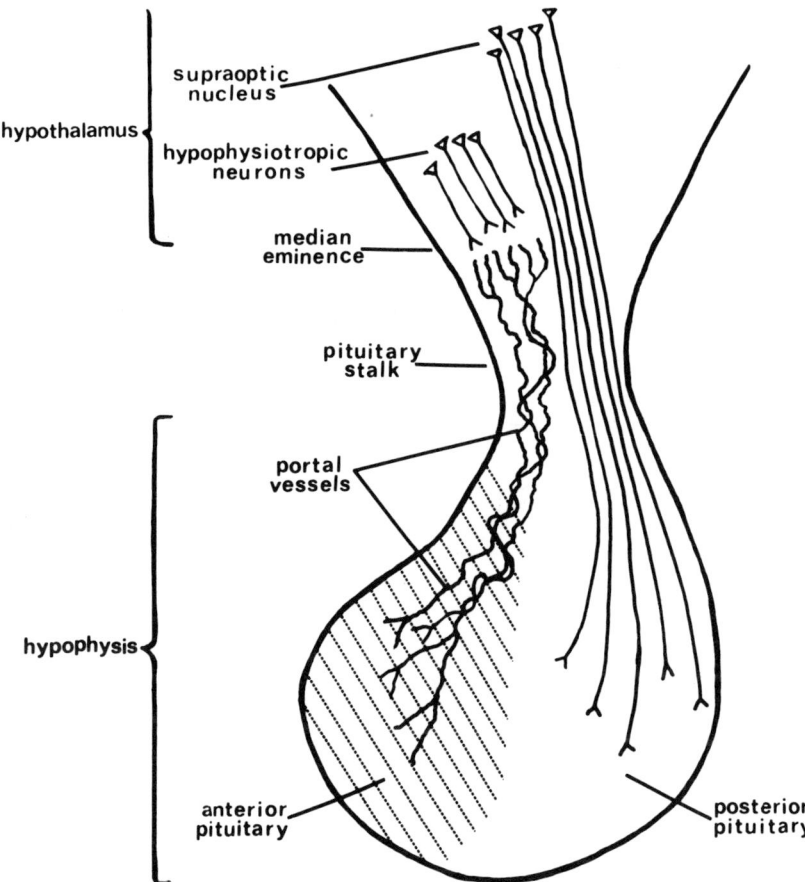

Figure 6.1 The hypothalamus-pituitary complex.

adenohypophysis. The hypophysiotropic neurons are in every way analogous to those which terminate in the neurohypophysis. They release their specific hormones in response to electrical stimulation of their cell bodies. In this way activity of neurons in the hypothalamus can regulate the activity of peripheral organs including endocrine glands (Figure 6.2).

The release of the pituitary hormones is controlled by complicated feedback mechanisms. The secretion of the neurohypophyseal releasing hormones is inhibited by the corresponding adenohypophyseal trophic hormones. This *short-loop feedback* is partly mediated by generally circulating ACTH, growth hormone, etc., but the most important control is direct

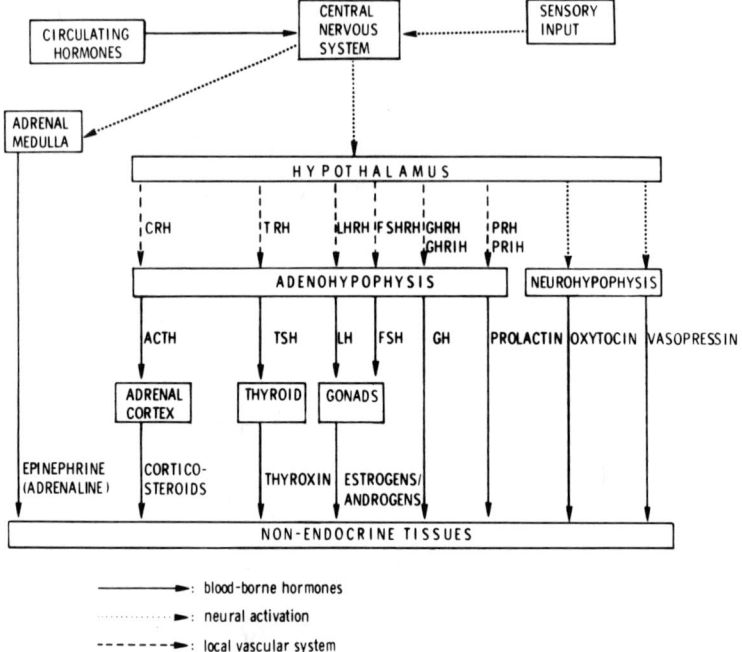

Figure 6.2 Neuroendocrine interrelationships. ACTH, adrenocorticotrophic hormone; CRH, corticotrophin releasing hormone; FSH, follicle-stimulating hormone; FSHRH, follicle-stimulating hormone releasing hormone; GH, growth hormone; GHRH, growth hormone releasing hormone; GHRIH, growth hormone release-inhibiting hormone; LH, lutenizing hormone; LHRH, lutenizing hormone releasing hormone; PRH, prolactin releasing hormone; PRIH, prolactin release-inhibiting hormone; TRH, thyrotropin releasing hormone; TSH, thyroid-stimulating hormone. FSHRH and LHRH may be chemically identical.

feedback in the local venous circulation from the adenohypophysis to the median eminence. For the pituitary hormones acting on endocrine glands, there is also a *long-loop feedback* via the peripherally produced hormones. Thus the corticosteroids released from the adrenal cortex in response to ACTH themselves inhibit the secretion not only of ACTH but also of corticotrophin releasing hormone (CRH). Similar feedback mechanisms operate for the estrogens, progesterone and thyroxin. Circulating hormones may directly control the direction and extent of brain metabolism. Steriod hormones have been shown to bind to specific hypothalamic sites and to increase the rate of synthesis of enzymes involved in the production of neurotransmitters (e.g., tryptophan hydroxylase). Gonadal steroids if implanted into precisely defined cerebral areas are able to modify the sexual behavior of an animal. Other effects of hormones on the nervous system are discussed in Chapter 9.

The way in which emotional conditions can influence endocrine states is suggested by several examples in which mental state alters pituitary function. Deprivation dwarfism, a condition associated with emotional stress in children, results in stunted growth. If such children are placed in a less stressful environment, normal growth may resume and this can be correlated with increased blood levels of growth hormone. Thus the environment can apparently significantly affect the production of growth hormone releasing hormone (GHRH). In the adult, mental stress can lead to hyperthyroidism (excess activity of the thyroid). Interestingly, this condition can be treated by thyroxin administration which inhibits the production of thyrotropin releasing hormone (TRH) by a feedback mechanism. Psychic trauma frequently causes menstrual disturbances in women, probably by changes in the levels of luteinizing hormone and follicle-stimulating hormone releasing hormones.

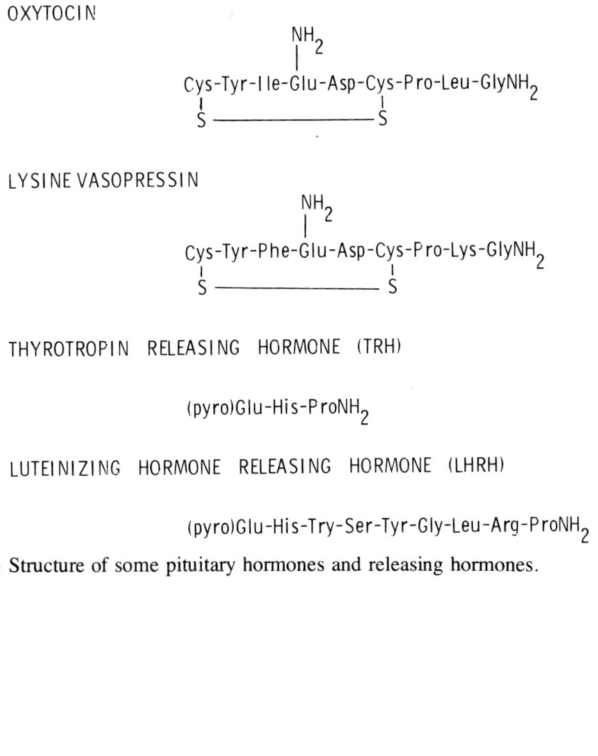

OXYTOCIN

$$\text{Cys-Tyr-Ile-Glu-Asp-Cys-Pro-Leu-GlyNH}_2$$
with NH_2 on Asp, and S—S bridge between the two Cys residues.

LYSINE VASOPRESSIN

$$\text{Cys-Tyr-Phe-Glu-Asp-Cys-Pro-Lys-GlyNH}_2$$
with NH_2 on Asp, and S—S bridge between the two Cys residues.

THYROTROPIN RELEASING HORMONE (TRH)

$$\text{(pyro)Glu-His-ProNH}_2$$

LUTEINIZING HORMONE RELEASING HORMONE (LHRH)

$$\text{(pyro)Glu-His-Try-Ser-Tyr-Gly-Leu-Arg-ProNH}_2$$

Figure 6.3 Structure of some pituitary hormones and releasing hormones.

Releasing hormones are biologically active in extremely small amounts. They are all small, heat-stable peptides containing between three and twelve amino acid residues.[9] The structures of two releasing factors are known and each begins with a cyclized glutamate residue and has a terminal proline (Figure 6.3). These peptides may be synthesized as proteins on ribosomes but there is some evidence that TRH and possibly LHRH may be synthesized like glutathione by peptide synthetases.[31]

The trophic hormones and growth hormone of the anterior pituitary are all small proteins with molecular weights ranging approximately from 4,000 to 30,000. TSH, LH and FSH are glycoproteins and each contains two distinct subunits. One of these subunits is very similar for all three hormones, though they are synthesized in separate cells. Oxytocin and vasopressin are transported in granules from the hypothalamus to the neurohypophysis tightly bound to specific proteins, the neurophysins. Neurophysin I binds oxytocin and neurophysin II binds vasopressin. The neurophysins are low molecular weight, acidic proteins whose synthesis is very tightly coupled to that of their respective hormones. It is not known whether the neurophysins are synthesized separately or whether they are synthesized together with the peptide hormones as one chain which is subsequently split, in the way that proinsulin is split to form the two polypeptide chains of insulin. Upon secretion, the neurophysins are released along with their respective hormones. Antisera to the neurophysins have proved useful in assaying the release of oxytocin and vasopressin, especially since it is very difficult to produce antisera to the hormones themselves. The releasing factors for the hormones of the anterior pituitary are transported axonally in free form, not bound to carrier proteins.

The liberation of neurohypophyseal factors is contolled by the firing rate of the appropriate neurosecretory neurons. The stimuli for the secretion of posterior pituitary hormones and releasing factors may differ. Secretion of releasing factors is effected by neural activation of critical hypothalamic neurons. Vasopressin release is also controlled by osmoreceptors within the hypothalamus. A correlation has been clearly shown between the rate of vasopressin secretion and the electrical activity of the hypothalamic neurons of the supraoptic nucleus. Norstrom and Sjostrand have shown that the transport of ^{35}S-labeled proteins from the supraoptic nucleus to the hypothalamus is increased by dehydration.[32] Neurons in this region are sensitive to the osmotic pressure of the blood.

Neurohypophyseal vasopressin appears to be heterogeneous and only a small proportion of it is rapidly releasable. There are many parallels between vasopressin and neurotransmitters with respect to synthesis, transport, storage and release. The trophic hormones of the anterior pituitary and releasing hormones have several common features:

1. They are released into the bloodstream and metabolically activate target cells.
2. The mechanism of target cell activation is binding of the hormone to the surface of the target cell.
3. Target cell activation has often been found to be preceded by an increased activity of the membrane-associated adenyl cyclase (p. 46), thus elevating the intracellular concentration of cyclic AMP.[4]
4. The increased cyclic AMP may activate the target cell by specifically enhancing aspects of its metabolism distinctive for that cell. For example, the elevation of cyclic AMP levels in certain cells within the anterior pituitary may result in an increased production of a specific trophic hormone, while elevation of the concentration of cyclic AMP in the adrenal cortex enhances corticosteroid production.

The mode of action of cyclic AMP is not fully understood, but there is much evidence that cyclic AMP plays an important protein role in protein phosphorylation.[4] Addition of phosphate to some enzymes (e.g., phosphorylase) may activate them. Phosphorylation of histones may cause them to become less basic and thus bind less firmly to DNA. By loosening the histone-DNA complex, new areas of DNA may become available for transcription. Thus cyclic AMP may act as a genetic derepressor and allow the elaboration of new messenger RNA's and thus the production of new proteins.

In contrast, the steroid hormones penetrate their target cells and bind to specific cytoplasmic receptor proteins. Cyclic AMP does not appear to play a role at this step. In the uterus, and possibly also in the brain, the steroid-receptor-protein complexes are transported to the nucleus and may then activate specific genes.

Summary

The classical concept of the nervous system was as the rapid effector arm of an organism, while the endocrine system was considered to be the long-term modulator of metabolism. In recent years it has become clear that neuronal and cellular activation have many common features and that nervous and endocrine mechanisms are essentially components of a single regulatory system. This system functions in a coordinated manner in the maintenance of homeostasis and in effecting tissue differentiation and activation.

Nerve tissue may regulate the genetic expression of many other tissues. This may occur directly by the release of substances from the synapse to innervated cells or indirectly by secretion of hormones into the bloodstream. These hormones may act upon specific target organs through the general circulation. Alternatively, neurohumors may be secreted into a local vascular system, as in the hypothalamus-pituitary, bringing about the release of the peptide hormones in the anterior pituitary.

The release of posterior pituitary hormones is controlled directly from the hypothalamus. Thus a relatively small number of fibers conduct a large amount of information directed toward the endocrine system. The release of each anterior-pituitary trophic hormone is regulated by a distinct neurohumoral releasing hormone liberated from nerve termini of the hypothalamus into the hypophyseal portal system. This portal system enables secretions from a single neuron to activate many cells in the anterior pituitary. The hormones of the anterior pituitary enter the general circulation and effect the release of peripheral hormones from the target tissues. These in turn stimulate the specific metabolism of other tissues. The hypothalamic centers which produce releasing hormones respond to the trophic hormones of the anterior pituitary and thus a chemical feedback system exists, regulating the levels of trophic hormones. It has been calculated that a thousand-fold amplification is possible between hypothalamic and pituitary hormone release and about another thousand-fold amplification occurs between pituitary trophic hormone and endocrine hormone release. Thus a small number of neurosecretory fibers may regulate a considerable proportion of total peripheral metabolism.

D. PROSTAGLANDINS[10]

Another class of hormone-like substances, the prostaglandins, is important for nervous system function. Prostaglandins were discovered by Von Euler as the factor in semen that caused smooth muscle to contract. Chemically they are a complex group of 20-carbon carboxylic acids based on cyclopentane. All native prostaglandins have a 13:14 trans double bond (Figure 6.4).

Prostaglandins are produced from arachidonic acid, following distortion or damage to cell membranes of any tissue. Thus they arise from such

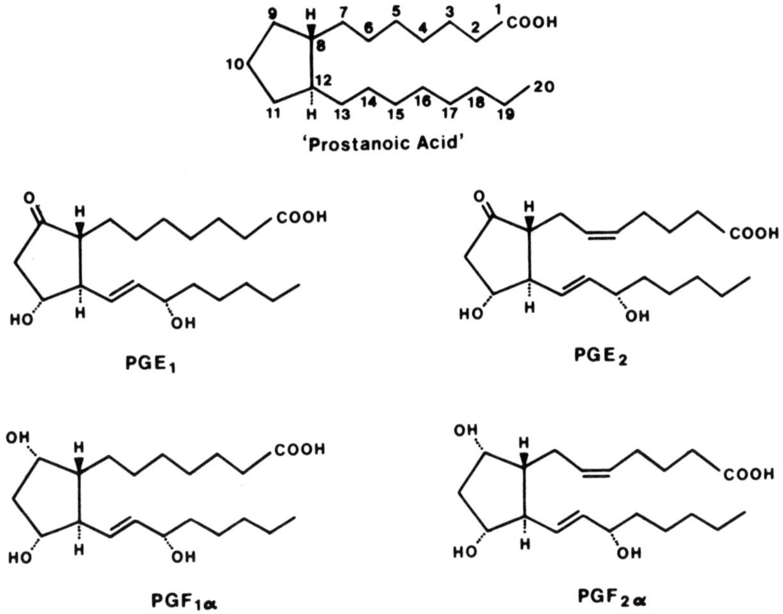

Figure 6.4 Structures of the principal prostaglandins.

treatments as nervous or hormonal stimulation, burns, scalds, wounds, osmotic shock, cold stress, inflammation, or the action of venoms, toxins, bradykinins or phospholipases. The tissue content of prostaglandins is very low, amounting to only a few times the amount released per minute in activated tissue. (Estimates of content may be erroneously high, since the act of homogenization itself initiates prostaglandin synthesis). The rate-limiting step in synthesis that is stimulated by the various treatments is unknown but may well be the release of arachidonic acid from membrane phospholipids. The synthesis and therefore the secretion of prostaglandins is severely inhibited by salicylate and acetylsalicylate (aspirin), which may account for the analgesic action of these drugs. Prostaglandins are rapidly inactivated by oxidation in tissues and in the bloodstream, one passage through the lungs being sufficient to totally inactivate normal physiological concentrations.

The bodily functions of prostaglandins include lowering of blood pressure, oxytocin-like activity and smooth muscle contractile activity, as well as roles in immunological and inflammatory responses. There also appears to be a specific activity associated with neurotransmission. Prostaglandins are synthesized postsynaptically following interaction of the neurotransmitter with the postsynaptic receptor; this is analogous to the interaction of hormones with cell-surface receptors, which also results in the secretion of prostaglandins. It is thought that prostaglandins are either released as a result of receptor binding and in turn activate adenyl cyclase, or released concomitantly with cyclase activation. In Purkinje cells, prostaglandins E_1 and E_2 (but not F_1 or F_2) block the inhibition of firing produced by norepinephrine but not cyclic AMP (p. 185). This is not a general effect on all norepinephrine receptor neurons, though it has been demonstrated in the pyramidal cells of the hippocampus. In the spinal cord, prostaglandin E_1 stimulates both the basal and presynaptically stimulated firing of motor neurons. Prostaglandins probably have both pre- and postsynaptic effects. The former most likely is by control of neurotransmitter secretion, possibly by an effect on calcium ions. Prostaglandins appear to be messengers, communicating locally between cells but not in the gross way that hormones do.

CHAPTER 6 REFERENCES

Reviews and General References

1. Gaze, R. M. *The Formation of Nerve Connections,* Academic Press, New York, 1970.
2. Jacobson, M. *Developmental Neurobiology,* Holt, Rinehart, Winston, New York, 1970.
3. Sidman, R. L. Cell-cell recognition in the developing central nervous system. In *The Neurosciences, Third Study Program* (Ed. F. O. Schmitt and F. G. Worden), M.I.T. Press, Cambridge, Mass., 1974, pp. 743 – 63.
4. Sutherland, E. W. Studies on the mechanism of hormone action. *Science* 177:401 – 08, 1972.
5. Cowan, W. M. Studies on the development of the avian visual system. In *Cellular Aspects of Neural Growth and Differentiation* (Ed. D. C. Pease), University of California, Los Angeles, 1971, pp. 177– 222.
6. Bondy, S. C., and Margolis, F. L. Sensory deprivation and brain development. The avian visual system as a model. In Brain and Behaviour Research, Monograph Series Vol. 4 (Ed. J. Bureš, E. R. John, P. G. Kostjuk, and L. Pickenhain), Gustav Fischer Verlag, Jena, 1971.
7. Guth, L. Trophic effects of vertebrate neurons. *Neurosci. Res. Prog. Bull.* 7:1 – 73, 1969.
8. Ganong, W. F. Brain mechanisms regulating the secretion of the pituitary gland. In *The Neurosciences, Third Study Program* (Ed. F. O. Schimitt and F. G. Worden), M.I.T. Press, Cambridge, Mass., 1974, pp. 549 – 63.
9. Schally, A. V., Arimura, A., and Kastin, A. J. Hypothalamic Regulatory Hormones. *Science* 179:341 – 50, 1973.
10. Kahn, R. H., and Lands, W. E. M. *Prostaglandins and cyclic AMP,* Academic Press, New York, 1973.

Literature Cited

11. Sperry, R. W. Effect of 180° rotation of the retinal field on visuomotor coordination. *J. Exp. Zool.* 92:263–79, 1943.
12. Jacobson, M., and Baker, R. E. Development of neuronal connections with skin grafts in frogs: behavioural and electrophysiological studies. *J. Comp. Neurol.* 137:121–42, 1969.
13. Barbera, A. J., Marchase, R. B., and Roth, S. Adhesive recognition and retinotectal specificity. *Proc. Nat. Acad. Sci. U.S.A.* 70:2482–86, 1973.
14. Fayet, G., and Lissitzky, S. Cyclic 3′,5′-adenosine monophosphate-mediated follicular reorganization of isolated thyroid cells in culture. *FEBS Letters* 11:185–88, 1970.
15. Fifková, E. Changes in the visual cortex of rats after unilateral deprivation. *Nature* 220:379–80, 1968.
16. Freeman, R. D., Mitchell, D. E., and Millodot, M. A neural effect of partial visual deprivation in humans. *Science* 175:1384–86, 1972.
17. Hubel, D. H., Wiesel, T. N. Receptive fields and functional architecture of monkey striate cortex. *J. Physiol.* 195:215–43, 1968.
18. Cleland, B. G., Dubin, M. W., and Levick, W. R. Simultaneous recording of input and output of lateral geniculate neurones. *Nature, New Biol.* 231:191–92, 1971.
19. Blakemore, C., and Mitchell, D. E. Environmental modification of the visual cortex and the neural basis of learning and memory. *Nature* 241:467–68, 1973.
20. Changeux, J. P., Kasai, M., and Lee, C. Y. Use of a snake venom toxin to characterize the cholinergic receptor protein. *Proc. Nat. Acad. Sci. U.S.A.* 67:1241–47, 1970.
21. Albuquerque, E. X., Warnick, J. E., Tasse, J. R., and Sansone, F. M. Effects of vinblastine and colchicine on neural regulation of the fast and slow skeletal muscles of the rat. *Exp. Neurol.* 37:607–34, 1972.
22. Mommaerts, W. F. H. M., Buller, A. J., and Seraydarian, K. The modification of some biochemical properties of muscle by cross-innervation. *Proc. Nat. Acad. Sci. U.S.A.* 64:128–33, 1969.
23. McComas, A. J., Sica, R. E. P., and Currie, S. Muscular dystrophy: evidence for a neural factor. *Nature* 226:1263–64, 1970.
24. Hironaka, T., and Miyata, Y. Muscle transplantation in the aetiological elucidation of murine muscular dystrophy. *Nature, New. Biol.* 244:221–23, 1973.
25. Lentz, T. L. Nerve trophic function: *in vitro* assay of effects of nerve tissue on muscle cholinesterase activity. *Science* 171:187–89, 1971.
26. Loewenstein, W. R. Membrane junctions in growth and differentiation. *Fed. Proc.* 32:60–64, 1973.
27. Giller, E. L., Schreier, B. K., Shainberg, A., Fisk, H. R., and Nelson, P. G. Choline acetyl transferase activity is increased in combined cultures of spinal cord and muscle cells from mice. *Science* 182:588–89, 1973.
28. Korr, I. M., Wilkinson, P. N., and Chornock, F. W. Axonal delivery of neuroplasmic components to muscle cells. *Science* 155:342–45, 1967.
29. Hydén, H. Dynamic aspects on the neuron-glia relationship — a study with microchemical methods. In *The Neuron*, Elsevier Press, Amsterdam, 1967, pp. 179–219.
30. Clark, R. B., and Perkins, J. P. Regulation of adenosine 3′5′-cyclic monophosphate concentration in cultured human astrocytoma cells by catecholamines and histamine. *Proc. Nat. Acad. Sci. U.S.A.* 68:2757–60, 1971.
31. Reichlin, S., and Mitnick, M. Biosynthesis of hypothalamic hypophysiotropic factors.

In *Frontiers in Neuroendocrinology, 1973*. (Ed. W. F. Ganong and L. Martini), Oxford University Press, London, 1973, pp. 61–88.
32. Nörstrom, A., and Sjöstrand, J. Effect of salt-loading, thirst and water-loading on transport and turnover of neurohypophyseal proteins of the rat. *J. Endocrinol.* 52:87 – 105, 1972.

VII. The Biochemistry of Neural Stimulation

Before one can approach the complex problem of the biochemistry of behavior, some of the biochemical effects of nervous stimulation should be understood. This may permit the distinction between chemical events associated with neural transmission per se, and those that may be more specifically associated with the *information* conveyed. There are probably subtle chemical changes associated with conduction which underly the eventual storage of the information. This chapter is concerned with the effect on neural tissue of either direct or indirect electrical stimulation.

A. ELECTRICAL STIMULATION OF NERVOUS TISSUE

i) Energy Metabolites and Convulsions

From what is known about the mechanism of neuronal conduction, impulse transmission can be expected to be associated with a neuronal loss of K^+ and a gain of Na^+. ATP will then be used by the ion pumps in order to restore the ion concentrations, and this will in turn increase the respiratory rate to produce more ATP (see Figure 2.2). These processes occur both in isolated nerves and in preparations of brain tissue that are stimulated.

McIlwain has studied these phenomena in thin slices of brain tissue which when incubated under appropriate conditions display a metabolism similar to that observed *in vivo*[1,2]. He has examined the effect of electrical stimulation on the ion content, and the use of substrates by the slices. Such stimulation produces electrical responses (including action potentials under appropriate conditions) and a concomitant loss of K^+ and an uptake of Na^+ into the slices. After the cessation of stimulation, normal ionic gradients are rapidly reestablished in the presence of adequate supplies of glucose and oxygen. Electrical stimulation of brain slices may also result in lactate production from glucose (anaerobic glycolysis). In the living animal, convulsions or hyperactivity also increase brain lactate, but the increased systemic production of lactate by muscles complicates the interpretation of such data. The major drawback of the use of slices is the lack of blood supply, so that the nutrient supply to and waste-product elimination from the slice can only take place by diffusion from the incubation medium. Slices also have the following disadvantages: (1) they gain water and swell during incubation; (2) when they are incubated in media containing physiological extracellular K^+ concentrations, the concentration of K^+ in the slices is never as high as that in the native tissue; (3) in order to maintain adequate oxygenation of the interior of the slice, incubation must be carried out with a high and somewhat toxic oxygen concentration.

Electroconvulsive shock treatment (ECS) is carried out by applying an electrical current to the brain through suitable electrodes. This provokes an electrical discharge known as a brain seizure, which is the result of large numbers of neurons throughout the brain firing repeatedly, and to some extent synchronously. During the seizure the overall firing rate of cerebral neurons is much greater than in the normal state. If the brain seizure is severe enough, it will result in bodily convulsions in which repeated, and often violent, muscular activity occurs. The convulsions may often restrict respiration and/or blood flow to the brain. This causes the brain to become anoxic and its ATP is depleted. Calculations have shown that anoxia is not the only reason for the depression of ATP levels and the brain seizure itself provokes a vastly increased demand for energy (four-fold by one estimate).[6] This increase presumably reflects the increased neural activity during the seizure. Its magnitude indicates the high energy requirement of neuronal conduction. In agreement with this it has been shown that there is depression of ATP following brain seizures that do not result in behavioral convulsions (subconvulsive electroshock).[7] The CO_2 and lactate produced by electrical activity within the brain cause vasodilation. These chemicals then operate a feedback mechanism (autoregulation) which alters the rate of nutrient supply in response to local changes of metabolic activity in specific brain areas.

It is not clear whether electroconvulsive shock is an appropriate model for the study of electrical stimulation. However, most of the data collected with ECS agree very well with that obtained using slices or chopped tissue. The changes of energy metabolites discussed above may merely reflect the increased metabolic demand resulting from increased neural activity, and it is not known whether these changes themselves are capable of producing the more permanent effects that underlie adaptation.

The nature of the chemical trigger for convulsions has attracted the attention of many investigators.[8-10]. Often there is a decrease in the concentration of brain ATP immediately preceding the convulsions, and for many years it was thought that the decrease in ATP or in other high-energy metabolites might trigger the convulsions. However, seizures are observed with some convulsants (Metrazol and methionine sulfoximine) without a prior fall in ATP and, conversely, falls in ATP are observed (e.g., with electroshock and secobarbitone anesthesia) that do not lead to convulsions.[11] Another trigger that has been considered is ammonia. Increases in cerebral ammonia content are associated with hypoxia, ischemia and convulsions; the ammonia presumably derives from the catabolism of purines and possibly amino acids. Also, high doses of ammonium salts are convulsive. Yet, the correlation between ammonia levels and the convulsive state is poor,[9] in particular since the minimum convulsant dose of ammonium salts causes a sixty-fold increase in brain ammonia, very much higher than observed with other convulsants.

Current ideas favor the activity of γ-aminobutyric acid (GABA) as a physiological anticonvulsant. GABA not only is an inhibitory neurotransmitter of considerable importance in the brain, but also has anti-excitatory effects on neurons (pp. 76, 143). In this respect it is opposed by glutamate as well as by aspartate and possibly acetylcholine. There is an excellent correlation between the susceptibility to convulsions and the brain concentration of GABA, or, perhaps better, the ratio of GABA to glutamate.[10] Low GABA is associated with a high susceptibility, and vice versa. Injections of GABA, either systemic or intracranial, have proved remarkably effective in preventing the convulsive action of a number of agents, including freeze-lesions, glutamate, pentylenetetrazole, aluminum oxide and high-pressure oxygen.[10] As a result, it has been speculated that elevation of

GABA may be the physiological mechanism for the termination of convulsions.

Inhibition of the formation of GABA may produce a convulsive state. Pyridoxal phosphate is an essential cofactor for glutamic acid decarboxylase (GAD), the enzyme used to synthesize GABA. Thus in vitamin B_6 deficiency the brain concentrations of pyridoxal phosphate and GABA are depressed, which may be the reason for the seizure-prone state. In agreement with this, derivatives of pyridoxal phosphate that inhibit GAD are convulsants *in vivo*.[10] Conversely, elevations of GABA inhibit convulsions. Compounds such as amino-oxyacetic acid that inhibit GABA-transaminase, the enzyme that destroys GABA, have some anti-convulsant effects.

While the evidence for the anticonvulsant activity of GABA and its possible physiological role is good, the commonly used anticonvulsants do not affect GABA. The barbiturates, such as phenobarbital, interfere with conduction. Probably the anticonvulsant drug diphenylhydantoin (Dilantin) acts similarly. The effect of carbonic anhydrase inhibitors is most likely concerned with reducing extracellular K^+, thus preventing any trend to depolarization.

Increases in cyclic AMP are also associated with convulsions, and though this may be a secondary effect (see p. 185) administration of cyclic AMP and its derivatives may cause convulsions. It has therefore been suggested that elevated cyclic AMP might be the convulsive trigger.[12]

ii) Neurotransmitter Substances

Electrical stimulation that results in synaptic transmission will deplete the presynaptic store of neurotransmitter. The synthesis of neurotransmitters is under feedback control, so that any loss of neurotransmitter is rapidly replaced by new synthesis. This feedback control is normally mediated by end-product inhibition of one of the synthetic enzymes. For example, tyrosine hydroxylase is inhibited by norephinephrine.

Measurable depletion of neurotransmitters by repeated stimulation has been difficult to demonstrate (p. 117). It may be that the total presynaptic store of neurotranmitters is not available for immediate release. Those stores (vesicular or otherwise) that are particularly close to the presynaptic membrane may be in an activated state ready to be released. These activated stores may then become depleted without detectable depletion in the total stores. This kind of mechanism would explain the data obtained on the specific radioactivity of released neurotransmitters (p. 118). It would also provide a mechanism for synaptic habituation, in which repeated stimulation of a synapse reduces the effectiveness of the stimulation (as measured by the magnitude of the postsynaptic potential). Depletion of releasable transmitter stores may result in the release of decreased amounts of neurotransmitter. Such an effect would readily be reversed as more neurotransmitter was synthesized or more stable stores were mobilized.

Longer-term effects on neurotransmitter synthesis may be mediated by enzyme induction and repression.[13,14]. The drug reserpine interferes with the storage of catecholamines and results in their depletion. Reserpine induces an increase in the rate of catecholamine synthesis from tyrosine, and also in the activity of the enzyme tyrosine hydroxylase (TH) in the adrenals, sympathetic ganglia and brain stem. Cycloheximide and actinomycin D prevent the reserpine-induced increase of TH in the superior cervical ganglion. It is therefore likely that these long-term changes involve the synthesis of new enzyme (enzyme induction), especially since reserpine treatment increases the incorporation of amino acids into protein in the adrenals, liver and superior cervical ganglion.[13]

$$\text{tyrosine} \xrightarrow{\text{TH}} \text{DOPA} \xrightarrow{\text{DOPA-dC}} \text{dopamine} \xrightarrow{\text{DBH}} \text{norepinephrine}$$

L-DOPA, the product of tyrosine hydroxylase, blocks the effect of reserpine on the adrenals. Thus the enzyme induction could be due to the release of a feedback control caused by the low levels of catecholamines. In accordance with this, 6-hydroxydopamine, which destroys sympathetic terminals, also induces tyrosine hydroxylase. Moreover, L-DOPA alone decreases the activity of TH, yet this effect does not occur in the presence of inhibitors of the decarboxylase that converts L-DOPA to dopamine. Inhibitors of dopamine-β-hydoxylase do not prevent the L-DOPA effect and themselves depress TH. This might implicate dopamine as the active repressor of TH. However, phenoxybenzamine, which is a postganglionic blocker, also induces TH. A common effect of reserpine, 6-hydroxydopamine and phenoxybenzamine is the impairment of postganglionic sympathetic neurotransmission. Because of the feedback systems operating in the sympathetic nervous system, this will increase preganglionic activity (cholinergic). Thus the increase in TH activity may, in part, be secondary to the increased preganglionic neural input. That this is the case is also suggested by the observation that the effect of reserpine on TH activity in the adrenals and superior cervical ganglion is prevented by cutting the preganglionic nerve or by ganglionic (cholinergic) blocking agents. Furthermore, in the adrenals, acetylcholine, in the presence of eserine (a cholinesterase inhibitor), stimulates TH. Thus cholinergic reception may be the transynaptic effector.[13,14]

Dopamine-β-hydroxylase (DBH), another enzyme used in catecholamine synthesis, undergoes some changes similar to TH. Reserpine increases the activity of DBH in the adrenals and sympathetic ganglia but not in the brain. Decentralization of the adrenals or sympathetic ganglia prevents the reserpine-induced increase of DBH, as does cycloheximide. In the adrenals, reserpine increases the incorporation of amino acids into DBH molecules separated by immunoabsorption. Using the superior cervical ganglion isolated in organ culture, high levels of K^+ are sufficient to stimulate DBH activity. The total aromatic amino acid decarboxylase activity is unaffected by reserpine, but the activity of specific dopamine decarboxylase (p. 132) has not yet been studied.

Increased sympathetic activity thus results in increased catecholamine synthesis. This probably occurs at first by the removal of the end-product inhibition of tyrosine hydroxylase by catecholamines. However, long-term changes apparently involve the induction of new molecules of tyrosine hydroxylase and dopamine-β-hydroxylase. What is the mechanism of this effect? Thoenen and his co-workers, who performed all the above-mentioned work, have also shown that the increases of TH induced by reserpine in heart and sciatic nerve occur with delays that suggest the supply of the new enzymes from the nerve cell body by axoplasmic transport.[13] However, the amount of enzyme in the axons is insufficient to account for the observed increase at the terminals. Further, cycloheximide prevents the appearance of new enzymes at the terminals even when administered *after* the increase of enzyme activity in the cell bodies. Since cycloheximide has not been observed to interfere with axoplasmic flow, Thoenen concludes that the major part (85 percent) of the change at the terminals is due to local synthesis of new enzyme. To account for the delay in reserpine-induced increase of TH, they postulate that some factor arrives by axoplasmic flow to initiate the process. It is difficult to reconcile this conclusion with the rather limited protein synthetic capacity of the nerve terminal (p. 148).

The ganglia of the sympathetic nervous system seem likely to find extensive use as models for the study of the effects of neural activity on the metabolism of neurotransmitters and other compounds. The synthesis of the preganglionic transmitter acetylcholine is also increased when the superior cervical ganglion is stimulated by reserpine. As in the case of the postganglionic neurotransmitter, induction of the synthetic enzyme (choline acetylase) is responsible for this increase.[15] The mechanism of these inductions may involve cyclic AMP, since the cyclic nucleotide induces tyrosine hydroxylase in the adrenal medulla and superior cervical ganglion.[14]

iii) RNA

The idea that RNA might be involved in neural stimulation was suggested by Hydén in the 1940's. He demonstrated that mild stimulation by exercise resulted in increases in the RNA content of spinal ganglion neurons, but prolonged stimulation by exercising to exhaustion resulted in a decreased RNA content.[16] Similar effects were observed with direct electrical stimulation. From these experiments arose the concept that mild stimulation of nerves increases their RNA content, whereas strong or prolonged stimulation decreases it. Hydén suggested that electrical activity in the neurons in some way consumes RNA, and that this RNA can be replaced rapidly by transfer of RNA or RNA precursors to the neurons from the surrounding glia. Thus a temporary increase in neuronal RNA may be observed. However, if the stimulation were excessive, both the neuronal and glial stores of RNA would become depleted and the neuronal RNA content would fall. Working independently, Pevzner has been able to verify the predicted changes in neuronal and glial RNA in a number of different systems.[17] These results, however, were all obtained using cytospectrophotometric assays, in which the RNA content of the cells on microscope slides was estimated by ultraviolet absorption using a microscope. Unfortunately, there are many technical problems with such assays and their validity is not universally accepted, so that confirmation of these results using other analytical methods is highly desirable.

Geiger found that mild stimulation of the brain via the brachial plexus (20 cycles per second for 20 seconds) resulted in an 8 percent decrease in the nucleic-acid nitrogen content of cerebral cortex.[18] Electroconvulsive shock (ECS) has also been shown to decrease brain RNA content. More recent attempts to show a change in brain RNA content following ECS have been unsuccessful, or have found only small changes in the nuclear fraction.[19] Since nuclear RNA turns over very rapidly (p. 58), this decrease may be related to the depression of ATP levels caused by the ECS, which would limit RNA synthesis from nucleoside triphosphates without affecting their rates of degradation. ECS does severely depress the incorporation of radioactive uridine into RNA, but it is unclear whether this may be taken as a measure of RNA synthesis.[19] Though electrical stimulation of cortical slices also depresses uridine incorporation into RNA,[20] this may again be related to the depressed ATP levels caused by the stimulation.

Several workers have shown that stimulation of single cells may increase the incorporation of [^{3}H]uridine into RNA. Stimulation of the isolated abdominal ganglion of *Aplysia* resulted in such an increase in the large, R2 cells.[21] Not only was this increase proportional to the number of stimuli, but the stimuli needed to be presynaptic. Antidromic stimulation did not produce the biochemical response, which may therefore have been initiated by neurotransmitter reception rather than depolarization of the cell.[22] Stimulation of the ganglion did not change the incorporation of [^{3}H]uridine into the immediate nucleotide precursors (UMP, UDP and UTP), so that the effect was considered to indicate a real change in the synthesis of RNA.[23] However, Wilson and Berry subsequently reported that the effect was only observed when the uridine concentration in the incubation medium was high, and that with low concentrations no increase of radioactive RNA was observed.[24] They concluded that the effect may have been due to some undefined effect on nucleotide metabolism, but the effects of uridine on the system are currently in dispute.[25]

Stimulation also resulted in an increase of the incorporation of radioactive uridine into RNA of the superior cervical ganglion.[26] This increase was evoked by electrical stimulation or by administration of the preganglionic neurotransmitter acetylcholine, but not in the presence of cholinergic blocking agents or by antidromic stimulation. The concentration of uridine used in the medium was not reported. An increase of RNA synthesis following stimulation would, however, agree well with the reported increase in RNA content of the ganglion following reserpine treatment of the intact animal.[27]

Stimulation of the hippocampus either electrically or with K$^+$ has been reported to increase its RNA content. This effect may be related to the reported effects of behavioral treatments on brain RNA metabolism (see p. 207).

iv) Protein

The biosynthesis of protein has not proved as responsive to stimulation as that of RNA. Electrical stimulation of cortical slices decreased the incorporation of amino acids into protein, though it stimulated their uptake into the tissue.[28] Similarly, in a number of studies ECS inhibited amino acid incorporation and decreased the polyribosome content of brain.[19] All of these phenomena may well have been secondary to the depression of ATP or to the disturbance of cation balance. Electrical stimulation of isolated nerves has not generally resulted in increased amino acid incorporation. Stimulation of the R2 neuron of *Aplysia* under conditions that increased the uridine incorporation into RNA was without effect on the incorporation of amino acids into protein.[24] Similarly, in a study of the stimulation of dorsal roots of spinal cord *in vitro* no effect on amino acid incorporation was found.[29] Stimulation of the superior cervical ganglion *in vitro* initially increased [U-^{14}C] valine incorporation into protein but shortly afterwards decreased it.[30] In contrast, work with the isolated squid giant axon showed an increased amino acid uptake into protein with electrical stimulation.[31] However, most of the protein synthesis in this system occurs in the glial sheath and there may be transport of this material into the axoplasm. In fact, transport of intact proteins into the axon was increased by electrical stimulation.[32] Nevertheless, in the sympathetic nervous system *in vivo*, increases of protein synthesis and of specific enzymes have been observed in response to stimulation (p. 182).

Modifications of proteins subsequent to neural activity have also been reported. Prolonged stimulation (twenty minutes) of the brain via the sciatic nerve caused spectrophotometric changes in proteins of brain homogenates. These may have corresponded to an increase in sulfhydryl groups and conformational changes involving ionizable groups.[33] Recently, it was reported that ECS decreased the ability of synaptosomal plasma membranes to be phosphorylated *in vitro*.[34] This may reflect changes in the conformation of membrane constituents.

v) Cyclic Nucleotides

There has been considerable interest lately in the relationship between neurotransmission and cyclic nucleotides. Electrical stimulation of cortical slices has long been known to elevate their cyclic AMP content.[35] Electroconvulsive shock also elevates brain cyclic AMP concentrations. After decapitation, the brain cyclic AMP concentation rises rapidly while the ATP concentration falls. Adenosine in very low concentrations (10 μM) elevates the concentration of cyclic AMP in cerebral cortex slices by up to thirty-fold. Thus the rise in cyclic AMP that follows ECS or death may be mediated by a small amount of free adenosine liberated from the phosphorylated adenine nucleotides during the anoxia.[36] Curiously, the stimulation of adenyl cyclase by electrical stimulation or adenosine is blocked by theophylline.[35] Theophylline is ordinarily regarded as an inhibitor of the phosphodiesterase and would be expected to potentiate cyclic AMP increases, which it does in the case of the stimulation by the neurotransmitters (see below).

Local electrical stimulation in the brain elevates cyclic AMP, and local application of cyclic AMP alters the firing rate of some cells. Bloom and his co-workers have studied these phenomena extensively in cerebellar Purkinje cells.[37] These cells receive an inhibitory input from the locus coeruleus, in which norepinephrine is thought to be the neurotransmitter. Stimulation of the locus coeruleus hyperpolarizes Purkinje cells in a characteristic way and decreases their spontaneous firing rate. These effects may be mimicked precisely by the application of norepinephrine or cyclic AMP to the surface of Purkinje cells. Since norepinephrine will elevate the concentration of cyclic AMP in cerebellar slices, it is suggested that the electrical consequences of synaptic input to Purkinje cells may be mediated by intracellular cyclic AMP. In this way cyclic AMP would be performing its function as an intracellular second messenger (p. 171).

There are other indications of the important role of cyclic AMP in the nervous system. The concentration of adenyl cyclase is the highest in the brain of any mammalian tissue examined. It is membrane-bound and largely in the synaptosomal fraction. Cyclic AMP phosphodiesterase is also exceptionally concentrated in brain, and again partially concentrated in the synaptosomal fraction. Histochemical studies have indicated that it is concentrated in the postsynaptic region, very closely associated with the postsynaptic thickening at most cerebellar synapses. Preparations of brain adenyl cyclase are stimulated *in vitro* by norepinephrine and dopamine. Norepinephrine-stimulated adenyl cyclase activity has been found in cultured glial tumor cells as well as in neuroblastoma cells (p. 114). Thus if the extrapolation of the results derived from tumor studies to the intact brain is valid, catecholamine-sensitive cyclases may be present both in glia and in neurons.

There is also evidence for the involvement of cyclic AMP in synaptic transmission in the peripheral nervous system. Greengard and his co-workers have shown that preganglionic stimulation of the superior cervical ganglion elevates its cyclic AMP content.[38] This effect may be mimicked by dopamine, which also produces the characteristic hyperpolarizing response seen on preganglionic stimulation. The effect of dopamine on cyclic AMP concentration and on the membrane potential is prevented by α-adrenergic blocking agents. Phosphodiesterase inhibitors such as theophylline tend to increase intracellular levels of cyclic AMP and to potentiate the effects of dopamine. Further, cyclic AMP applied to the ganglion produces the same characteristic membrane potential changes. These results were interpreted to indicate that a dopaminergic interneuron has an inhibitory input to the postganglionic nerve, and that the slow IPSP caused by dopamine reception is mediated by a postsynaptic increase in the cyclic AMP within the nerve.[38]

Somewhat similar results have been obtained in the abdominal ganglion of *Aplysia*. Preganglionic electrical stimulation of the ganglion elevated the cyclic AMP content of the ganglion (measured radioactively).[39] This increase was blocked by concentrations of Mg^{2+} that inhibit the release of neurotransmitters, and was not observed when the ganglion was stimulated by glutamate (which would not involve synaptic activity). Cyclic AMP elevations were also produced by the direct application to the ganglion of serotonin and dopamine, but not by carbachol (an acetylcholine analogue), glutamate, norepinephrine or histamine.[39] The effects of dopamine and serotonin were not blocked by high concentrations of Mg^{2+}. The deduction, then, is that it is the reception of the neurotransmitter that results in the elevation of cyclic AMP.

There is thus evidence that the reception by postsynaptic cells of catecholamine and indoleamine neurotransmitters may elevate cyclic AMP concentrations in those cells, and that this elevation of cyclic AMP may be responsible for postsynaptic potential changes in the cells. Similarly, there is evidence that reception of acetylcholine at certain muscarinic receptors, in brain, heart, intestinal smooth muscle, and the superior cervical ganglion, is associated with an elevation of cyclic GMP.[40] In contrast to cyclic AMP, cyclic GMP depolarizes nerve cells and is generally excitatory. The effect of these cyclic nucleotides may not be limited to electrical potential changes but more sophisticated or more permanent chemical changes may also occur.

The mechanism of the cyclic AMP effects on the polarization of the membrane may be related to activation of protein kinases and consequent increased phosphorylation of proteins. Synaptosomal plasma membranes contain several phosphorylated proteins[41] and the phosphorylation state of these proteins is influenced by ECS[34] or behavioral treatments (p. 216). Phosphorylation of a protein is very likely to change its conformation and, if the protein is part of the membrane structure, changes in the ion permeability might result. Following ECS, an increased permeability to K^+ occurs, together with a change in the phosphorylation of synaptosomal membrane proteins.[42] In the toad bladder it has been shown that the reception of vasopressin results in a stimulation of adenyl cyclase and a reduction in the phosphate content of the only membrane protein that is phosphorylated. This change is apparently due to the activation by cyclic AMP of a specific phosphoprotein phosphatase. The change in protein phosphorylation is correlated with an increased Na^+ permeability. One might speculate on an analogous molecular basis for the postsynaptic changes in brain.

The effect of prostaglandins on these processes is of considerable interest. Bloom has shown that prostaglandins E_1 and E_2 (but not $E_{1\alpha}$, $E_{2\alpha}$, $F_{1\alpha}$ or

$F_1\beta$) selectively block the electrical response of Purkinje cells to stimulation of the locus coeruleus or to the administration of norepinephrine.[37] However, the effect of cyclic AMP on Purkinje cells is not blocked. Similarly, prostaglandin E_1 blocks the postganglionic effects of preganglionic stimulation or of dopamine addition on the superior cervical ganglion.[38] Prostaglandins appear to be acting here essentially as hormones controlling synaptic transmission. The interesting feature is that they do not appear to act on or mimic the neurotransmitters themselves (as do many psychoactive drugs), but exert their effect by modifying the effects of neurotransmitter reception by the postsynaptic cell.

Intracellular cyclic AMP appears to be compartmented and effects of neurotransmitters on cyclic AMP may be associated with certain small metabolically responsive pools of cyclic AMP. When cerebral cortex slices are prelabeled with adenine, the addition of histamine or adenosine causes large increases in the radioactivity of cyclic AMP but no change in gross cyclic AMP concentrations. If labeled adenosine is used rather than adenine, such increases in the specific activity of cyclic AMP are not observed.[43,44] Thus, only a small pool of ATP may be involved in this response, and adenine but not adenosine has access to this pool. It is not known whether this pool has a synaptosomal location. Adenine is incorporated into nucleotides by adenine phosphoribosyltransferase, whereas adenosine is phosphorylated by the action of adenosine kinase (p. 44). Adenine phosphoribosyltransferase may thus be specifically associated with the small pools that are precursors to cyclic AMP.

Many compounds, including dopamine, norepinephrine, serotonin, histamine, and adenosine, will stimulate brain cyclic AMP levels. Since the effects of many such compounds are additive, they are probably not mediated through a common receptor. In fact, the effects of selective blocking agents indicated the existence of separate receptors for histamine, the catecholamines, serotonin and adenosine.[43] Such additivity also suggests that different pools of adenine nucleotides could be involved. It is possible that these pools correspond to neurons with different receptor specificities.

vi) Inositol Phosphatides

Electrical activity in the brain and sympathetic nervous system may result in an increase in the labeling of inositol phospholipids by radioactive phosphate. In the superior cervical ganglion, preganglionic electrical stimulation of the ganglion *in vitro* increased the phosphatidyl inositol (PI) labeling.[45] Larrabee has reported that such changes are associated with the reception of acetylcholine by postsynaptic neurons, since they are mimicked by the application of carbachol and the effect of stimulation may be blocked by atropine or tubocurarine. The increase of phospholipid labeling was probably not associated with axonal conduction, since it was not elicited by antidromic stimulation of the ganglion and was not observed in stimulated nerve trunks.[45]

Schacht and Agranoff have shown that acetylcholine increased phosphate incorporation into phosphoinositides of isolated brain synaptosomes, and that this effect was blocked by atropine.[46] There was no parallel increase of labeling of inositol phosphatides when radioactive ^{14}C precursors of the diglyceride (the fatty acid, arachidonic acid) or inositol were used. Following the addition of acetylcholine to synaptosomes, concentrations of the di- and triphosphoinositides (DPI and TPI) were slightly decreased, but this effect was not specific for acetylcholine, since it was not blocked by atropine and also occurred with addition of free choline. They suggest that the specific effect of acetylcholine is to increase the hydrolysis of phosphatidic acid (PA) to diglyceride, which is rate-limiting for PI synthesis. The released diglyceride forms a specific pool associated with the membranes. Accelerated PA synthesis from this diglyceride will result in increased labeling of PI from $[^{32}P]$phosphate, but not from labeled diglyceride or inositol. A nonspecific effect of acetylcholine is an increased degradation of TPI to DPI, and DPI to PI, by the phosphomonoesterases. The phosphodiesterases are not involved, since no increase of soluble inositol phosphates was observed.[46] The pathways involved are illustrated in Figure 7.1 (see also p.

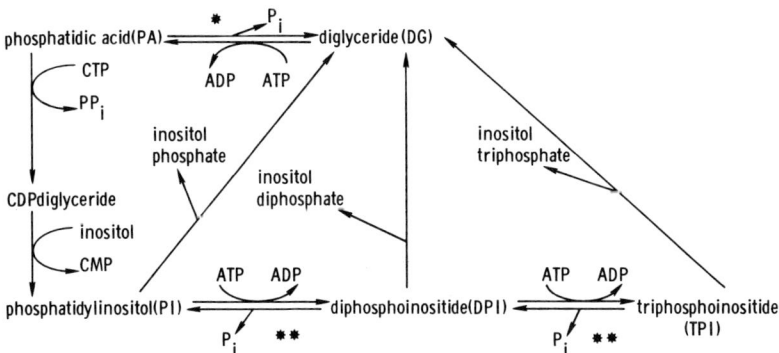

Figure 7.1 Metabolism of inositol phosphatides. *Phosphatidic acid phosphohydrolase, suggested by Schacht and Agranoff[46] to be specifically activated by acetylcholine. **Phosphomonoesterases, suggested by Schacht and Agranoff to be non-specifically activated.

84). These changes in inositol phosphatides may also be related to temporary alterations in the properties of the postsynaptic membrane.

B. SENSORY DEPRIVATION AND STIMULATION

Sensory input to the brain can be modified in a number of ways. These range from complete deafferentation of specific regions to electrical and sensory stimulation. For example, in the visual system activity in the optic nerve may be terminated by extirpation of the eye, light stimulation may be prevented by maintaining animals in total darkness, or patterned light may be removed by corneal occlusion or eyelid suture. Activity in the optic nerve may also be modified by the use of electrical stimulation, patterned images, flashing lights, etc. Non-ablative procedures have the advantage over surgical approaches in that they are less traumatic and more closely resemble normal physiological variations of nervous input to the brain. Milder procedures may also be reversible, enabling the permanence of any changes observed to be assessed. Moreover, surgical deafferentation prevents not only the transmission of electrical activity but also the migration of chemicals within nerve cells. Thus deafferented cerebral sensory areas are deprived of axonally migrating substances that may be important for their function (see Chapter 6).

i) Short-Term Studies

The long-term effects of sensory deprivation of the brain are the cumulative results of a series of chemical processes. Sensory deprivation frequently leads to metabolic disruption of specific cerebral areas. In time these changes result in major changes of chemistry and morphology. With the use of radioisotopes, rapid changes in metabolic activity that precede major changes of the concentration of chemicals can be detected.

Several studies have indicated decreased rates of protein and RNA synthesis after periods of visual deprivation. Such effects have been found in cerebral regions primarily innervated by the optic nerve, and also in indirectly innervated areas such as the cerebral hemispheres. Most retinal ganglion cells respond to changes in the intensity of illumination rather than to continuous light or darkness. Thus exposure of the eye to a flickering light is likely to maximize activity within the optic nerve. In monkeys, stimulation of the eye with a rhythmically flickering light has been reported to increase the rate of incorporation of radioactive precursors into protein in the occipital cortex, while the incorporation of precursors into RNA was unaffected.[3] Similarly, rats that were housed in darkness for three days and then exposed to light for fifteen minutes exhibited increases of the incorporation of leucine into occipital cortex over unexposed controls.[47] Increases were also observed in the proportion of ribosomes found in polyribosomes and in the protein synthetic activity of the ribosomes *in vitro*, and were seen in all areas of cortex, not just visual cortex. Studies of the first exposure of rats to light have shown more complex results. In the first two hours of exposure there was an increase in $[4,5\text{-}^3\text{H}]$lysine incorporation in primary and secondary visual areas, but this was followed by a prolonged decrease. Recently, the increase of lysine incorporation has been shown to be confined to specific protein bands separated by polyacrylamide gel electrophoresis, and to the neuronal fraction.[48] To what extent the neuronal-specific location accounts for the protein band specificity remains to be assessed.

In all of these studies, the specific radioactivity of the precursors was determined a considerable while after isotope administration at the time when the animal was killed for assay of radioactivity protein or RNA. However, the radioactivity of the precursors may rise very rapidly and reach a peak very shortly after their injection. The total incorporation of radioactivity into macromolecules is related to the integral of the specific radioactivity of the precursor pool over the entire incorporation period. Experimentally this can best be estimated by determining the precursor specific radioactivity at a series of time points during the incorporation period.

Working without the use of radioactive tracers, Hydén found that vestibular stimulation of the rat by rotation resulted in changes in the base composition of RNA of neurons in the vestibular nucleus.[49] The results were consistent with a transport of RNA from the glia to the neurons. Olfactory stimulation of the catfish by morpholine has likewise been reported to result in alterations of the base composition of the RNA of the olfactory bulb.[4]

Recent data have shown that suture of the eyelid in the chick resulted in approximately a 10 percent fall of cerebral blood supply both to contralateral primary optic regions (optic lobes) and to the contralateral cerebral hemispheres that are secondarily innervated by the sutured eye.[5] These effects can be detected within twenty minutes of eyelid suture. Conversely, upon first exposure of one eye of the chick to patterned light, cerebral blood flow through the contralateral hemispheres, optic lobe and thalamus rose significantly within five minutes.[50] The uptake of chemicals into the brain from the blood can be selectively modified in response to sensory input. Thus in the monocularly sutured chick there is a specific increase in the uptake of tyrosine, but not choline in the cerebral hemisphere and optic lobe innervated by the sutured eye.[51] Large changes in blood supply may also occur in response to activity within cerebral motor areas as well as sensory areas. In man, during vigorous arm work, the velocity of blood flow through the area of the motor cortex effecting this is increased by 40 percent.[52]

Such increases in blood supply to specific cerebral regions may increase the rate of delivery of isotopes and account for apparent changes in the rate of macromolecular synthesis. Nevertheless, the vascular changes that produce an increase in the supply of nutrients to particular areas of the brain may reflect a local elevation of metabolic processes. Thus changes in the incorporation of radioactive precursors into macromolecules, while very poor estimates of real rates of synthesis, may reflect changes in anabolic activity.

ii) Long-Term Studies

Visual deprivation

An extreme form of visual deprivation which does not involve surgery is the housing of animals in complete darkness. Dark maintenance may result in the retarded or improper development of behavioral and physiological responses. These include imprinting in chicks, the appearance of the visual evoked potential in the rat, and the maintenance of REM sleep in the young macaque.[5] In dark-reared mice, a reduction in dendritic spines in the occipital cortex has been described. At the biochemical level, light deprivation may reduce the development of normal levels of acetylcholinesterase in the chick.[5] However, dark maintenance undoubtedly has many physiological consequences, including changes in the endocrine and nutritional states which may cause widespread metabolic changes. Diurnal rhythms of neurotransmitters such as acetylcholine and serotonin are presumably disrupted. Thus the mechanisms underlying the chemical, anatomical and behavioral changes caused by dark maintenance are difficult to determine.

Occlusion of the eye with an opaque contact lens or eyelid suture eliminates the transmission of patterned information. This procedure can be carried out monocularly so that comparisons between paired optic regions within a single animal can be made. Differences found between the two sides must then be directly due to the experimental manipulation, rather than the secondary effects resulting from systemic humoral variations. Three weeks after monocular eyelid suture of newly hatched chicks, a small but significant reduction in weight of the cerebral hemisphere contralateral to the sutured eye is seen relative to the paired ipsilateral hemisphere.[5] When monocularly sutured chicks were dark-maintained, no such asymmetry was apparent. The contralateral cerebral hemisphere is secondarily innervated by the sutured eye but receives no direct innervation from the optic tract. Visual deprivation may thus cause deficits in secondarily innervated areas, and this impairment may be widespread and involve nonvisual areas of the brain.

Monocular suture in rats resulted in a loss of spines from the apical dendrites of the pyramidal cells of the visual cortex. It also caused a diminished perikaryon size in the neurons of the lateral geniculate nucleus. The loss of dendritic spines could be reversed by the restoration of patterned vision.[5] Monocular suture in cats produces more severe changes in the contralateral geniculate than does binocular suture. This has been attributed to binocular competition.[53] It is of interest that in the *secondary* visual areas, the effect of monocular eyelid suture is often as severe as the effect of unilateral enucleation.

Another form of visual deprivation is the restriction of input to a given pattern such as vertical or horizontal bars. When reared in an environment of alternate black and white vertical bands, kittens appeared blind to similar horizontal bands; if the kittens were reared with horizontal bands, they appeared blind to vertical ones.[54] The nature of early visual experience may thus influence the response to pattern of visual cortex neurons in cats (p. 160). To be meaningful, chemical studies of such alterations of visual afferent patterns would have to be conducted on a single cell basis, but none have yet been reported.

CHAPTER 7 REFERENCES

Reviews and General References

1. McIlwain, H. *Chemical Exploration of the Brain: A Study of Cerebral Excitability and Ion Movement.* Elsevier Press, Amsterdam, 1963.
2. McIlwain, H., and Bachelard, H. S. Metabolic, ionic and electrical phenomena in separated cerebral tissues. In *Biochemistry and the Central Nervous System,* Churchill Livingstone, London, 1971, pp. 61–97.
3. Talwar, G. P., and Singh, U. B. Excitation. In *Handbook of Neurochemistry,* Vol. 6 (Ed. A. Lajtha), Plenum Press, New York, 1971, pp. 29–61.
4. Rappoport, D. A., Trieff, N. M., O'Heeron, M. K., Benignus, V. A., and Benton, R. G. Chemosensory stimulation. In *Handbook of Neurochemistry,* Vol. 6 (Ed. A. Lajtha), Plenum Press, New York, 1971, pp. 1–28.
5. Bondy, S. C., and Margolis, F. L. *Sensory Deprivation and Brain Development. The Avian Visual System as a Model.* In *Brain and Behaviour Research,* Monograph Series

Vol. 4 (Ed. J. Bureš, E. R. John, P. G. Kostjuk, and L. Pickenhain). Gustav Fischer Verlag, Jena, 1971.

Literature Cited

6. King, L. J., Lowry, O. H., Passonneau, J. V., and Venson, V. Effects of convulsants on energy reserves in the cerebral cortex. *J. Neurochem.* 14:599 – 611, 1967.
7. Dunn, A. The dependence of brain ATP content on cerebral electroshock current. *Brain Research* 61:442 – 45, 1973.
8. Tower, D. B. *Neurochemistry of Epilepsy.* Charles Thomas, Springfield, Ill., 1960.
9. Wolfe, L. S., and Elliott, K. A. C. Chemical studies in relation to convulsive conditions. In *Neurochemistry,* 2nd ed. (Ed. K. A. C. Elliot, I. H. Page, and J. H. Quastel), Charles Thomas, Springfield, Ill., 1962, pp. 694 – 727.
10. Lovell, R. A. Some neurochemical aspects of convulsions. In *Handbook of Neurochemistry,* Vol. 6 (Ed. A. Lajtha), Plenum Press, New York, 1971, pp. 63 – 102.
11. Collins, R. C., Plum, F., and Posner, J. Energy and epilepsy. *Science* 170:1430 – 31, 1970.
12. Walker, J. E., Lewin, E., Sheppard, J. R., and Cromwell, R. Enzymatic regulation of adenosine 3',5'-monophosphate (cyclic AMP) in the freezing epileptogenic lesion of rat brain and in homologous contralateral cortex. *J. Neurochem.* 21:79 – 85, 1973.
13. Thoenen, H., and Oesch, F. New enzyme synthesis as a long-term adaptation to increased transmitter utilization. In *New Concepts in Neurotransmitter Regulation* (Ed. A. J. Mandell), Plenum Press, New York, 1973, pp. 33 – 52.
14. Thoenen, H. Trans-synaptic enzyme induction. *Life Sciences* 14:223 – 35, 1974.
15. Oesch, F., and Thoenen, H. Increased activity of the peripheral sympathetic nervous system: induction of choline acetyltransferase in the preganglionic cholinergic neurone. *Nature* 242:536 – 37, 1973.
16. Hydén, H. Dynamic aspects on the neuron-glia relationship. A study with microchemical methods. In *The Neuron,* Elsevier Press, Amsterdam, 1967, pp. 179 – 219.
17. Pevzner, L. Z. Macromolecular changes within neuron-neuroglia unit during behavioral events. In *Macromolecules and Behavior,* 2nd ed. (Ed. J. Gaito) Appleton-Century-Crofts, New York, 1972, pp. 335 – 58.
18. Geiger, A. Chemical changes accompanying activity in the brain. In *Metabolism of the Nervous System* (Ed. D. Richter), Pergamon Press, London, 1957, pp. 245 – 56.
19. Dunn, A., Giuditta, A., Wilson, J. E., and Glassman, E. The effect of electroshock on brain RNA and protein and its possible relationship to behavioral effects. In *The Psychobiology of Convulsive Therapy* (Ed. M. Fink, J. McGaugh, S. Kety, and T. A. Williams), Winston & Sons, Wash ngton, D.C., 1974, pp. 185 – 97.
20. Orrego, F. Synthesis of RNA in normal and electrically stimulated brain cortex slices *in vitro. J. Neurochem.* 14:851 – 58, 1967.
21. Berry, R. W. Ribonucleic acid metabolism of a single neuron: correlation with electrical activity. *Science* 166:1021 – 23, 1969.
22. Kernell, D., and Peterson, R. P. The effect of spike activity versus synaptic activation on the metabolism of ribonucleic acid in a molluscan giant neurone. *J. Neurochem.* 17:1087 – 94, 1970.
23. Berry, R. W., and Cohen, M. J. Synaptic stimulation of RNA in the giant neuron of *Aplysia californica. J. Neurobiol.* 3:209 – 22, 1972.
24. Wilson, D. L., and Berry, R. W. The effect of synaptic stimulation on RNA and protein metabolism in the R2 of soma of *Aplysia. J. Neurobiol.* 3:369 – 79, 1972.

25. Peterson, R. P., and Erulkar, S. D. Parameters of stimulation of RNA synthesis and characterization by hybridization in a molluscan neuron. *Brain Research* 60:177 – 90, 1973.
26. Gisiger, V. Triggering of RNA synthesis by acetylcholine stimulation of the postsynaptic membrane in a mammalian sympathetic ganglion. *Brain Research* 33:139 – 46, 1971.
27. Jarlstedt, J., and Dahlström, A. Changes in RNA-content of sympathetic ganglion cells of reserpine-pretreated rats. *Neuropharmacology* 11:447 – 50, 1972.
28. Orrego, F., and Lipmann, F. Protein synthesis in brain slices. *J. Biol. Chem.* 242:665 – 71, 1967.
29. Jethmal, E., and Koenig, E. Effect of electrical stimulation of nerve roots on amino acid incorporation into axonal protein *in vitro*. *Nature, New Biol.* 241:28 – 29, 1973.
30. Banks, P. The effect of preganglionic stimulation on the incorporation of L-[U-^{14}C] valine into the protein of the superior cervical ganglion of the guinea pig. *Biochem. J.* 118:813 – 18, 1970.
31. Guiditta, A., Dettbarn, W.-D., and Brzin, M. Protein synthesis in the isolated giant axon of the squid. *Proc. Nat. Acad. Sci. U.S.A.* 59:1284 – 87, 1968.
32. Giuditta, A., D'Udine, B., and Pepe, M. Uptake of protein by the giant axon of the squid. *Nature, New Biol.* 229:29 – 30, 1971.
33. Ungar, G., and Romano, D. V. Sulfhydryl groups in resting and stimulated rat brain; their relationship with protein structure. *Proc. Soc. Exptl. Biol. Med.* 97:324 – 26, 1958.
34. Appel, S. H., and Locher, C. Changes in synapse membrane protein phosphorylation following electroconvulsive shock. *Neurology* 23:410, 1973.
35. McIlwain, H. Regulatory significance of the release and action of adenine derivatives in cerebral systems. *Biochem. Soc. Symp.* 36:69 – 85, 1972.
36. Sattin, A. Increase in the content of adenosine 3',5'-monophosphate in mouse forebrain during seizures and prevention of the increase by methylxanthines. *J. Neurochem.* 18:1087 – 96, 1971.
37. Bloom, F. E., Hoffer, B. J., and Siggins, G. R. Central noradrenergic receptors: localization, function and molecular mechanisms. In *New Concepts in Neurotransmitter Regulation* (Ed. A. J. Mandell), Plenum Press, New York, 1973, pp. 223 – 38.
38. McAfee, D. A., and Greengard, P. Adenosine 3',5'-monophosphate: electrophysiological evidence for a role in synaptic transmission. *Science* 178:310 – 12, 1972.
39. Cedar, H., and Schwartz, J. H. Cyclic adenosine monophosphate in the nervous system of *Aplysia californica*. II. Effect of serotonin and dopamine. *J. Gen. Physiol.* 60:570 – 87, 1972.
40. Goldberg, N. D., O'Dea, R. F., and Haddox, M. V. Cyclic GMP. In *Advances in Cyclic Nucleotide Research*, Vol. 3 (Ed. P. Greenberg and A. Robinson), Raven Press, New York, 1973, pp. 155 – 223.
41. Ueda, T., Maeno, H., and Greengard, P Regulation of endogenous phosphorylation of specific proteins in synaptic membrane fractions from rat brain by adenosine 3',5'-monophosphate. *J. Biol. Chem.* 248:8295 – 305, 1973.
42. Escueta, A. V., and Appel, S. H. The effects of electroshock seizures on potassium transport within synaptosomes from rat brain. *J. Neurochem.* 19:1625 – 38, 1972.
43. Daly, J. W., Huang, M., and Shimizu, H. Regulation of cyclic AMP levels in brain tissue. *Adv. Cyclic Nucleotide Research* 1:375 – 87, 1972.
44. Schultz, J., and Daly, J. W. Cyclic adenosine 3'5'-monophosphate in guinea pig cerebral cortical slices. *J. Biol. Chem.* 248:843 – 52, 1973.
45. White, G. L., and Larrabee, M. G. Phosphoinositides and other phospholipids in sym-

pathetic ganglia and nerve trunks of rats. Effects of neuronal activity and inositol analogs [δ- and γ-hexachlorocyclohexane(lindane)] on [^{32}P]-labelling, synaptic transmission and axonal conduction. *J. Neurochem.* 20:783–98, 1973.

46. Schacht, J., and Agranoff, B. W. Interaction of cholinergic agents with phospholipid metabolism in guinea pig cortex synaptosomes. In *Neurochemistry of Cholinergic Receptors* (Ed. E. de Robertis and J. Schacht), Raven Press, New York, 1974, pp. 121–29.
47. Appel, S. H., Davis, W., and Scott, S. Brain polysomes: response to environmental stimulation. *Science* 157:836–38, 1967.
48. Rose, S. P. R., Sinha, A. K., and Broomhead, S. Precursor incorporation into cortical protein during first exposure of rats to light; cellular localization of effects. *J. Neurochem.* 21:539–46, 1973.
49. Hydén, H. RNA in brain cells. In *The Neurosciences: A Study Program* (Ed. G. C. Quarton, T. Melnechuk, and F. O. Schmitt), The Rockefeller University Press, New York, 1967, pp. 248–66.
50. Bondy, S. C. The regulation of regional blood flow in the brain by visual input. *J. Neurol. Sci.* 19:425–32, 1973.
51. Bondy, S. C., and Purdy, J. Selective regulation of the blood-brain barrier by sensory input. *Brain Research.* 76:542–545, 1974.
52. Olesen, J. Contralateral focal increase of cerebral blood flow in man during arm work. *Brain* 94:635–46, 1971.
53. Guillery, R. W. The effect of lid suture upon the growth of cells in the dorsal lateral geniculate nucleus of kittens. *J. Comp. Neurol.* 148:417–22, 1973.
54. Blakemore, C., and Mitchell, D. E. Environmental modification of the visual cortex and the neural basis of learning and memory. *Nature* 241:467–68, 1973.

VIII. The Biochemical Basis of Behavior

Why do we think that behavior has a biochemical basis? The important aspect of behavior in higher organisms is the ability to adapt. This behavioral plasticity cannot be explained in terms of electrical activity alone; presumably, it has a chemical basis and is also probably chemically controlled. The idea of a chemical involvement is reinforced by the knowledge that certain behaviors that we regard as mental illnesses are associated with chemical disturbances of the body and brain, and that drugs may specifically alter behavior.

Much of behavior is conditioned by previous experience and the memory thus acquired. On the other hand, much is inherited, presumably by genetic control of the make-up of the nervous system. Though distinction between the genetic and environmental factors is not always easy, this chapter is generally concerned with the latter. The available evidence indicates a chemical basis for learning and memory. This does not necessarily mean that the information content of memory resides in the structure of specific molecules located in the brain. To understand the necessity for a chemical basis for learning, some neurophysiological properties of the brain must be understood.

The nervous system works electrically. This is evidenced from the electrical excitability of neurons, the transmission of electrical impulses throughout the body, the recorded electrical activity of the brain (electroencephalogram, EEG,) and the way in which this activity varies in response to stimuli. The brain is often thought of as a miniature but complex computer with individual neurons as connecting wires. The complexity of this computer arises both from the multiplicity of connections (synapses) in the brain (at least 10^9) and from the fact that each neuron apparently acts as an integrator of its own electrical inputs. Moreover, the connections themselves are not passive and may function variably. Thus both the synapses and the entire neurons are capable of processing electrical information and making decisions. Furthermore, the activity of an individual neuron is influenced by those surrounding it, with or without synaptic connections. Many, if not most, CNS neurons are not electrically insulated by myelin, and the surrounding glia may respond to the electrical state of the neurons. These interactions need not be mediated by synaptic contacts; postsynaptic potential changes, especially those in the perikaryon, may be transmitted by volume conduction. The brain waves are as much comprised of these potential changes as they are of action potentials. These waves may be very clearly defined, indicating the synchronous change in potential, and perhaps firing, of many thousands of neurons. In this way steady rhythms occur, which may persist for several seconds or longer. Thus volume conduction and mass interaction confound ideas of the brain merely as a complex electronic wiring pattern. Nevertheless, brain function may still be considered at the electrical level.

But what happens when the brain learns? The behavioral change involved in learning presumably requires a change in electrical circuitry. These connectivity changes are necessary whether the brain is conceived in terms of simple circuitry or as a holograph. Generally, they are thought to involve an alteration in the processing of impulses by synapses or neurons. It is unlikely that long-term memory resides in persisting electrical patterns (reverberating circuits), because interference with the electrical activity of the brain (including flattening of the EEG by anoxia or low temperature) does not interfere with most memories, although it may impair the more recent ones. Thus the changes must have a chemical basis even though they may also be regarded as electrical. What kind of chemical changes could be involved? Minor local changes could alter the conduction properties of the synaptic membrane. Alternatively, major structural changes could occur, such as the formation of a new synapse or the destruction of a preexisting one.

In the relationship of chemistry to behavior there are several interfaces. At the sensory level, cues from the environment are transduced by the sensory receptors into electrical signals. In motor processes electrical impulses

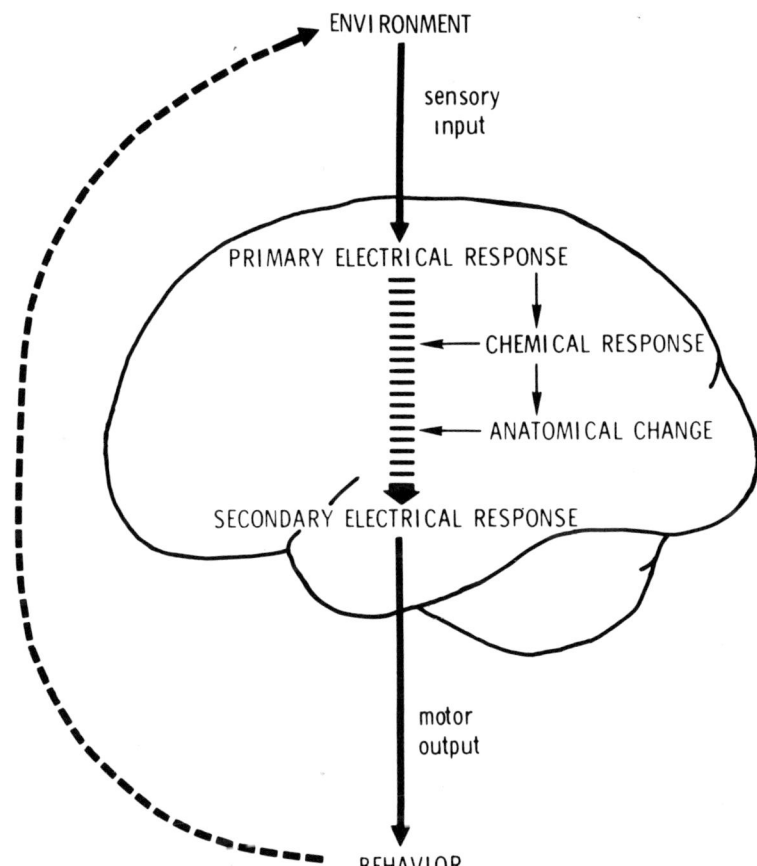

Figure 8.1 Information processing by the brain. The primary electrical response due to the sensory input is processed by the brain according to the prevailing circuitry and electrical and chemical states, to produce the motor output which is behavior. Chemical responses to either the sensory input or the processing may, in the long term, result in anatomical changes, thus altering the circuitry.

are transduced into the muscular contractions that constitute the behavior of the animal. Between these processes occur the cerebral events that are so poorly understood (Figure 8.1). The primary electrophysiological response of the brain to the sensory input is processed by the electrical circuitry to result in the motor output. However, the sensory input will also trigger chemical responses such as alterations of the metabolism of particular cells and possibly the secretion of hormones. These chemical responses may profoundly affect the electrical activity of the brain and hence the motor output. Neurotransmission is subject to pharmacological manipulation and is most likely affected by hormones and other physiological chemicals. Thus the response to stimuli known as behavior involves complex integrative processes in the brain. It is likely that in the long term the combined effects of the electrical and chemical responses result in anatomical changes which alter the electrical processing. This then may be the basis of long-term memory.

A. EXPERIMENTAL APPROACHES

In the study of the biology of behavior there are serious problems in the design of adequate experimental controls and consequent difficulty in determining the significance of any differences observed. In experimental situations a single stimulus may precipitate a cascade of events which may ultimately alter almost all the funcitons of the organism. Thus analysis requires the painstaking task of dissecting out the intricate sequence of events and their interrelationships.

The problem of the biochemistry of behavior may be approached in two distinct ways. The first is to modify animal behavior and observe any corresponding biochemical changes. The second is to use treatments that affect brain chemistry and to observe the resultant effect on the behavior. Neither of these approaches is particularly easy nor particularly conclusive. Proof of a specific biochemical change as the basis of a behavior will require a large number of unrelated experiments. Using either approach, there are a very large number of possible metabolites and treatments to be studied. Deciding where to start is essentially guesswork. The best that can be hoped for is that the guesses will be guided by the information available from all fields concerning the way in which the nervous system functions. Past guesses have yet to be brought to fruition, and some unfortunate errors have been made. Very careful research is needed in this very difficult area.

Before leaving this general discussion we feel it appropriate to comment on an important aspect of research in the chemistry of behavior. The interest in understanding brain chemistry is often justified in terms of designing pharmacological therapies for brain disorders or for "improving" normal brain function. While drug therapy may be important for the alleviation of certain mental disorders, pharmacological solutions have certain dangers. An obvious problem is the opportunity given to governments or individuals to manipulate thought or mood. The dangers of manipulation by drugs should be considered in the same context as the social and political manipulation for which it may substitute.

A second, less obvious aspect may also be potentially dangerous: the claim that mental illness is *caused* by a change in brain chemistry. While this is certainly true for genetic disorders and those maladies induced by drugs or toxins, the chemical changes associated with other disorders may only be secondary or symptomatic. This may be especially true for schizophrenia and depression. While a chemical change may be the immediate cause of the behavioral change, the underlying cause can be environmental or social. The danger is that chemical changes encourage pharmaceutical treatments, which need not be appropriate for socially induced ills. If at all possible the disease should be treated rather than its symptoms. Social diseases require social remedies.

B. LEARNING AND MEMORY

The chemistry of learning and the molecular basis of memory have commanded a great deal of attention in recent years. The problem is a difficult one and many pitfalls have been encountered. The major practical difficulty has been to simultaneously satisfy the requirements of the behavior and the biochemistry in the same experiment, but difficulties have also arisen within the two disciplines because they were not adequately developed to answer the kinds of questions involved in these experiments. Many of the experiments that have been performed were weak in either the biochemistry or the behavior, or sometimes both. Simple collaboration by experts in the two fields is not enough, since it is now apparent that the research has problems of its own and that experiments are best performed by workers having a full understanding of both the biochemical and the behavioral problems and limitations.

Memory is though to persist in the arrangement of neuronal connections and in the individual electrical properties of particular neurons. Chemical events are necessary, both to support the electrical function by producing energy and pumping ions and to build and maintain the anatomical structure. Furthermore, as explained above, chemical events are also necessary to allow the occurrence of changes in the electrical circuitry. It is the nature of *these* chemical events that is of interest. The idea of molecules with specific information content is currently in disrepute, since none of the necessary transductions have been shown to occur and there are no plausible models to support the idea.

In common with other behaviors, there are two general approaches to the biochemistry of learning:[1]

1. Biochemical changes that occur while animals learn are studied and attempts made to associate the changes with the learning per se. The shortcomings of this approach are considerable.[1,2] Of the many possible chemicals that may be involved, the correct ones must be selected and studied in the correct place at the correct time. Then there is the possibility that the changes may be too small or too localized to be detected. The process of memory formation almost certainly involves at least several metabolic steps. One is therefore seeking not single changes, but pathways, which may have to be elucidated in their entirety for real understanding to be possible. Another problem is that of specificity. The learning phenomenon is a complex one and, aside from factors controlling receptivity such as attention and motivation, sensory input is necessary. In animals, because of the lack of verbal communication, learning and the existence of memory may only be inferred by observing behavioral responses. This in turn involves motivation and other emotional factors, besides performance and memory retrieval. It is common to refer to these factors as nonspecific and to attempt to dissociate them from learning itself. This task is not only difficult; it may be futile. If one removes the ''nonspecific'' components, the learning may not occur. The problem is not technical but conceptual. If memory is considered to be the association of ideas, then the physical connection linking the ideas *is* the memory. As such, it cannot exist in the absence of either the sensory stimulus or the behavioral output. Looked at in this way, ''nonspecific'' factors appear more specific.

2. Treatments that alter memory processes are studied in the hope of finding a common mechanism. The problem is to find treatments of sufficient chemical specificity. If several treatments that block memory formation have a common biochemical effect, then it is likely that this biochemical process is involved in memory. However, proof can never be obtained in such a way, since no treatment will have a single effect and there will un-

doubtedly be secondary chemical consequences of the primary effect. The only proof attainable by this technique is that a particular metabolic reaction is *not* involved if total inhibition of it has no effect on learning.

Fortunately, the shortcomings of these two approaches to the biochemistry of learning are to some extent distinct, so that the approaches complement each other.

i) Agents That Affect Learning

Much of what we know about learning and memory stems from the use of treatments that disrupt memory processes, particularly electroconvulsive shock and the inhibitors of protein synthesis. ECS, when administered under appropriate conditions shortly after an experience, can prevent the formation of a memory that can be retrieved the following day or later, but does not prevent immediate retrieval. These, and similar results with other convulsants and with inhibitors of protein synthesis, are the basis of the consolidation hypothesis.[3] Essentially this hypothesis states that the learning experience initiates a process of consolidation of itself into a permanent or long-term memory. ECS may interrupt the early stages of this consolidation, but the process shortly becomes refractory to the treatment. Immediate or short-term memory is not affected by ECS and is thus different in nature. While this hypothesis is not universally accepted, considerable experimental support for it exists.[4] It initiated the idea that immediate, short-term memory is electrical, whereas long-term memory is chemical. This is false. It is unlikely that the severe electrical disturbances produced by ECS would not disrupt the electrical activity, but even flattening of the EEG by ischemia does not affect short-term memory. Thus short-term memory may also have a chemical basis, albeit of a different nature. It may be that short-term memory involves a rapid chemical change such as the phosphorylation of a membrane protein (perhaps at a synapse or synapses), whereas long-term memory involves the synthesis of new molecules, possibly structural macromolecules (see Figure 8.2).

Probably the important effect of ECS is the brain seizure; the presence of this alone without bodily convulsions is sufficient to produce amnesia. The biochemical effects of ECS are numerous and several possible explanations of the amnestic effect have been suggested, including the observed inhibition of protein synthesis and disturbances of neurotransmitter metabolism.[5,6] However, following ECS there is a severe depression of brain ATP concentrations, presumably as a result of the greatly accelerated energy demand

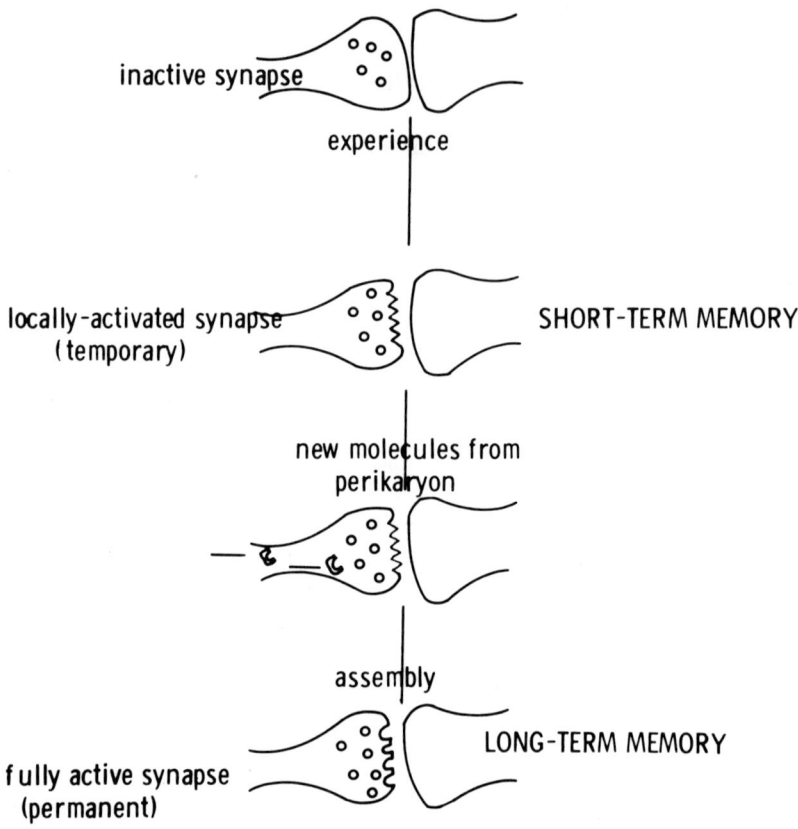

Figure 8.2 Hypothetical synaptic mechanisms for short- and long-term memory. A temporary change involving minor modifications of presynaptic membrane macromolecules could alter the properties of the synapse so that a short-term memory is formed. Long-term memory may be formed when newly-synthesized macromolecules arrive from the cell body to permanently alter the properties of the synapse.

by ion pumps (p. 78). This important metabolic change may have such diverse effects that meaningful analysis is impossible. Furthermore, structural tissue damage may occur as a result of the seizure, since temporary morphological changes have been observed in the brain following ECS.[7] If such damage were selective for those synaptic contacts that were active at the time of the seizure, this could explain the specificity of the effect for recently learned experiences. This specificity of ECS for recent memory is not absolute, and older memories may also be lost, but the probability is less.

The other treatment that has been studied extensively is the inhibition of protein synthesis by drugs such as puromycin, cycloheximide and acetoxycycloheximide.[8] These drugs have all been shown to cause amnesia in experimental animals, but problems have arisen regarding the specificity of the effects. In particular, puromycin has been shown to have side effects, some of which may be due to its pyrimidine structure, which resembles cyclic AMP, and some to the release of puromycyl peptides from the polyribosomes. These effects include glycogen degradation, local brain seizures and mitochondrial swelling.[1,5] Nevertheless, a range of protein synthesis inhibitors including anisomycin and streptovitacin are also amnestic.[9] The drugs must be used in sufficient concentration to inhibit protein synthesis by about 90 percent for significant amnesia effects to be detected. To explain the high inhibition of protein synthesis necessary to impair memory formation, it has been argued that much redundancy exists in the information stores of the brain, an idea reinforced by the demonstration that memory in overtrained animals is less affected by cycloheximide.[10] It has also been suggested that there are sites of protein synthesis particularly resistant to the inhibitors, because of either limited access of the drugs or inherent resistance to the inhibitors of a particular class of ribosomes.[5] The important factor may be the integrity of the polyribosomal structures. Since control of gene expression may in part be exerted at the polyribosome level, the active polyribosomes may be synthesizing protein in accordance with a program determined by the history of that cell. Polyribosomes are disrupted by puromycin (and by ECS) but only to a lesser extent by cycloheximide.[11]

In view of the central importance of protein in cell function, it is scarcely surprising that severe inhibition of protein synthesis affects memory. Even if we accept that the amnestic effects of puromycin and cycloheximide are due to inhibition of protein synthesis, this does not bring us close to the identification of the particular proteins involved. The reduction of the synthetic rate of any molecule essential for the normal functioning of the cell may result in an impairment of memory, but this does not help to locate the mechanisms *specific* for memory formation.

Other agents that disrupt memory include anoxia, carbon dioxide and ouabain.[5,12] The metabolic consequences of these are so profound that it would indeed be surprising if they were not amnestic. Thus they are of little or no use in elucidating the processes crucial to the formation of memory. More significantly, cytosine arabinoside, an inhibitor of DNA synthesis, and 8-azaguanine, an inhibitor of RNA synthesis, do not impair memory formation in rats. However, actinomycin D, while not amnestic in rats, is amnestic in goldfish.[13] Actinomycin D is highly toxic and its amnestic effects may be due to general malaise rather than a specific inhibition of brain RNA synthesis. The same criticism applies to α-amanitin, which is also amnestic and highly toxic.[14] However, camptothecin, an inhibitor of ribosome assembly which is not particularly toxic, is amnestic in goldfish.[15] These conflicting results suggest that DNA synthesis is not immediately necessary for the formation of memory, but that RNA synthesis may be.

Drugs that facilitate memory are potentially more useful, since they may reveal the rate-limiting steps in the memory consolidation process. (A stimulation of a step that is not rate-limiting would not be expected to show an overall effect.) The widely reported effect of magnesium pemoline in enhancing memory has not withstood close inspection, though it may have some behavioral effects.[13] The reported enhancement of memory following the feeding of RNA may at least in part have been due to placebo effects or the correction of nutritional defects. Two other compounds have recently excited interest, since they apparently facilitate learning. These are strychnine,[16] which in high doses is a lethal convulsant, and lysine vasopressin,[17] a naturally occurring pituitary peptide. Strychnine, when administered in doses that facilitate learning, increases brain RNA content.[18]

ii) Biochemical correlates of learning[1,13]

The basis of memory must be stable and long-lasting. This may mean that the molecules directly involved in the memory must themselves be stable, but it is just as likely that the stability resides in a self-regenerating system of which the molecules form a part. For example, if the storage of a memory required the formation of a new synapse, it would be possible for all the molecules that constitute the synapse to be replaced, but, provided the synapse itself remained, the memory might still remain intact. Since it has been difficult to conceive that small molecules exclusively could form the basis of stable changes, macromolecules have been the favorite targets for study. This notion has been strengthened by the important structural role of macromolecules, especially as membrane components but also because of their intimate role in gene expression both as repositories of the genetic code and as regulators of its expression.

What sort of chemical changes could be responsible for the formation of memory? Minor changes in components of the synaptic membrane could alter the connectivity between contacting neurons and form the basis of short-term memory. Possibilities include changes in the membrane proteins such as phosphorylation, alkylation, acylation or glycosylation, or the addition of sialic acid to gangliosides. Such changes could occur very rapidly indeed, producing conformational changes that would be relatively stable. Long-term changes might involve structural changes, e.g., in synaptic contacts or the branching of neuronal processes. These might require gene activation and the flow of new materials from the perikaryon along the axon or dendrite. An important question is whether long-term memory is a more permanent fixation of the short-term changes (as in the model in Figure 8.2). Unfortunately, no definitive evidence exists to indicate whether long-term memory is dependent on short-term memory. Thus we do not know which pathway is correct in the diagram below.

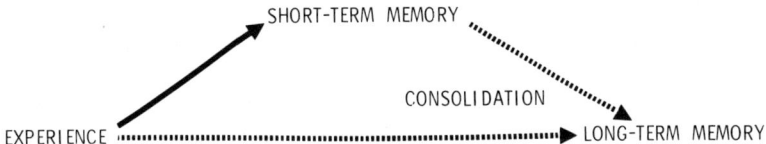

RNA

The discovery that molecules of nucleic acids contained genetic information encoded in their base sequences excited the prospect for a similar role in information storage in the brain. Consequently, the RNA metabolism of brain has been extensively studied in relation to learning, and has proved to be unusually responsive to environmental stimulation.

The initial impetus for these studies arose from Hydén's observations that associated neural activity with changes in the nucleic acid content of neurons, studied both histologically and, later, cytospectrophotometrically. Convinced that the important changes must occur in individual cells, Hydén set about developing techniques for the microdissection of single cells and the analysis of their RNA, not only in gross amount but also by base composition and molecular size. Using these techniques he found consistent changes in the base composition of RNA of rat vestibular neurons and Deiter's nucleus, associated with the learning of a wire-balancing task.[19] Reciprocal changes were found between the neurons and their surrounding glia, suggesting the transfer of RNA from the latter to the former and thus providing support for the neuronalglial-unit hypothesis (p. 165). Hydén was criticized by psychologists regarding the specificity of the effect for learning. Also vestibular stimulation by a thermal gradient between the eardrums of rabbits was found to produce a similar biochemical response.[20]

Hydén also explored another learning task in which rats learned to retrieve food pellets from a device that only permitted the use of one paw. He forced the animals to use the paw opposite to that which they used initially when no preference was exerted. In this reversal-learning situation, animals exhibited RNA base changes in pyramidal cells of the CA3 region of the hippocampus, similar to those observed previously in the Deiter's nucleus cells.[19] The significance of this effect is difficult to evaluate since the "learning" is the acquisition of a motor task. The validity of the evidence for glial-neuronal transfer has been questioned, since microdissected neurons are essentially only cell bodies; the dendrites and axons are included in the glial fraction. Thus a redistribution of RNA in the neuron could account for the results without intercellular transfer.[21] Furthermore, the RNA was hydrolyzed for the base composition studies using hydrochloric acid, which seriously degrades some of the bases (especially cytidine and adenine) and necessitates the use of correction factors larger than the effects observed. Nevertheless, the results are evidence of a brain response to the environment and, because radioactive compounds were not used, are free of some of the problems inherent in tracer studies.

There have been many reports of relatively large effects of training on the incorporation of radioactive precursors into brain RNA.[13] In contrast to the results of Hydén, changes have been found either in the whole brain or in rather large anatomical regions. Serious problems exist in relating changes of precursor incorporation to changes in the synthesis of macromolecules. The incorporation obviously depends on the amount (or, more accurately, the specific radioactivity) of precursor available. This will be determined both by the delivery to the tissue through the bloodstream and by the uptake into the cell, as well as by the activity of synthetic and catabolic processes. To complicate matters, these factors are likely to be different for the various cells in the sample, and may even be different for separate parts of the same cell (e.g., dendrites and soma, nucleus and cytoplasm). Further, the processes are all kinetic and will vary throughout the incorporation period. These factors collectively constitute the *precursor pool problem*. There is no way of adequately compensating for all these factors with the use of radioisotopes. However, differential effects (e.g., between RNA species) are more convincing. Also, the effects seen with radioactive isotopes may be confirmed subsequently with quantitative measurements not involving the incorporation of labeled precursors. Despite the limitations of the tracer technique, it is capable of revealing small changes of rate that would be undetectable in gross amount. Radioactive tracer methods also greatly facilitate the biochemical analysis and permit several compounds to be studied in the same experiment.

A further problem is the blood-brain barrier. Many precursors will not enter the brain from the bloodstream. Intracerebral injections have the disadvantage that tissue damage is produced, which together with the anesthesia generally used can impair learning. In addition, intracerebrally injected materials may be unevenly and variably distributed. For example, intraventricularly injected uridine is concentrated in cells adjacent to the ventricles near the injection site. Variations in this distribution may produce misleading results.

Another consideration is the specificity of the precursor. If the injected tracer is the precursor of only one type of macromolecule, then there are less competing demands on the pool and the results are less susceptible to artifact. In theory any of the four bases or their nucleosides or nucleotides, or phosphate could be used as a precursor of RNA. In practice, the free bases and nucleotides and phosphate are very poorly taken up by the brain and phosphate is very nonspecific, being incorporated into a variety of biochemicals. Uridine has been the preferred precursor since it is not directly used for DNA synthesis. However, it is converted in the brain to cytidine, which is a DNA precursor. Furthermore, both nucleosides will be incorporated into RNA and changes in the extent of the conversion of uridine to cytidine will affect the net incorporation.

Glassman and Wilson, and their co-workers, reported an increase of the incorporation of radioactive uridine into RNA of brain but not liver during avoidance training of mice.[13] A sophisticated series of behavioral controls suggested that the effect was specifically related to novel learning. However, the effect was not specific for any species of RNA separated by sucrose gradients or polyacrylamide gel electrophoresis. In their experiments they examined the radioactivity in free uridine nucleotides, determined as UMP, to control for the variability in the cellular uptake of the intraventricularly injected uridine. More recent studies from the same laboratory, using quantitative techniques for the recovery of RNA and UMP and intraperitoneal or subcutaneous uridine injection, suggest that the major effect is not an increase in the radioactivity of the total RNA but a decrease in that of UMP.[22] This decrease may be related to a concomitant increase in the uridine diphosphate sugar derivatives which constitute over one-third of the free uridine nucleotides in brain. Thus a specific behavioral change formerly thought to be in RNA may in fact be an alteration in RNA precursor metabolism.

Changes in the incorporation of radioactive uridine into polyribosome-associated RNA have been observed by several groups. The RNA associated with polyribosomes accounts for less than 10 percent of the radioactivity in brain RNA at the times after uridine injection used in the experiments described above, so that a change in this type of RNA would not have been detected in measurement of the total RNA radioactivity. However, a close replication of the studies of the Glassman group indicates that the effect was at least in part explicable by an increase in the proportion of ribosomes aggregated into polyribosomes.[23]

Shashoua has used a subtle technique to detect changes in RNA type by administering [^{3}H]orotic acid as a precursor of RNA.[24] Orotic acid will be incorporated into RNA both as uridine and cytidine nucleotides, and thus a change in the ratio of radioactivity in these two nucleotides in the RNA may reflect a change in the type of RNA synthesized. (For example, the uridine-cytidine ratio for messenger RNA is higher than that for ribosomal RNA.) In goldfish that learned to swim upside down, changes were detected in the brain RNA uridine-cytidine ratio, but not in that of the free nucleotide precursors. However, elevated CO_2 concentrations in the aquarium water can produce similar changes in goldfish brain RNA and in the free precursor nucleotides.[25] Consequently, alterations of precursor nucleotide metabolism may have influenced the incorporation into RNA. This may be true for other studies that have used radioactive precursors to detect changes of RNA metabolism. Since both purine and pyrimidine nucleotides are known to respond to stimuli such as ECS, and since many are psychoactive (barbiturate drugs are analogues of uracil), it may be that all the reported changes in RNA synthesis in reality reflect responses of the volatile metabolism of nucleotides. Unfortunately, if precursor metabolism is altered, it is difficult to determine whether there are also changes in RNA metabolism.

Those studies that have chemically determined changes in RNA are exempt from this criticism. Thus Izquierdo and his co-workers have demonstrated changes in the concentration of hippocampal RNA in rats following avoidance training, electrical stimulation of the fornix producing hippocampal theta rhythms or stimulation of the brain with concentrations of potassium salts.[26] These interesting observations deserve replication.

Aside from the base composition studies of Hydén, several workers have examined brain RNA for qualitative changes, concomitant with behavioral modification. An important technique for this is DNA-RNA hybridization. There are many problems in interpreting results obtained with this technique, notably those involving concentration differences between different RNA and DNA sequences.[27] Moreover, if the RNA is radioactively labeled *in vivo*, the technique suffers from all the problems inherent in the use of tracer radioisotopes. However, it is possible to circumvent many of these problems either by labeling the RNA *in vitro* or by the use of radioactive DNA. Using *in vitro* labeled brain RNA, an apparent increase in gene expression was observed in cats that learned a visual discrimination task. This effect was observed only on the side of the (split) brain that could be considered to have learned the discrimination (K. A. Bonnet, unpublished observations).

Another approach to the problem of precursor pools has been used by Bateson and Rose, and their co-workers, in studies of imprinting in chicks.[28] Imprinting is the phenomenon in which the newborn chick fixates on the first object it perceives, treating it subsequently as a mother object. Rose showed that the imprinting to a flashing light is accompanied by an increase in the incorporation of $[^3H]$uracil into RNA in the forebrain roof of the chicks. To determine whether the effect truly involved an increase in RNA synthesis, the activity of the brain RNA polymerase was measured *in vitro*. The activity of the enzyme isolated from the forebrain roof, but not the other brain regions tested, was increased in chicks that were imprinted. The relationship between *in vitro* RNA polymerase activity and *in vivo* RNA synthesis is not clear, since the former operates at only a small fraction of the rate of the latter, and many factors including availablility of template DNA affect *in vitro* polymerase activity. Nevertheless, this finding suggests that the increased uracil incorporation observed is not a precursor pool artifact and represents increased RNA synthesis. However, the effect may have been triggered by arousal or visual stimuli. It is also debatable whether imprinting is an appropriate model for learning. In fact, it has recently been shown that when one eye of a chick is exposed to an important stimulus (food), there is an increase in blood flow through the optic lobes and cerebral hemispheres contralateral to this eye.[29] This effect is independent of the intensity of the incident light.

The data discussed above on the possible role of RNA in learning and memory are inconclusive. On the one hand, it is clear that the significance of many reports must be reevaluated in the light of recent studies on RNA precursors. On the other hand, we cannot rule out the involvement of RNA in these processes; indeed, there are data which indicate such a role. We must also consider the possibility that the disturbances of nucleotide metabolism may be *caused* by changes in RNA metabolism. We may also ask why the concentration and composition of RNA and its synthesis from radioactive precursors are so sensitive to behavioral treatments. One possibility is that in the brain nucleotides may be extensively involved in the synthesis of carbohydrates, glycoproteins, glycolipids and lipids. High proportions of the free nucleotides of cytosine and uracil are found as nucleotide-carbohydrate derivatives. Another salient point is that many psychoactive drugs are analogues of bases or nucleotides. Orotic acid and UMP may affect learning,[30] as may nicotine and purine metabolites.[31] Answers to these questions will need much very careful research.

Protein

The classical metabolic role of RNA suggests that changes in RNA synthesis should be accompanied by changes in protein synthesis. While these have been sought extensively, changes in the rate of the incorporation of radioactive amino acids into protein correlated with learning have rarely been found. In an early study, Altman and Das observed an increase in the incorporation of [^{3}H]leucine into brain protein in exercised rats as compared to controls.[32] However, this effect was not apparent when the rats had been preadapted to the exercise. The authors interpreted the change to be a nonspecific reaction to the stress of the experience. In the rat a decreased [4,5-^{3}H]lysine incorporation was observed in response to exercise.[33] Changes of amino acid incorporation in response to light exposure were discussed on p. 191. Small increases of the incorporation of [^{3}H]leucine were also detected radioautographically in the neuronal nuclei of the hippocampus during avoidance conditioning of rats.[34]

Hydén reported that training rats in the handedness-reversal task, described above, also results in changes of protein synthesis in pyramidal cells of the CA3 region of the hippocampus on the side contralateral to the paw used.[35] The incorporation of [^{3}H]leucine into three specific acidic protein bands, including that due to S-100, separated by polyacrylamide microgel electrophoresis, was increased. This effect was not seen in animals that were completely familiar with the task (thirty days' training). In his earlier reports of this phenomenon, Hydén did not give any details of the effect observed on the total protein of the cells, nor of any proteins other than his three bands, so that we do not know whether the effects were selective. More recently using the same behavioral situation, he has reported increases of leucine incorporation into the total protein of large areas of entorhinal cortex and septum when both sides of the brain were pooled.[36] In other experiments performed in his laboratory, increases of specific radioactivity were detected in all subcellular fractions (except perikaryal mitochondria) of the hippocampus, but not of cerebral cortex.[37] Hydén has now reported than when *intraperitoneal* (rather than intracranial) injections of [^{3}H]leucine were used, training resulted in a *decreased* incorporation into protein of all brain regions, but the hippocampus was less affected than the other regions studied.[38] These results are very difficult to relate to the earlier ones and Hydén did not attempt it.

Rose observed an increase of [4,5-^{3}H]lysine incorporation into protein in the forebrain roof of chicks during imprinting. Thus the apparent change in RNA synthesis discussed above was in this case paralleled by an apparent increase in protein synthesis.[8] However, others have found that the response to imprinting stimuli is unimpaired by prior injection of inhibitors of protein synthesis (cycloheximide and puromycin).[39]

Some recent data may help to explain many of the earlier observations on the incorporation of amino acids into brain proteins in relation to behavioral experience. Using subcutaneously injected [4,5-^{3}H]lysine as a precursor, mice trained in an active avoidance situation showed increased incorporation into brain protein compared with quiet controls.[40] Similar effects were observed with [4,5-^{3}H]leucine and [1-^{14}C]leucine. The effect was not, however, specific for the training and could be elicited by exposure to the sound or electric footshock involved in the training procedure. The magnitude of the effect decreased markedly on successive days of training — especially in the liver, which also showed the biochemical response. These results display all the characteristics of a stress response, especially since the lysine incorporation decreases as the animal habituates to the stressful experience. Injection of ACTH into intact animals elicited a biochemical response similar to that of the behavioral treatments. However, mice that had had their adrenal glands removed also showed a response to footshock treatment. It is possible, therefore, that pituitary ACTH may change the incorporation of amino acids into both brain and liver proteins in the absence of intermediate adrenal activity.

These data are consistent with those of Altman and many of the other studies mentioned above. The important question is whether the biochemical effects are really nonspecific or incidental by-products of the stress. All learning involves an element of stress. The brain responds to novelty, which it interprets as stress, by secreting a hormone that prepares the body for stress. The fact that this hormone itself directly affects brain metabolism suggests a significance for the brain. The stress-induced secretions may function by adapting the brain to cope with the experience, just as they do for the other bodily organs. This could take the form of an increased readiness to process the information or store it as memory. In this view of learning, the brain has two functions: first, it acts as a receptor and integrator of sensory information, which, if determined as novel, results in a stress response leading to the secretion of ACTH; second, it adapts by storing the information of that experience, a process facilitated by the hormones released in the stress response.

Support for this concept comes from the work of De Wied.[41] Hypophysectomized rats (those that have had their pituitaries removed) do not generally learn as well as intact animals. De Wied has shown that the ability of hypophysectomized rats to learn normally may be restored by ACTH. This effect occurs even in adrenalectomized animals and thus cannot be attributed to adrenal steroids. It was also produced by $ACTH_{4-10}$, a heptapeptide fragment of ACTH which has no effect on the adrenals. Furthermore, ACTH facilitates the acquisition of one active avoidance task in intact rats. Biochemical sutdies have shown that the restored ability of hypophysectomized rats to learn is paralleled in the brain stem by a restoration to normal levels of RNA content, the proportion of ribosomes found as polyribosomes and the incorporation of amino acids into protein.[42] This suggests that the continued presence of ACTH may be necessary to maintain the brain in a state in which it can learn optimally.

Another pituitary peptide, lysine vasopressin, has an effect on learning similar to that of ACTH. Flexner, in his studies with mice, found that the puromycin-induced amnesia could be prevented by the administration of corticotrophin gel. Since purified ACTH was inactive but desglycinamide lysine vasopressin was active, he now considers the activity of the crude gel preparation to have been due to vasopressin contamination.[43]

Another effect may be accounted for by the activity of a pituitary peptide. It had been reported that the acquisition of a dark avoidance response could be transferred from a trained to a naive newt by transplanting the forebrain.[44] This effect has now been attributed to melanocyte stimulating hormone (MSH) secreted by the pituitary in the trained animals (see also p. 218). MSH is released by newts and many other animals, including rodents, in response to stress. The N-terminal amino acid sequences of β-MSH and ACTH are identical.

The choice of precursor amino acid and the mode of its administration are critical in studies of precursor incorporation into protein. Many amino acids have diverse functions especially in the brain, and many are poorly taken up by brain tissue. Leucine, a favorite precursor for the study of protein synthesis, is extensively metabolized to glutamate, aspartate and other catabolites, whether administered peripherally or intracerebrally. Tritiated compounds are frequently degraded to yield tritiated water. This effect is apparently largely peripheral (perhaps hepatic), since it is very small when tritiated compounds are administered intracerebrally. Degradation to water may be extensive: in mice, 40 percent of the ^3H found in the brain ten minutes after subcutaneous injection of $[4,5-^3H]$lysine is in water;[40] for $[5-^3H]$uridine the figure is 87 percent after forty-five minutes. If samples are dried, this tritiated water is not detected and it is not a problem since it is so diluted at the doses normally used that no detectable incorporation into macromolecules occurs. It is advisable not to use mixed (DL) isomers, as the catabolism of the D-isomer may confuse the results. Amino acids labeled with ^{14}C in only the 1-position (α-carboxyl carbon atom) are useful since catabolism normally involves decarboxylation with consequent loss of the radioactivity as $^{14}CO_2$.[45] Nevertheless, ^{14}C from L-$[1-^{14}C]$leucine is soon incorporated into a variety of other compounds. L-$[4,5-^3H]$lysine appears to be a good precursor. It is readily taken up into the brain following peripheral or central injections, and is rapidly incorporated into protein, probably because the free lysine pool of brain is small. Sixty minutes after subcutaneous or intraperitoneal injection, the radioactivity in the brain, aside from that in water, is essentially all in lysine either free or in protein.[33,40] These factors greatly simplify the necessary biochemical procedures and controls, and reduce the possibility of artifact.

It is desirable that the results of any radioactive tracer experiment be confirmed by an independent method. In the case of protein synthesis, examination of the proportion of ribosomes aggregated into polyribosomes is a useful adjunct.[5] The approach of seeking selective changes in particular protein species may partly counter problems of the precursor pool. In addition, it may indicate the actual proteins changed, and, presumably, therefore important to the experience. If proteins are made from the same pool at the same time, they should have the same specific radioactivity. However, the existence of separate metabolic compartments in the brain is a complicating factor. Glial and neuronal proteins from the same brain region may not be comparable since they do not share a common pool and could thus be differentially affected.

Glycoproteins, glycolipids and phosphoproteins

Since glycoproteins are located on the outer surface of neuronal plasma membranes, and synapses are especially rich in them, it has been speculated that they might play a role in behavioral adaptation. Glycoproteins need not be synthesized *de novo*, but carbohydrates might be added to preexisting proteins or the carbohydrate attachments of preexisting glycoproteins might be modified. Such simple modifications, which might rapidly be accomplished, could form the basis of short-term memory. Nevertheless, there are relatively few studies on glycoproteins in relation to learning. In a limited study, Bogoch reported the appearance of new glycoproteins in the brains of pigeons that had learned a discrimination task some months previously.[46] Other workers have not found alterations in the synthesis of glycoproteins from radioactive glucose or glucosamine during learning.[1,47] A recent study suggests that the synthesis of fucosyl glycoproteins is sensitive to the environment in a rather complex way. The odor of electrically footshocked mice stimulates the incorporation of $[^3H]$ fucose, whereas footshock itself decreases the incorporation. This effect was found not only in brain, but also in liver and plasma.[48]

The synaptic location of gangliosides and some of their other properties (see p. 89 and p. 147) has suggested a role in plasticity. Recently, an increase in the synthesis of gangliosides from $[1-^3H]$ glucosamine without a concomitant change in glycoproteins was detected in mice during avoidance training.[47]

Proteins may be phosphorylated in a simple one-step reaction. The phosphorylation will result in a marked change in the properties of the protein. This process could then produce a very rapid and relatively stable chemical change. A study of the phosphorylation of nuclear proteins during training revealed that the phosphorylation with radioactive phosphate of the nonhistone proteins of rat brain was increased, whereas that of the histones was decreased.[47] The increased phosphorylation occurred on serine residues of the nonhistone proteins and was also observed, without the use of radioisotopes, as an increased proportion of phosphorylated serine in the protein. However, the effect was not specific for learning and was observed whenever the rat was reexposed to many aspects of the training experience, but was not seen in similarly treated untrained rats.[49] These changes in phosphorylation could conceivably result in changes in gene expression.

An increased phosphorylation of synaptosomal proteins with radioactive phosphate was also observed in mice during active avoidance training.[47] The effect was seen only in the protein fraction of synaptosomes and not in any other subcellular fraction. Unlike the nuclear protein phosphorylation, the effect was apparently specific for a novel training experience. It is likely that both of these protein phosphorylation changes are initiated by cyclic AMP, since all the known cellular actions of cyclic AMP are mediated by changes of protein phosphorylation. The increased phosphorylation of synaptosomal proteins might well be associated with the effect of neurotransmitters on cyclic AMP metabolism (see p. 186).

Neurotransmitters

Interference with the activity of several neurotransmitters has been reported to impair learning. Since pathways involving most, if not all, neurotransmitters are likely to be involved in complex mental processes, this result is hardly unexpected. Depletion of catecholamines (e.g., with reserpine) has been shown to impair conditioned responses in the rat.[50] There also seems to be an increased turnover of norepinephrine associated with such responses. However, there is no indication that the catecholamines play any specific role in storing the memory of the conditioned responses. In contrast, high concentrations of serotonin may be amnestic, possibly by interfering with protein synthesis.[6] A more specific role in learning has been postulated for acetylcholine. Depending on the time adminstered after initial training, antagonists may facilitate or inhibit learning. Cholinergic antagonists may also block retention of training. Deutsch has interpreted these results to indicate the involvement of specific cholinergic synapses in learning.[51] Much more work is need to establish this, but even if confirmed, these data tell us little about the mechanisms involved in establishing memory.

iii) Memory transfer

There has been considerable interest over the last decade in the possibility that the memory of specific experiences might be transferred from one animal to another by pharmacological means. A large number of reports indicate that extracts from the brains of animals trained to perform particular tasks have the ability to confer the memory of the training on a second animal, sometimes even of a different species. Initially, workers in this field considered the active principle to be RNA, but more recently the emphasis has been on peptides that may have contaminated the RNA extracts. Ungar, the foremost proponent of this work, has published the sequence of an undecapeptide, scotophobin, extracted from the brains of rats trained to avoid the dark.[52] He has also reported that synthetic scotophobin is fully active. Considerable controversy surrounds these striking claims.[53]

Perhaps the most remarkable aspect of the transfer effect is the apparent ability of the active molecule to affect the brain following intraperitoneal or intracranial injections. If memory resides in specific molecules in specific cells in the brain, then the transport of the active molecule to its correct location is a remarkable feat. Ungar prefers to consider that scotophobin can specifically facilitate certain synapses, thus producing the "learning." It is important to realize that in these experiments one cannot demonstrate memory per se, but only infer its presence from an alteration of behavior or an increased rate of learning of the task. The nature of Ungar's training paradigm and the fact that scotophobin is a peptide suggest that it might be a physiological hormone with a behavioral effect far less specific than that claimed. Indeed, it has recently been reported that α-melanocyte stimulating hormone (α-MSH) can induce a similar behavioral response in axolotls, and that this effect explains previously reported transfer effects in this animal (P. P. Giorgi and D. Samuel, unpublished observations). Ungar has indicated the transfer of a number of different responses in several species and that the peptide factors involved are different, but he has not yet published sufficient details of these other effects to allow assessment of this important claim.

C. ENVIRONMENTAL ENRICHMENT

Many workers have compared the effect of enriched or impoverished environments on morphological and neurochemical parameters. Essentially, an enriched environment comprises many animals in a cage, with many toys and ample exposure to visual, auditory and social stimulation. Deprived or impoverished animals are kept either alone or in pairs in dark, otherwise empty cages, in quiet settings. It is presumed that the animals reared in an enriched environment will be exposed to more stimuli and learn more.

Pronounced behavioral, morphological and biochemical differences have been noted after exposure of the rats to these different environments for several weeks following weaning. Rats raised in enriched environments learned behavioral tasks more readily and displayed increased cortical weight and thickness.[54] This latter effect was explained by an increase in the number of glial cells with no change in the number of neurons. The total *amount* of cortical DNA, RNA and protein was increased, but while the DNA *concentration* was decreased slightly, there was no change in the RNA or protein concentration. Thus the increase of the RNA:DNA ratio was a rather sensitive index of the change. These results were interpreted to indicate an increase in the mean size of cells together with a small increase in the number of glial cells in the enriched animals.

The incorporation of precursors into RNA was not different in the two groups of animals, but recent data show that an increased proportion of the DNA is hybridizable to the brain RNA from environmentally enriched animals.[55] This may indicate increased gene expression. In rats exposed to the enriched environment for seven days following weaning, the incorporation of amino acids into protein in all subcellular fractions of both hippocampus and cortex was increased relative to environmentally impoverished controls.[56] No changes in specific proteins of hippocampal nuclei or synaptosomes were detected by gel electrophoresis. At later times increased amino acid incorporation was confined to synaptosomal fractions. The changes in synaptosomes were paralleled by morphological changes, detectable in the electron microscope. In the third layer of the cortex of enriched animals, the number of synaptic thickenings was decreased but the average length of the thickening was increased.[57] The calculated net effect was a larger total area of synaptic contact. An increased dendritic branching has also been reported in occipital cortex using Golgi staining.[58] In environmentally enriched rats, both cholinesterase and acetylcholinesterase activities were increased in cortical and subcortical regions, but no change was observed in hexokinase.[54]

The relationship of these observations to the learning process is difficult to evaluate. Some of them at least are apparently reversible, although environmentally enriched animals do not return to the levels of the impoverished ones. The effects are apparently not due to stress, nor solely to visual stimulation, since blinded animals also respond to an enriched environment. However, it is possible that effects are mediated by the endocrine system, though they are still found in hypophysectomized rats.[54]

D. AFFECTIVE DISORDERS AND SCHIZOPHRENIA

There have been many attempts to associate mental or nervous disorders with defects of the metabolism or function of specific neurotransmitters. Notable in this respect are the association of certain defective dopaminergic pathways with Parkinson's disease and the recent finding of a deficiency in GABA metabolism in Huntington's chorea (p. 143). Likewise, the biogenic amines have been associated with the affective disorders, mania and depression. Most of the brain neurons containing the catecholamines have their cell bodies in the brain stem. Their axons descend into the caudal stem and spinal cord and ascend ventrally to the mesencephalon, diencephalon and cortex.[59] There are two major ascending noradrenergic pathways in the brain, both of which originate in the medulla and pons. The ventral pathway innervates mainly the hypothalamus and the preoptic area, while the dorsal pathway, which originates in the locus coeruleus, innervates the cortex and hippocampus. Similarly, there are two principal dopaminergic pathways: the nigrostriatal pathway referred to above, and a mesolimbic pathway which originates in the mesencephalon and runs rostrally to innervate the nucleus accumbens and the olfactory tubercle. The serotonin-containing fibers originate in the Raphé areas and run rostrally in the medial forebrain bundle to the septum and amygdala.[59] All three amines have been implicated in the affective disorders, but the best evidence relates to norepinephrine.

The catecholamine theory of affective disorders suggests that depression is associated with a deficit of norepinephrine, and mania with an NE surfeit. The evidence arises primarily from the clinical effects of several drugs:

1. Monamine oxidase inhibitors, which elevate brain concentrations of amines, are antidepressants.

2. The depressant drug reserpine depletes both norepinephrine and serotonin, but the depressant effects of reserpine can be reversed by DOPA.

3. The tricyclic antidepressants (e.g., amitryptyline) block the re-uptake of NE and thus potentiate its action.

4. The amphetamines, which are stimulants, potentiate NE activity, possibly in several different ways.

5. The anti-manic drug lithium may facilitate re-uptake of NE.

Thus, in all cases, drugs that are antagonistic to NE are depressant especially in mania, and those that potentiate NE alleviate depression. Though this evidence favors an important role for norepinephrine, it is likely that serotonin may also be involved.[60] Whether or not the gross activity state of these amines plays any role in regulating mood in "normal" individuals remains to be determined.

The chemistry of schizophrenia is very much confused. Older theories concentrated on the hallucinatory aspects and postulated the formation of hallucinogenic substances in the brains of schizophrenics.[61] However, hallucinations are not omnipresent in schizophrenia and when present are more often auditory than visual like those induced by the known hallucinogens. There have been numerous reports of unusual substances in the urine of schizophrenics, notably indoleamine derivatives, but none of these has ultimately been found to correlate well with schizophrenia.[61] Most researchers now believe that the catecholamines are involved. A favorite theory is that there is a defect in the dopamine pathways. This is based on the finding that phenothiazines, which are the best drugs for the treatment of schizophrenia, increase dopamine turnover and that there is a good correlation among the various phenothiazines between this activity and their therapeutic value. Moreover, several antipsychotic drugs cause an increase in the CSF of homovanillic acid, a catabolite of DA.[62] Stein, however, has postulated that the primary defect in schizophrenics is in the catecholamine pathways involved in reward. He argues that schizophrenia is due to a lack of directed drive, and has convincingly shown that norepinephrine is involved in self-stimulation, regarded as a model system for the study of reward. More recently, he has extended these findings to show that human schizophrenics are deficient in dopamine-β-hydroxylase, the last enzyme in the pathway for the formation of NE.[63] There was no deficiency in monamine oxidase or catechol-O-methyl transferase, but choline acetylase was also decreased. It is possible that both theories are correct and that blockade of DA is the best way to correct the imbalance caused by the deficiency of NE. The involvement of NE in reward systems would explain its implication in many behavioral studies, e.g., those in learning and memory (p. 217).

E. SLEEP

Despite the apparent necessity in mammals for prolonged periods of sleep, its physiological role is still largely a matter of speculation; it is apparently unnecessary for regenerative or repair processes of the body. It seems most likely that sleep fulfills a requirement of the central nervous system because it occurs only in animals that have a highly developed central nervous system, because it principally affects CNS function, and because it is associated with distinctive neurophysiological activity (EEG) in the brain.

Biochemical studies of sleep are somewhat meager, partly because of the difficulty of conducting experiments. Moreover, the significance of many of the biochemical studies of sleep is hard to evaluate because of its apparent heterogeneous nature. Electrophysiologically, there are two major states of sleep: slow-wave sleep and paradoxical (REM) sleep. Paradoxical sleep is an electrophysiologically hyperactive state associated with rapid eye movements (hence REM) and certain characteristic alterations of muscular tone. It is probable that the biochemistry associated with these two sleep states is distinct, and that biochemical analyses need to be correlated with concurrent electrophysiological recordings.

Early physiological studies revealed the surprising fact that the metabolic rate of the brain is not significantly depressed during sleep; the rates of oxygen consumption and glucose oxidation were not measurably altered. Now that sleep states can be distinguished, it seems that there is probably a slight decrease in the metabolic rate during slow-wave sleep, but an increase during REM sleep. These observations underline the close association between cerebral metabolic rate and electrophysiological activity. The state of the high-energy metabolites of the brain during sleep is controversial. A general consensus indicates that during sleep there are small increases in the ratio of ATP to ADP and in the concentration of creatine phosphate, but it has not been established whether the measured differences reflect the real situation *in vivo,* or whether the cerebral metabolism of sleeping animals responds more slowly to the shock of the killing procedures. The idea that sleep is characterized by increased cerebral anabolic activity has received some support. The diurnal rhythm in the incorporation of radioactive lysine into brain protein in rats peaks early in the sleep period.[64] However, the peak concentration of brain nuclear RNA, RNA polymerase activity and the incorporation of $[^3H]$uridine into RNA occurs in the waking part of the cycle.[65] During sleep the activity of succinoxidase is increased in neurons of the caudal reticular formation, with a reciprocal decrease in the glial activity of the enzyme.[19]

An increased incorporation of radioactive phosphate into protein has been observed in immature and adult rats during sleep. This effect has been attributed to an increase in a specific phosphoprotein in which the phosphate is probably linked to a histidine residue. The significance of these results is now difficult to evaluate, since the increased incorporation of ^{32}P did not occur when the rats had been acclimatized to the apparatus in which they were allowed to sleep.[66]

There has been some interest in the presence of sleep-inducing substances in the CSF and cerebral venous blood. Classical studies, including parabiosis, had indicated the presence of such substances, but the results have not always been confirmed. The most well-developed series of experiments are those of Pappenheimer[67] and Monnier.[68] Pappenheimer has shown that the CSF of sleep-deprived goats is soporific when infused intraventricularly into goats or rats. The active substance (Factor S) is dialyzable and is not identifiable with serotonin, GABA, glutamate, γ-hydroxybutyrate, butyrolactone, or cyclic 3′,5′AMP.[67] The CSF apparently also contains another active principal, Factor E, which is excitatory and probably a peptide. Pappenheimer suggests that sleep and wakefulness are balanced by the activity of these two factors. Monnier has isolated a Delta factor from the CSF or cerebral venous blood of rabbits following electrical stimulation of hypothalmic "sleep centers." The Delta factor is also soporific on intraventricular infusion and its chemical identity has been vigorously pursued. It appears to be a peptide containing approximately seven amino acids.[68]

It is not clear how these sleep factors relate to the elegant neurophysiological studies of Jouvet[69,70] and others. This work has indicated a close relationship between serotonin and sleep in cats. Lesions of the Raphé nuclei in the brain stem cause insomnia. The Raphé nuclei contain more than 90 percent of the brain serotonin and depression of this neurotransmitter with p-chlorophenylalanine (pCPA) is also insomnic. Slow-wave sleep is affected more than REM sleep. If the pCPA block is circumvented by administering 5-hydroxytryptophan, sleep returns. Jouvet showed that there is a good correlation between the serotonin concentration in the Raphé nuclei and sleep during both the depletion and the recovery phases.[69] However, other workers have reported that when pCPA is administered chronically the ability to sleep is recovered without a concomitant rise in serotonin.[71]

Wakefulness is affected by catecholamines. The drug α-methyl-p-tyrosine (αMpT), which blocks catecholamine synthesis, causes decreased activity and wakefulness. These defects are all reversed by administration of DOPA. Amphetamines which normally increase activity are ineffective in the presence of αMpT. Reserpine, which also depletes catecholamines, depresses activity as well. An oversimplified generalization is that wakefulness is promoted by catecholamines and sleep by serotonin.[70]

REM sleep may also involve catecholaminergic pathways. Jouvet has shown that locus coeruleus lesions in the cat suppress REM sleep and deplete forebrain norepinephrine. It is important to realize that REM sleep is to some extent dependent on slow-wave sleep, which always precedes REM sleep, so that the amount and proportion of REM sleep is not independent of the amount of slow-wave sleep.[70] Jouvet has found that lesions of certain nuclei within the Raphé area suppress REM sleep, whereas others have no effect. He suggests that REM sleep is under the control of serotoninergic, catecholaminergic and cholinergic mechanisms. In such a complex system it is obviously impossible to interpret the effects of the often conflicting results of gross pharmacological manipulations (e.g., the suppression of REM sleep by MAO inhibitors).

Jouvet has been criticized for the nonspecificity of his rather large lesions and for his simplistic approach. The latter criticism is unfair, since the existence of a clearly defined hypothesis has both stimulated research in the area and provided experimentally testable deductions. A most important piece of evidence for his theories would be the demonstration that stimulation of the Raphé nuclei augments slow-wave sleep, and that stimulation of the locus coeruleus augments REM sleep.

Unfortunately, the results that have been obtained from the cat do not seem to apply to other experimental animals and man. In humans catecholamines appear to suppress and serotonin appears to augment REM sleep.[72] Hopefully, improved techniques, including localized application of drugs and more discrete stimulation, will resolve these problems.

CHAPTER 8 REFERENCES

Literature Cited

1. Entingh, D., Dunn, A., Wilson, J. E., Glassman, E., and Damstra-Entingh, T. Biochemical approaches to the biological basis of memory. In *Handbook of Psychobiology* (Ed. M. S. Gazzaniga and C. Blakemore), Academic Press, New York, 1974.
2. Horn, G., Rose, S. P. R., and Bateson, P. P. G. Experience and plasticity in the central nervous system. Is the nervous system modified by experience? Are such modifications involved in learning? *Science* 181:506–14, 1973.
3. McGaugh, J. L., and Dawson, R. G. Modification of memory storage processes. *Behav. Sci.* 16:45–63, 1971.
4. Deutsch, J. A. Electroconvulsive shock and memory. In *The Physiological Basis of Memory*, Academic Press, New York, 1973, pp. 113–24.
5. Dunn, A., Guiditta, A., Wilson, J. E., and Glassman, E. The effect of electroshock on brain RNA and protein synthesis and its possible relationship to behavioral effects. In *The Psychobiology of Convulsive Therapy* (Ed. M. Fink, J. McGaugh, S. Kety, and T. A. Williams), Winston & Sons, Washington, D.C., 1974, pp. 185–97.
6. Essman, W. B. *Neurochemistry of Cerebral Electroshock*, Spectrum Publications, Flushing, NY., 1973.
7. Aleksandrovskaya, M. M., and Kruglikov, R. I. Effect of electroshock on memory and glio-neuronal relationships in rat brain. *Dokl. Akad. Nauk. SSSR* 197:1216–17, 1971.
8. Chapouthier, G. Behavioral studies of the molecular basis of memory. In *The Physiological Basis of Memory* (Ed. J. A. Deutsch), Academic Press, New York, 1973, pp. 1–25.
9. Flood, J. F., Bennett, E. L., Rosenzweig, M. R., and Orme, A. E. The influence of duration of protein synthesis inhibition on memory. *Physiol. Behav.* 10:555–62, 1973.
10. Barondes, S. H., and Cohen, H. D. Delayed and sustained effect of acetoxylcyclohex-imide on memory in mice. *Proc. Nat. Acad. Sci., U.S.A.* 58:157–64, 1967.
11. MacInnes, J. W., Luttges, M. W. Interaction of puromycin and cycloheximide with electroconvulsive shock in producing alterations of brain polyribosomes. *J. Neurochem.* 19:2889–92, 1972.

VIII. The Biochemical Basis of Behavior

12. Mark, R. F., and Watts, M. E. Drug inhibition of memory formation in chickens. *Proc. R. Soc. Lond. B.* 178:439–64, 1971.
13. Glassman, E. The biochemistry of learning: an evaluation of the role of RNA and protein. *Ann. Rev. Biochem.* 38:605–46, 1969.
14. Thut, P. D., Hruska, R. E., Kelter, A., Mizne, J., and Lindell, T. J. The effect of α-amanitin on passive and active avoidance acquisition in mice. *Psychopharmacologia* 30:355–68, 1973.
15. Neale, J. H., Klinger, P. D., and Agranoff, B. W. Camptothecin blocks memory of conditioned avoidance in the goldfish. *Science* 179:1243–45, 1973.
16. Dawson, R. G., and McGaugh, J. L. Drug facilitation of learning and memory. In *The Physiological Basis of Memory* (Ed. J. A. Deutsch), Academic Press, New York, 1973, pp. 77–111.
17. Bohus, B., Ader, R. and de Wied, D. Effects of vasopressin on active and passive avoidance behavior. *Hormones and Behavior* 3:191–97, 1972.
18. Nasello, A. K., and Izquierdo, I. Effect of learning and of drugs on the ribonucleic acid concentration of brain structures of the rat. *Exptl. Neurol.* 23:521–28, 1969.
19. Hydén, H. Biochemical changes accompanying learning. In *The Neurosiences, A Study Program* (Ed. G. C. Quarton, T. Melnechuk and F. O. Schmitt), Rockefeller University Press, New York, 1967, pp. 765–71.
20. Jarlstedt, J. Functional localization in the cerebellar cortex studied by quantitative determination of Purkinje cell RNA. *Acta Physiol. Scand.* 67:Suppl. 271, pp. 1–24, 1966.
21. Rose, S. P. R. In *Applied Neurochemistry* (Ed. A. N. Davison and J. Dobbing), Blackwell Scientific Publications, Oxford, 1968, p. 351.
22. Entingh, D., Damstra-Entingh, T., Dunn, A., Wilson, J. E. and Glassman, E. Brain uridine monophosphate: reduced incorporation of uridine during avoidance learning. *Brain Research* 70:131–38, 1974.
23. Uphouse, L. L., MacInnes, J. W. and Schlesinger, K. Effects of conditioned avoidance training on polyribosomes of mouse brain. *Physiol. Behav.* 8:1013–18, 1972.
24. Shashoua, V. E. RNA metabolism in goldfish brain during acquisition of new behavioral patterns. *Proc. Nat. Acad. Sci., U.S.A.* 65:160–67, 1970.
25. Baskin, F., Masiarz, F. R., and Agranoff, B. W. Effect of various stresses on the incorporation of [^{3}H]orotic acid into goldfish brain RNA. *Brain Research* 39:151–62, 1972.
26. Izquierdo, I. Hippocampal physiology: experiments on regulation of its electrical activity, on the mechanism of seizures, and on a hypothesis of learning. *Behav. Biol.* 7:669–98, 1972.
27. Bishop, J. O. Interpretation of DNA-RNA hybridization data. *Nature* 224:600–03, 1969.
28. Bateson, P. P. G., Horn, G. and Rose, S. P. R. Effects of early experience on regional incorporation precursors into RNA and protein in the chick brain. *Brain Research* 39:449–65, 1972.
29. Bondy, S. C., Lehman, R. A. and Purdy, J. L. Visual attention affects brain blood flow. *Nature* 248:440–41, 1974.
30. Matthies, H. Biochemical regulation of synaptic connectivity. In *Memory and Transfer of Information* (Ed. H. P. Zippel). Plenum Press, New York, 1973, pp. 531–47.
31. Essman, W. B. Drug effects and learning and memory processes. *Adv. Pharmacol. Chemotherapy.* 9:241–330, 1972.
32. Altman, J., and Das, G. D. Behavioral manipulations and protein metabolism of the brain: effects of motor exercise on the utilization of leucine-H^3. *Physiol. Behav.* 1:105–08, 1966.

33. Tiplady, B. Brain protein metabolism and environmental stimulation, effects of forced exercise. *Brain Research* 43:215–25, 1972.
34. Beach, G., Emmens, M., Kimble, D. P., and Lickey, M. Autoradiographic demonstration of biochemical changes in the limbic system during avoidance training. *Proc. Nat. Acad. Sci., U.S.A.* 62:692–96, 1969.
35. Hydén, H., and Lange, P. W. Protein changes in nerve cells related to learning and conditioning. In *The Neurosciences, Second Study Program* (Ed. F. O. Schmitt), Rockefeller University Press, New York, 1970, pp. 278–89.
36. Hydén, H., and Lange, P. W. Protein synthesis in limbic structures during change in behavior. *Brain Research* 22:423–25, 1970.
37. Levitan, I. B., Ramirez, G., and Mushynski, W. E. Amino acid incorporation in the brains of rats trained to use the non-preferred paw in retrieving food. *Brain Research* 47:147–56, 1972.
38. Hydén, H., and Lange, P. W. Protein changes in different brain areas as a function of intermittent training. *Proc. Nat. Acad. Sci., U.S.A.* 69:1980–84, 1972.
39. Gervai, J., and Csányi, V. The effects of protein synthesis inhibitors on imprinting. *Brain Research* 53:151–60, 1973.
40. Rees, H. D., Brogan, L. L., Entingh, D. J., Dunn, A. J., Shinkman, P. G., Damstra-Entingh, T., Wilson, J. E., and Glassman, E. Effect of sensory stimulation on the uptake and incorporation of radioactive lysine into protein of mouse brain and liver. *Brain Research* 68:143–56, 1974.
41. de Wied, D. Pituitary-adrenal system hormones and behavior. In *The Neurosciences, Third Study Program* (Ed. F. O. Schmitt and F. G. Worden), M.I.T. Press, Cambridge, Mass., 1974, pp. 653–66.
42. Gispen, W. H., and Schotman, P. Pituitary-adrenal system, learning and performance: some neurochemical aspects. *Prog. Brain Res.* 39:453–58, 1973.
43. Lande, S., Flexner, J. B., and Flexner, L. B. Effect of corticotropin and desglycinamide[9]-lysine vasopressin on suppression of memory by puromycin. *Proc. Nat. Acad. Sci., U.S.A.* 69:558–60, 1972.
44. Hershkowitz, M., Segal, M., and Samuel, D. The acquisition of dark avoidance by transplantation of the forebrain of trained newts *(Pleurodeles waltl)*. *Brain Research* 48:366–69, 1972.
45. Banker, G., and Cotman, C. W. Characteristics of different amino acids as protein precursors in mouse brain: advantages of certain carboxyl-labeled amino acids. *Arch. Biochem. Biophys.* 142:565–73, 1971.
46. Bogoch, S. Brain glycoproteins and learning: new studies supporting the "sign-post" theory. In *Current Biochemical Approaches to Learning and Memory*, (Ed. W. B. Essman and S. Nakajima) Spectrum Publications, New York, 1973, pp. 147–57.
47. Dunn, A., Entingh, D., Entingh, T., Gispen, W. H., Machlus, B., Perumal, R., Rees, H. D. and Brogan, L. Biochemical correlates of brief behavioral experiences. In *The Neurosciences, Third Study Program* (Ed. F. O. Schmitt and F. G. Worden), M.I.T. Press, Cambridge, Mass., 1974, pp. 679–84.
48. Damstra-Entingh, T., Entingh, D., Wilson, J. E. and Glassman, E. Environmental stimulation and fucose incorporation into brain and liver glycoproteins. *Pharmacol. Biochem. Behav.* 2:73–8, 1974.
49. Machlus, B., Entingh, D., Wilson, J. E., and Glassman, E. Brain Phosphoproteins: the effect of various behaviors and reminding experiences on the incorporation of radioactive phosphate into nuclear proteins. *Behav. Biol.* 10:63–74, 1974.

50. Seiden, L. S., Brown, R. M., and Lewy, A. J. Brain catecholamines and conditioned behavior: mutual interactions. In *Chemical Modulation of Brain Function* (Ed. H. C. Sabelli), Raven Press, New York, 1973, pp. 261–75.
51. Deutsch, J. A. The cholinergic synapse and the site of memory. In *The Physiological Basis of Memory*, Academic Press, New York, 1973, pp. 59–76.
52. Ungar, G. Evidence for molecular coding of neural information. In *Memory and Transfer of Information* (Ed. H. P. Zippel), Plenum Press, New York, 1973, pp. 317–41.
53. Stewart, W. W. Comments on the chemistry of scotophobin. *Nature* 238:202–9, 1972.
54. Rosenzweig, M. R., Bennett, E. L., and Diamond, M. C. Chemical and anatomical plasticity of brain: replications and extensions, 1970. In *Macromolecules and Behavior*, 2nd ed. (Ed. J. Gaito), Appleton-Century-Crofts, New York, 1972, pp. 205–77.
55. Uphouse, L. L. *Developmental Psychobiology*, in press.
56. Levitan, I. B., Mushynski, W. E., and Ramirez, G. Effects of environmental complexity on amino acid incorporation into rat cortex and hippocampus *in vivo*. *J. Neurochem.* 19:2621–30, 1972.
57. Møllgard, K., Diamond, M. C., Bennett, E. L., Rosenzweig, M. R., and Lindner, B. Quantitative synaptic changes with differential experience in rat brain. *Int. J. Neurosci.* 2:113–27, 1971.
58. Volkmar, F. R., and Greenough, W. T. Rearing complexity affects branching of dendrites in visual cortex of the rat. *Science* 176:1445–47, 1972.
59. Ungerstedt, U. Stereotaxic mapping of the monoamine pathways in the rat brain. *Acta. Physiol. Scand.* 82(Suppl. 367):1–48, 1971.
60. Kety, S. S. Brain amines and affective disorders. In *Brain Chemistry and Mental Disease* (Ed. B. T. Ho and W. M. McIsaac), Plenum Press, New York, 1971, pp. 237–44.
61. Denber, H. C. B. Some current biochemical theories concerning schizophrenia. In *Biochemistry of Brain and Behavior* (Ed. R. E. Bowman, and S. P. Datta), Plenum Press, New York, 1970, pp. 171–205.
62. Matthysse, S. Schizophrenia: relationship to dopamine transmission, motor control, and feature extraction. In *The Neurosciences, Third Study Program* (Ed. F. O. Schmitt and F. G. Worden), M.I.T. Press, Cambridge, Mass., 1974, pp. 733–37.
63. Wise, C. D., and Stein, L. Dopamine-β-hydroxylase deficits in the brains of schizophrenic patients. *Science* 181:344–47, 1973.
64. Richardson, K., and Rose, S. P. R. A diurnal rhythmicity in incorporation of lysine into rat brain regions. *Nature, New Biol.* 233:182–84, 1971.
65. Merritt, J. H., and Sulkowski, T. S. Rhythmicity of RNA polymerase activity and RNA levels in nuclei of rat cerebral cortex. *J. Neurochem.* 17:1327–28, 1970.
66. Reich, P., Geyer, S. J., Steinbaum, L., Anchors, M., and Karnovsky, M. L. Incorporation of phosphate into rat brain during sleep and wakefulness. *J. Neurochem.* 20:1195–205, 1973.
67. Pappenheimer, J. R., Miller, T. B., and Goodrich, C. A. Sleep-promoting effects of cerebrospinal fluid from sleep-deprived goats. *Proc. Nat. Acad. Sci., U.S.A.* 58:513–17, 1967.
68. Schoenenberger, G. A., Cueni, L. B., Monnier, M., and Hatt, A. M. Humoral transmission of sleep. VII. Isolation and physical-chemical characterization of the "sleep inducing factor delta." *Pflugers Arch.* 338:1–17, 1972.
69. Jouvet, M. Biogenic amines and the states of sleep. *Science* 163:32–41, 1969.
70. Jouvet, M. The role of monoamines and acetylcholine-containing neurons in the regulation of the sleep-waking cycle. *Erg. der Physiol.* 64:165–307, 1972.

71. Barchas, J., Dement, W., Ferguson, J., Cohen, H., and Henriksen, S. Effect of chronic treatment with parachlorophenylalanine (PCPA) on brain serotonin and behavior. *Fed. Proc.* 29:747 Abs., 1970.
72. Wyatt, R. J. *et al.* Brain catecholamines and human sleep. *Nature* 233:63–65, 1971.

IX. Development of the Brain

Maturation of the brain involves the appearance of a specialized chemistry and morphology in tissue that embryonically appears rather undifferentiated.

The development of the brain occurs as a complex sequence of highly coordinated events.[1] Figure 9.1 illustrates the sequence for the chick; the general pattern is similar for other species. Several factors interact in establishing the ultimate level of efficacy that is attained by the mature brain. These can be grouped as genetic, humoral and impulse-related factors.

Early development

The division of cells destined to become neurons ceases early in neurogenesis. These neuroblasts then undergo a series of complex migrations that are genetically determined. At the end of this phase, extensive outgrowth of neuronal processes occurs. These young neurons already display an enhanced capacity to accumulate K^+. The metabolism of nerve tissue changes from glycolytic to aerobic, while the concentrations of cytochrome oxidase and succinic dehydrogenase rise.

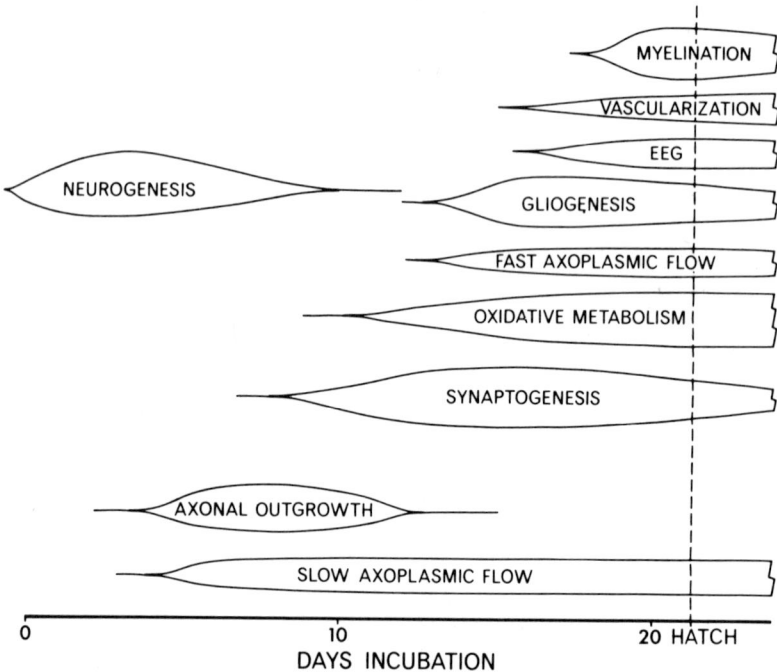

Figure 9.1 Relative time of appearance of various properties of chick brain.

The middle stage of development

The concentration of many components characteristic of nerve tissue rises sharply. Such components include the glial-specific S-100 protein, the neuronal-specific 14.3.2 protein and many enzymes associated with neurotransmitter metabolism, including acetylcholinesterase, choline acetylase, monoamine oxidase and glutamic acid decarboxylase. The intracellular concentration of glutamic, aspartic and γ-aminobutyric acids rises, while that of most free amino acids decreases. The concentration of neurotransmitters such as acetylcholine, norepinephrine and dopamine also rises, as does that of gangliosides. The character of the gangliosides changes as well, since young brain is higher in G_{T1} and G_{D1b} and lower in G_{D1a} and G_{M1} than mature brain.

These changes coincide with critical morphological and physiological developments such as the appearance of mature synapses and spontaneous electrical activity within neurons. The ability of prostaglandin E_1 or adenosine to elevate intracellular cyclic AMP levels in rat brain cell suspensions appears at this time.

The pentose phosphate pathway appears to be maximally active in immature tissue, and several enzymes associated with this pathway, such as glucose-6-phosphate dehydrogenase, decline as maturation proceeds.

Later development

As the rate of cell division and the outgrowth of processes falls, the rates of DNA, RNA and protein synthesis also fall. During early development the brain is supplied with nutrients largely by diffusion. The growing brain becomes increasingly dependent on its vascular supply and capillaries rapidly invade the nervous tissue mass. Initially, substances can readily pass from the capillaries into the brain, but later the ability of many compounds to be transported from the blood is severely reduced. The appearance of a blood-brain barrier coincides with astroglial maturation. It is around this time that metabolic compartmentation (p. 47) becomes increasingly apparent in the brain. In most species, during development, the dry weight of the brain increases from 10 percent to approximately 20 percent of the wet weight.

The enzymes involved in the formation and breakdown of myelin constituents appear relatively late. These include enzymes of cerebroside and sulfatide metabolism. Immature myelin significantly differs in composition from adult myelin.

A. GENETIC FACTORS

The genetic potential of the developing brain underlies its ultimate possibilities and sets limits on the effect of the other factors that may influence cerebral development. Tissue culture studies have shown that much of the early differentiation of the neuron is genetically preprogrammed and can take place independently of the influences of bodily hormones.

Embryonic brain cells derived from neurological mutants may show abnormal development in tissue culture (p. 158). Many severe neurological diseases of humans have a genetic origin. Such diseases may be characterized by the absence or deficiency of key synthetic or (more frequently) degradative enzymes. Ultimately, abnormalities may occur in the microscopic appearance and chemical composition of the brain, though this need not necessarily occur. Some genetic disorders may involve malfunction of the whole body and nerve tissue may be affected to a variable extent. Defects may involve the faulty metabolism of a wide range of chemicals including specific amino acids, carbohydrates, porphyrins, mucopolysaccharides or nucleotides. These may secondarily result in varying degrees of mental retardation. For example, porphyria is an autosomal genetic disease characterized by an overproduction in the liver of δ-aminolevulinic acid. This molecule is a porphyrin precursor whose high concentration in the plasma causes central autonomic and peripheral neuropathy. Another class of genetic disorders involves the disturbed metabolism of compounds largely or solely confined to nerve tissue (such as constituents of myelin). In such cases, the nervous system is the primary target and effects on nonnervous tissue may be secondary. However, the secondary lesions may be more striking than the primary defect. Several diseases involving dystrophy of muscle tissue are thought to be of neuronal origin and caused by the imperfect supply of materials along the axon to the muscle. The locus of the genetic defect leading to the wasting of the muscle may then originate in the spinal cord.

Glycosphingolipid metabolism is especially vulnerable to genetic errors. In humans an enzyme deficiency mutation is known for almost every step in the degradative pathway of these compounds (Figure 4.8). No effective treatment exists at present for defects with their focal origin within nerve tissue. However, several genetic diseases affecting amino acid or carbohydrate metabolism can be treated by dietary modification. Examples of this are phenylketonuria (p. 31) and galactosemia, which involves a galactose-1-phosphate uridyl transfererase deficiency. Thus galactosemic patients are unable to effectively metabolize galactose which may, if ingested in sufficient amounts, cause toxic symptoms.[2] However, if such patients are maintained on a galactose-low diet (by restriction of milk and milk-product foods), toxic symptoms can be completely avoided. In both diseases the developing brain is the most vulnerable. Galactosemia, if untreated, will lead to severe brain damage, as well as damage to a variety of other organs such as the kidney, the liver and the eye.

The Lesch-Nyhan syndrome is a sex-linked recessive disease occuring only in males. The defect is the absence of an enzyme involved in purine metabolism: hypoxanthine-phosphoribosyl transferase. This enzyme converts the purine bases hypoxanthine and guanine to the nucleotides by the addition of ribose phosphate (Figure 2.10). Clinical features of Lesch-Nyhan syndrome include mental retardation, the passing of uric acid stones through the urinary tract, arthritis and nephropathy. Patients exhibit a very characteristic self-mutilating and aggressive behavior. When freed from restraint, they appear terrified and may inflict painful injury on themselves. The relationship between this sterotyped behavior and the biochemical lesion is unknown. It is interesting that individuals with only 5 percent of the normal level of hypoxanthine-phosphoribosyl transferase, while suffering from many clinical manifestations of Lesch-Nyhan disease, do not exhibit neurological or behavioral abnormality.[3]

Uric acid metabolism is also related to intellectual function. A number of studies have found a significant correlation between serum uric acid levels and higher cerebral functions such as intelligence and mental ability. Gout is a disease characterized by uric acid deposition in the bones. The precise enzyme abnormality leading to gout is not known. Probably a variety of defects involving excessive production or decreased breakdown of uric acid cause the disease. The incidence of gout among prominent men appears to be considerably greater than that in the whole population (where it occurs in about 1 in 2000 people).

Many genetic abnormalities have recently been found to involve a microscopically demonstrable deviance from the normal chromosomal complement. Mental retardation or abnormality is almost universally found in individuals with aberrant chromosomes—perhaps because cerebral differentiation depends on genes from all the chromosomes. Down's syndrome, or mongolism, is the most common autosomal abnormality, occurring in about 1 per 700 live births. This disease is characterized by the presence of forty-seven rather than the usual forty-six chromosomes and a variety of anomalies including severe mental retardation.[4] However, no major diagnostic neuropathological picture is found. Such an abnormality of a significant fraction of the total genome may result in multiple enzyme defects and there may be an abnormal enzyme profile rather than the absence of specific enzymes.

Genetic composition can also affect cerebral performance in a more subtle way. There is evidence that crossbred lines of rats have more intellectual capacity than the inbred laboratory strains, which are less genetically heterogeneous.

B. HUMORAL FACTORS

Early in embryogenesis, endocrine glands become active in the secretion of hormones, and these may dramatically influence cerebral differentiation.[5]

It is during development that the brain is most vulnerable to the hormonal and nutritional milieu. The relationship between thyroid hormone (thyroxin) and the brain is somewhat unusual. In most tissues, the major effect of thyroxin is the quantitative modulation of the metabolic activity. However, in the brain the major effect of thyroxin is to enable appropriate cerebral development to occur. In the rat, thyroidectomy at birth leads to a reduced rate of brain growth. At the cellular level, this appears as a failure of normal protein accretion, and a severe retardation of myelination and dendritic arborization.[5] As a result, neuronal perikarya are unusually densely packed and there is a reduced number of axo-dendritic synapses. The deficit can be reversed initially by thyroxin administration, but soon becomes irreversible. Neurophysiological and behavioral impairment is manifested by a delay in the development of evoked electrical responses and maze-learning ability. Thyroid hormone deficiency in the young human results in irreversible cretinism. Unlike other tissues, the metabolic rate of the adult brain is not directly affected to a large extent by the absence of thyroxin. However, in the adult human, thyroid deficiency causes physical and mental sluggishness, but both somatic and cerebral functioning can be fully restored with thyroxin therapy. Excess thyroid activity (hyperthyroidism), in addition to accelerating bodily metabolism, may cause emotional and affective disorders related to hyperexcitability.

A primary biochemical step affected by thyroid hormone is the respiratory rate of mitochondria. The precise site of action within mitochondria is unclear but may involve a flavin-linked intermediate in electron transport. Stimulation of the rate of oxidative phosphorylation increases the production of ATP, and this in turn may increase the supply of energy available for many anabolic reactions such as protein synthesis. In view of its rather special relation to cerebral development, it is possible that thyroxin may also exert its effects by direct stimulation of other enzyme systems.

Some hormones may influence the metabolism of discrete brain areas: several steroids have been shown to bind to precise brain regions, especially within the hypothalamus. Behavioral changes may occur as a result of such binding and subsequent activation of specific neuronal circuits. Testosterone increases the incorporation of [^{3}H]uridine into RNA in certain cerebral loci, and when injected into ovariectomized female rats will cause an increase in and greater persistence of exploratory behavior.[7]

The close relationship between cerebral development and the humoral environment is also seen in the direct effects of malnutrition on the nervous system. Though malnutrition has less of a dramatic effect on brain weight than it does on total body weight, malnutrition during development results in a reduced rate of cell proliferation, cell growth and myelination. Both in the human and in the rat, postnatal malnutrition most severely affects those regions in which cells are dividing, such as the cerebellum. Fetal cerebral growth is dependent on the nutritional status of the mother, and optimal maturation requires adequate pre- and postnatal nutrition.

An inadequate maternal diet in combination with subsequent malnutrition may result in a greatly reduced brain weight. Infants weighing less than 2 kg at birth, who then died of malnutrition during the first year of life, had a 60 percent reduction in the total number of cells in the brain. As with hormones, inadequacies incurred during an early period cannot be compensated for in later life, while adult malnutrition does not normally result in cerebral damage. In human populations, protein and caloric insufficiency is often associated with vitamin deficiency, which by causing the improper function of a series of enzymes further handicaps the growth of the brain.

The delicate balance of nutrients needed for cerebral development is illustrated by the fact that excess oxygen can severely damage nerve tissue. Hyperoxygenation may reduce both capillary proliferation during growth and cerebral blood flow. These features in combination can markedly reduce the supply of nutrients to the brain. In addition, high oxygen levels tend to inhibit oxidative respiration in relation to the glycolytic rate. This may impede the elaboration of the carbon skeletons required for protein, lipid and nucleic acid synthesis, which are produced from the tricarboxylic acid cycle.

Special growth factors may also be needed for the elaboration of fully differentiated brain cells. This is suggested by the fact that denervation of brain regions before the onset of electrical activity may result in their hypoplasia (p. 159). The injection of peptides tagged with a fluorescent dye into a single cell in tissue culture leads rapidly to the appearance of fluorescence in adjoining similar cells. Experiments of this type have shown that cells are able to recognize each other as being of the same type, and that a consequence of this recognition is that the junction between them becomes permeable to molecules of weights up to 10,000. In contrast, tumor cells that do not appear to recognize adjacent cells do not exchange such molecules. This type of exchange between cells may play a role in bringing about the differentiation of neurons and their correct orientation in relation to each other (Chapter 6).

A protein essential for the maturation and maintenance of the sympathetic nervous system is known.[6] This nerve growth factor (NGF) has been prepared and purified from several sources, notably snake venom and mouse submaxillary gland. It has been shown to stimulate the outgrowth of fibers from cultured dorsal root ganglia of the chick embryo. NGF is dissociable into three types of subunits, all of which are needed for maximal expression of biological activity. Antisera to pure NGF when injected into young rats destroy the neurons of the sympathetic nervous system. Such "immunosympathectomized" animals are viable and useful in many investigations. NGF has little effect on the central nervous system, and no corresponding growth factor essential for differentiation of the central nervous system has yet been identified. Recently, a striking structural similarity between insulin and NGF was noted. These hormones exhibit considerable homology of amino acid sequence, suggesting a common evolutionary origin. Both hormones appear to activate responsive cells by binding to receptors present in the surface membrane of such cells. The similarity of these hormones is indicated by the fact that many neurons metabolically activated by NGF respond similarly to insulin.

Humoral factors may constitute a means of transmitting information between generations, in addition to genetic or learned transfer. Thus, grandpups of female rats that have had avoidance training are significantly more active than control rats.[8]

C. IMPULSE-RELATED FACTORS

At a certain stage of development the electrical activity of nerve cells becomes significant. The relationship between neuronal usage and cerebral growth was discussed in Chapter 7. Sensory input is clearly required for the complete development of many cerebral regions. Patterned sensory input is also needed for the elaboration of complex neuronal interconnection of certain regions. Just how sophisticated such patterning must be may vary from one area to another.

Gross random electrical activity may be harmful for cerebral maturation. When a single ECS treatment is given to young adult rats, no effect on the DNA, RNA or protein content of the brain is observed. However, if rats are given such treatment during the first ten days after birth, the subsequent increases of cerebral DNA, RNA and protein are reduced.[9] This impaired development (presumably of cell number and cell size) is also reflected in the retarded appearance of behavioral abilities such as visual placing. These observations parallel the known correlation between neonatal seizures and mental retardation in man.

IX. *Development of the Brain* 237

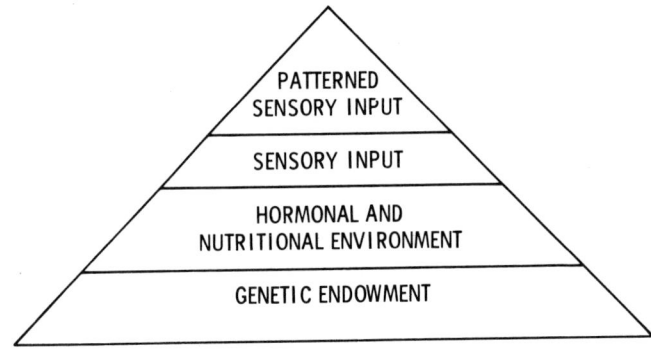

Figure 9.2 Parameters influencing attainable level of brain function.

The parameters that influence cerebral development are summarized in Figure 9.2. Each determinant is dependent on the adequacy of those below it.

However, such factors are not compartmentalized but interact in a complex manner. For example, studies on the development of bird song[10] have shown that the cheeping of chicks is inherited and not learned, while the chaffinch must learn its song from another chaffinch. At an intermediate level is the sparrow, which does not need to learn its song from another bird but can learn to sing if it is allowed to hear itself. Thus if the sparrow is deafened, it does not develop its typical song.

Genetic and maternal influences lay the basis for the capacity of the brain to respond to the environment.[11,12] The relative importance of genetic and environmental factors to the development of behavior varies not only with the species but also with the behavior. It may be that the greater effect of the environment in higher species reflects their more complex behavior. At present we cannot accurately assess the contributions of the two factors to complex attributes such as intelligence. A greater understanding of the chemistry of the brain may hasten this objective.

CHAPTER 9 REFERENCES

Reviews and General References

1. Benjamins, J. A., and McKhann, G. M. Neurochemistry of development. In *Basic Neurochemistry* (Ed. R. W. Albers, G. J. Siegel, R. Katzmann, and B. W. Agranoff), Little, Brown, Boston, 1972, pp. 269–98.

2. Kalckar, H. M., Kinoshita, J. H., and Donnell, G. N. Galactosemia: biochemistry, genetics, pathophysiology and developmental aspects. In *Biology of Brain Dysfunction*, Vol. 1 (Ed. G. E. Gaull), Plenum Press, New York, 1973, pp. 31–88.
3. Nyhan, W. L. Disorders of nucleic acid metabolism. In *Biology of Brain Dysfunction*, Vol. 1 (Ed. G. E. Gaull), Plenum Press, New York, 1973, pp. 265–300.
4. Hsu, L. Y. F., and Hirschhorn, K. Cytogenetic aspects of brain dysfunction. In *Biology of Brain Dysfunction*, Vol. 1 (Ed. G. E. Gaull), Plenum Press, New York, 1973, pp. 89–142.
5. Balázs, R., and Richter, D. Effects of hormones on the biochemical maturation of the brain. In *Biochemistry of the Developing Brain*, Vol. 1 (Ed. W. Himwich), Dekker, New York, 1973, pp. 253–356.
6. Angeletti, P. U., Angeletti, R. H., Frazier, W. A., and Bradshaw, R. A. Nerve growth factor. In *Proteins of the Nervous System* (Ed. D. J. Schneider), Raven Press, New York, 1973, pp. 133–154.

Literature Cited

7. Andrew, R. J., and Rogers, L. J. Testosterone, search behaviour and persistence. *Nature* 237:343–45, 1972.
8. Wehmer, F., Porter, R. H., and Scales, B. Pre-mating and pregnancy stress in rats affects behavior of grandpups. *Nature* 227:622, 1970.
9. Wasterlain, C. G., and Plum, F. Vulnerability of developing rat brain to electroconvulsive seizures. *Arch. Neurol.* 29:38–45, 1973.
10. Ploog, D. The relevance of natural stimulus patterns for sensory information processes. *Brain Research* 31:353–59, 1971.
11. Price, E. O., and Loomis, S. Maternal influence on the response of wild and domestic Norway rats to a novel environment. *Dev. Psychobiol.* 6:203–8, 1973.
12. Henderson, N. D. Brain weight increases resulting from environmental enrichment: a directional dominance in mice. *Science* 169:776–78, 1970.

APPENDIX

GLOSSARY

Action potential: A propagated reversal of the resting potential of an axon. It travels as wave or spike along the axon.

Activity (enzyme activity): The rate of catalysis of the particular enzymic reaction. A change in activity may be mediated by a change in the number of enzyme molecules or by a change in inhibitors or allosteric effectors.

Adenohypophysis (anterior pituitary): Endocrine gland formed from ectoderm of the roof of the mouth, containing nonneural cells which synthesize a number of hormones. The secretion of these hormones is under the control of releasing hormones (releasing factors) synthesized in the hypothalamus.

Afferent: A nerve that transmits impulses from the periphery to the CNS; a sensory nerve. It is also used to describe connecting neurons in the central nervous system that carry impulses *to* a nerve station.

Agonist: A drug that potentiates the activity of a hormone or neurotransmitter.

Allosteric enzyme: An enzyme that has a molecular binding site distinct from its catalytic one. The binding of *allosteric effectors* generally alters the catalytic activity of the enzyme. *Allosteric activators* increase the rate of catalysis; *allosteric inhibitors* decrease it.

Anabolism: The conversion of simple compounds to more complex ones by chemical processes in living organisms; the converse of catabolism.

Antagonist: A drug that blocks the action of a physiological hormone or neurotransmitter.

Astroglia, astrocytes: "Star-shaped" glial cells, in contact with neurons and often with long processes that may extend to the surface of blood vessels. There are two types of astrocytes: fibrous and protoplasmic. Since astroglia surround cerebral capillaries, they may constitute part of the blood-brain barrier. Astroglia frequently surround synapses and may segregate and chemically insulate the junctions. When the brain is lesioned, astroglia and microglia proliferate and may form glial scars.

Autoradiography: See *Radioautography*.

Autoregulation: The local regulation of vasodilation of capillaries by carbon dioxide and pH (see p. 24).

Autosomal: Associated with chromosomes other than the sex-chromosomes.

Axolemma: The external (plasma) membrane of the axon across which an ionic gradient is maintained.

Axon: A neuronal process that transmits action potentials to its distal termini. Each neuron generally possesses a single axon which may, however, be extensively branched. For the distinction between axons and dendrites, see *Dendrites* and Chapter 4.

Axon fan: The axonal equivalent of a dendritic tree, the spreading and area covered by axonal branching.

Axon hillock: The region of the nerve cell body in which the axon originates. In large neurons it is distinguished by the absence of ribosomes and an apparent funneling of neurotubules and neurofibrils from the cell body. The action potential is initiated at the axon hillock.

Catabolism: The conversion of complex compounds to more simple ones by chemical processes in living organisms; essentially synonymous with destruction or degradation; the converse of anabolism.

Catabolite: Any product of the catabolism of a particular chemical compound.

Dendrites: Neuronal processes which may be regarded as extensions of the neuronal perikaryon and contain similar organelles. They are distinguished from axons in that: (1) they have irregular contours such as spines protruding from their surfaces; (2) they may be highly ramified; (3) a neuron may contain many dendrites; (4) they are never ensheathed in myelin. (For a fuller discussion, see Chapter 4.)

Dendritic spines: The lateral projections of dendrites upon which axons from other neurons frequently synapse.

Efferent: A nerve that transmits impulses from the CNS to the periphery; a motor nerve. It is also used to describe connecting neurons in the CNS that carry impulses *from* a nerve station.

Electroencephalogram (EEG): The record of the changes of electrical potential detected by electrodes on or near the brain.

Encephalomyelitis: Inflammation of the brain and spinal cord.

Eukaryote (eucaryote): Cells possessing a clearly differentiated nucleus contained in a nuclear membrane.

Evoked potential: The electrical response recorded from the CNS due to stimulation of a peripheral sense organ or nerve.

Excitatory postsynaptic potential (EPSP): See *Postsynaptic potential.*

Exocytosis: The process by which substances enclosed in vesicles can cross membranes by fusing the vesicle membrane with the cell membrane (see Figure 5.2).

Ganglion: A knotlike mass comprising a group of nerve cell bodies, outside the CNS.

Glia (neuroglia): Nonneuronal cells specific to the nervous system. There are several types of glial (literally gluelike) cells, namely, astroglia, microglia, oligodendroglia and Schwann cells (see separate listings). Glial cells completely separate nerve cells from blood vessels and essentially constitute the matrix in which nerve tissue is suspended (see Chapter 1).

Gluconeogenesis: The production of glucose from tricarboxylic acid cycle intermediates.

Glycogenolysis: The breakdown of glycogen to its glucose subunits.

Glycolysis: The breakdown of sugars to simpler compounds; normally used to describe the catabolism of glucose to pyruvate. *Anaerobic glycolysis* refers to the conversion of glucose to lactate, which can occur in the absence of oxygen.

Golgi apparatus: A special configuration of the endoplasmic reticulum containing many cisternae but no ribosomes; known to have an important role in carbohydrate metabolism; considered a system for packaging molecules (e.g., neurotransmitters, proteins) into vesicles.

Golgi stain: A silver stain of great value in staining the fine dendritic and axonal extensions of the nerve cell. The method does not stain all neurons but fully stains those which are impregnated, though axons are occasionally not stained. This "all or none" property enables visualization of the dendritic tree of a single neuron against a relatively clear background.

Half-life: The time taken for half the molecules of a compound in a particular sample to be destroyed: the mean life-expectancy of a molecule. *Radioactive half-life* is the time required for half the radioactive atoms in a sample to decay.

Hybridization (nucleic acid hybridization, annealing): Permitting single-stranded molecules of nucleic acids (RNA or DNA) to combine into double-stranded structures in Watson-Crick base-pairs. The technique is used to compare the base sequences of nucleic acid molecules since only *complementary* sequences will hybridize efficiently (see p. 52).

Hyperplasia: Overdevelopment of tissue.

Hypoplasia: Defective development of tissue.

Hypoxia: Reduced oxygen content, especially of the blood.

Induction (enzyme induction): The process resulting in the synthesis of new enzyme molecules so that the total activity of the enzyme in the cell is increased. Enzyme induction requires the translation of messenger RNA sequences into the amino acid sequences of the protein, but may or may not require the transcription of new messenger RNA from the DNA.

Inhibitory postsynaptic potential (IPSP): See *Postsynaptic potential.*

Ischemia: Anemia caused by local or temporary restriction of the blood supply.

Isoenzyme, isozyme: Enzymes with the same catalytic activity that are molecularly distinct.

Macroglia: A collective term for astrocytes and oligodendrocytes, both of which, like the neuron, are of ectodermal origin.

Metabolism: The sum of the chemical processes occurring in living organisms; may be ascribed to the processes associated with a particular chemical compound.

Metabolite: Any product of metabolism.

Microfilaments (in nervous system): See *Neurofilaments.*

Microglia: Glial cells of mesodermal origin which enter the brain during its maturation. They are smaller than other glial cells. Microglia may undergo rapid proliferation in response to inflammatory or degenerative lesions of the nervous system. Under such conditions they turn into macrophages and have a phagocytic function.

Microtubules (in nervous system): See *Neurotubules.*

Myelin: A sheath around axons which insulates them chemically and electrically from their surroundings. The myelin sheath consists of a series of concentric membrane lamellae formed by glial cells wrapping themselves around the axon. Peripheral myelin is formed by Schwann cells and central myelin by oligodendroglia. The two forms are chemically distinct. (See Chapter 4.)

Nerve ending particle (NEP): See *Synaptosome.*

Neurilemma (neurolemma): The sheath derived from the Schwann cell which covers peripheral axons. In myelinated axons it surrounds the outer layer of the myelin sheath.

Neurites: The small neuronal extensions or sprouts that are the beginning of growth of new axons or dendrites.

Neurofibrils: Strands observed within neurons in the light microscope; thought to be aggregates of neurofilaments and neurotubules.

Neurofilaments: Filaments of about 100 Å diameter present in the cytoplasm, thinner than neurotubules but also tubular in structure. Like neurotubules they are found both in the cell body and in the nerve cell processes where they run longitudinally. Axonal neurofilaments appear more organized and may extend very close to synapses. They may play a role in transport phenomena and especially in neurite growth. They are disrupted by cytochalasin B.

Neuroglia: See *Glia.*

Neurohypophysis (posterior pituitary): Neural portion of hypophysis formed of the termini of hypothalamic neurons secreting oxytocin and vasopressin.

Neuropil: Areas of brain tissue containing intertwined and synapsing neuronal processes and glial cells, but not neuronal perikarya.

Neurosecretion: The release of a substance at the axonal terminus of a neuron.

Neurotrophy: The nutrition and maintenance of tissues by nervous influence.

Neurotropism: The tendency of nerves to grow toward specific peripheral locations.

Neurotubules: Long tubular elements of 200 Å to 260 Å in diameter found in large quantities in all regions of neurons; similar if not identical with the microtubules found in the nuclei of cells during mitosis. An outer dense layer surrounds a less dense core. Neurotubules are linearly arranged in axons and dendrites and run parallel to the axon length together with neurofilaments. Neurotubular protein binds colchicine or vinblastin rather specifically. They almost certainly play a role in axoplasmic transport (Chapter 4). Neurotubules may assume a twisted condition in certain pathological conditions such as Alzheimer's disease.

Nissl substance: Material staining intensely with acidic stains, uniquely found in neurons normally in the cell body but occasionally in dendrites. It consists of large collections of ribosomes associated with, but not predominantly attached to, folds of endoplasmic reticulum.

Node of Ranvier: The intervals between adjacent segments of the myelin sheath of both peripheral and central axons. The branching of myelinated axons always occurs at such a node. At these regions the axolemma is relatively unprotected.

Nucleus: A spheroid body within the cell containing the chromosomes within the nuclear membrane; also, a group of nerve cell bodies associated with a particular nerve tract in the CNS.

Oligodendroglia, oligodendrocytes: Glial cells responsible for the formation of the myelin sheath in the CNS. Oligodendroglia are found aligned in rows between axons in white matter and surround nerve cell bodies as satellite cells in gray matter.

Perikaryon: Literally, the area surrounding the nucleus, but often used to refer to the nerve cell body. It contains the Nissl substance and Golgi apparati, as well as mitochondria, ribosomes, neurofilaments and neurotubules.

Pinocytosis: The process in which substances outside the cell may be drawn inside by invaginating the cell membrane, eventually forming a vesicle containing the extracellular substance inside the cell (see Figure 5.2).

Plasma membrane: The membrane that encloses the cell, separating it from the extracellular space and other cells. It is chemically distinct in lipid and protein composition from other cell membranes.

Postsynaptic potential (PSP): Temporary changes in the voltage across the postsynaptic membrane caused by synaptic input. The potentials are generally observed in dendrites or the cell body. The potential changes may be transmitted electrically and therefore virtually instantaneously to other parts of the cell, but without an action potential. PSP's from different synaptic inputs may summate. PSP's that alter the voltage across the membrane toward a more easily excitable state (depolarized, generally a positive PSP) are termed excitatory (EPSP); those that alter the voltage away from excitability (hyperpolarized, generally a negative PSP) are termed inhibitory (IPSP).

Prokaryotes (procaryotes): Cells of the primitive (bacterial) type that do not possess a differentiated nucleus or nuclear membrane.

Radioautography: The detection of radioactivity by reaction of a photographic emulsion with emitted electrons; especially used with sections of tissue. Radioactive atoms in the tissue decay, producing a latent image in a thin film of photographic emulsion overlying the section. Development of the exposed emulsion produces visible silver grains, and in this way the location of radioactive molecules in tissue may be determined. The technique is capable of very high resolution with the use of the radioactive hydrogen isotope tritium (^{3}H) and the electron microscope.

Releasing factors (releasing hormones): Peptides synthesized in the *hypophysiotropic* areas of the hypothalamus, released into the portal circulation of the hypophysis at the median eminence. They are transported to the adenohypophysis, where they stimulate the secretion of anterior pituitary hormones. There are separate release factors for each hormone (except prolactin, which is under inhibitory control). (See p. 166).

Repression (enzyme repression): The prevention of the synthesis of new enzyme molecules.

Respiratory quotient (RQ): The molar ratio of carbon dioxide produced to oxygen consumed by a tissue or preparation.

Satellite cells: Cells encapsulating neuronal cell bodies, normally astroglia or oligodendroglia. They may play a role in the protection and nutrition of neurons.

Schwann cells: Glial cells surrounding peripheral axons. These cells repeatedly wrap the axon in a sheet of specialized plasma membrane forming myelin.

Soma: The cell body of a neuron.

Specific activity: The rate of catalytic activity of an enzyme expressed per unit of protein. Specific activity is often used loosely for *specific radioactivity*.

Specific radioactivity: The radioactive decay rate of a sample (disintegrations per unit time, or curies) divided by the amount of the sample (grams or moles).

Spike: See *Action potential*.

Synapse: A specialized junction between neurons; normally formed between an axon and another neuron or effector cell. Axonal synapses with neurons may be formed upon dendrites (axo-dendritic), nerve cell bodies (axo-somatic) or, more rarely, other axons (axo-axonal). However, dendro-dendritic, somato-dendritic and somato-somatic synapses have been observed. Synapses may also be formed with muscle fibers as neuromuscular synapses or junctions. Synapses may be chemical, electrical or mixed (i.e., both). (See Chapter 5.)

Synaptic vesicles: Vesicles found in axons especially close to the synapse. The vesicles may have differing morphologies but are normally the same in any one cell. They are thought to contain neurotransmitters.

Synaptosome (nerve-ending particle, NEP): A morphological fraction that can be prepared from homogenates of brain and consists of the torn-off synaptic terminals that have resealed to form particles. These particles contain synaptic vesicles and mitochondria, as well as the synaptic junction itself. Postsynaptic material, especially the postsynaptic (subsynaptic) membrane, may also be present to a variable extent. (See p. 121.)

Tubulin: The major protein constituent of neurotubules.

Turnover: The rate at which a chemical compound is synthesized and degraded.

Volume conduction: Conduction of electrical activity through the cells of the nervous system without necessarily precipitating action potentials or transynaptic transmission.

ABBREVIATIONS

Å	Angstrom unit
AcCoA	acetylcoenzyme A
ACh	acetylcholine
ACTH	adrenocorticotrophic hormone (corticotrophin)
ADP	adenosine 5′ diphosphate
ala	alanine
AMP	adenosine 5′ monophosphate
ATP	adenosine 5′ triphosphate
ATPase	adenosine 5′ triphosphatase
CDP	cytidine 5′ diphosphate
cer	ceramide
CMP	cytidine 5′ monophosphate
CMP-NANA	cytidine 5′ monophosphate N-acetylneuraminic acid
CNS	central nervous system
CoA	coenzyme A

COMT	catechol-O-methyltransferase
CRH	corticotrophin releasing hormone
CSF	cerebrospinal fluid
CTP	cytidine 5′ triphosphate
DA	dopamine
DBH	dopamine β-hydroxylase
DFP	di-isopropyl fluorophosphate (di-isopropyl phosphorofluoridate)
DG	diglyceride
DMI	desmethylimipramine
DNA	deoxyribonucleic acid
dNAD	deamino-NAD
DOPA	3,4-dihydroxyphenylalanine
DOPA-dC	3,4-dihydroxyphenylalanine decarboxylase
DPI	diphosphoinositide
EAE	experimental allergic encephalitis
EEG	electroencephalogram
ECS	electroconvulsive shock
EPSP	excitatory postsynaptic potential
FSH	follicle-stimulating hormone
FSHRH	follicle-stimulating hormone releasing hormone
GABA	γ-aminobutyric acid
GABA-T	γ-aminobutyric acid transaminase
GAD	glutamic acid decarboxylase
gal	galactose
galNAc	N-acetylgalactosamine
GDP	guanosine 5′ diphosphate
GH	growth hormone
GHRH	growth hormone releasing hormone
GHRIH	growth hormone release-inhibiting hormone
glu	glucose
GMP	guanosine 5′ monophosphate
GSH	glutathione (reduced)
GSSG	oxidized glutathione
GTP	guanosine 5′ triphosphate

5HIAA	5-hydroxyindole acetic acid
hnRNA	heterogeneous nuclear ribonucleic acid
hr	hour
5HT	5-hydroxytryptamine (serotonin)
5HTP	5-hydroxytryptophan
IMP	inosine 5′monophosphate
IPSP	inhibitory postsynaptic potential
L-DOPA	L-dihydroxyphenylalanine (= DOPA)
LH	luteinizing hormone
LHRH	luteinizing hormone releasing hormone
LSD	lysergic acid diethylamide
M	molar
MAO	monoamine oxidase
MEPP	miniature endplate potential
mM	millimolar
MPI	monophosphoinositide (phosphoinositol)
αMpT	α-methyl-p-tyrosine
mRNA	messenger RNA
MSH	melanocyte stimulating hormone
M.Wt.	molecular weight
NAD	nicotine adenine dinucleotide (formerly diphosphopyridine nucleotide, DPN, or coenzyme I)
NADP	nicotine adenine dinucleotide phosphate (formerly triphosphopyridine nucleotide, TPN, or coenzyme II)
NANA	N-acylneuraminic acid (sialic acid)
NE	norepinephrine (noradrenaline)
NGF	nerve growth factor
PA	phosphatidic acid
PAPS	3′phosphoadenosine-5′phosphosulfate
PAS	p-aminosalicylate
pCPA	p-chlorophenylalanine
P_i	inorganic orthophosphate
PNMT	phenylethanolamine-N-methyltransferase
PNS	peripheral nervous system

poly A	polyadenylic acid
poly C	polycytidylic acid
poly G	polyguanylic acid
poly U	polyuridylic acid
PP_i	inorganic pyrophosphate
PRH	prolactin releasing hormone
PRIH	prolactin release-inhibiting hormone (prolactin inhibiting factor)
PRPP	α-5-phosphoribosyl-1-pyrophosphate
PSP	postsynaptic potential
REM	rapid eye movement (sleep)
RNA	ribonucleic acid
RNP	ribonucleoprotein
rRNA	ribosomal ribonucleic acid
SAH	S-adenosylhomocysteine
SAM	S-adenosylmethionine
ser	serine
TH	tyrosine hydroxylase
TPI	triphosphoinositide
tRNA	transfer ribonucleic acid
TRH	thyroid stimulating hormone releasing hormone
TSH	thyroid stimulating hormone (thyrotropin)
tyr	tyrosine
UDP	uridine 5′diphosphate
UDPgal	uridine 5′diphosphate-galactose
UDPgalNAc	uridine 5′diphosphate-N-acetylgalactosamine
UDPglu	uridine 5′diphosphate-glucose
UMP	uridine 5′monophosphate.
UTP	uridine 5′triphosphate

ACTIONS OF COMMONLY USED DRUGS*

This section attempts to list the more commonly used metabolic inhibitors and to detail their principal activities and mechanism of action, where known.*

A. General inhibitors:

Drug	Property
Iodoacetate, iodoacetamide, N-ethylmaleimide, p-hydroxymercuribenzoate	bind to sulfhydryl groups forming alkyl derivatives (e.g., cysteine of proteins)

*For further details we recommend: (for therapeutic drugs) *The Pharmacological Basis of Therapeutics,* (Ed. L. S. Goodman and A. Z. Gilman) Macmillan, N.Y. 4th Edn. (1970); the series *Metabolic Inhibitors,* Volumes 1 to 4, (Ed. R. M. Hochster and J. H. Quastel) Academic Press, N.Y. (1963–1973); and *Fundamentals of Cell Pharmacology,* (Ed. S. Dikstein) Thomas, Springfield, Ill. (1973).

Drug	Property
di-isopropylphosphorofluoridate (DFP) (see also acetylcholine)	binds to hydroxyl groups (e.g., serine or threonine in proteins), interacts especially with enzymes that have serine in the active center
2,4-dinitrofluorobenzene (FDNB)	binds to amino groups forming dinitrophenyl derivatives (e.g., lysine and N-terminal amino acid of proteins)

B. Drugs that affect general metabolism:

Drug	Effect	Mechanism
cyanide, azide, carbon monoxide	inhibit respiration	combine with cytochromes inhibiting electron transport
amytal, antimycin A	inhibit respiration	inhibit electron transport
2,4-dinitrophenol	depresses ATP concentration	uncouples oxidative phosphorylation
oligomycin	depresses ATP concentration	inhibits oxidative phosphorylation
fluoride (see also cyclic nucleotides)	blocks glycolysis	inhibits enolase
fluoroacetate, fluorocitrate	blocks tricarboxylic acid cycle	inhibits aconitase
iodoacetate	blocks glycolysis	inhibits glycerol phosphate dehydrogenase
methionine sulfoximine	convulsant	inhibits glutamine synthetase and γ-glutamyl cysteine synthetase
ethionine (see also protein synthesis)	depresses ATP concentration	possibly by competing for methionine in S-adenosylmethionine formation
acetazolamide (Diamox)	inhibits CSF production, among other things	inhibits carbonic anhydrase
6-azauridine	depresses pyrimidine nucleotide content	inhibits orotic acid decarboxylase

C. Drugs that affect nucleic acid metabolism:

Drug	Effect	Mechanism
mitomycin C	inhibits DNA synthesis	binds to DNA
cytosine arabinoside	inhibits DNA synthesis	inhibits DNA polymerase as analog of substrate
actinomycin D	inhibits RNA synthesis	binds to guanine-rich sequences of double-stranded DNA
8-azaguanine	inhibits RNA synthesis	substitutes for guanine in RNA
α-amanitin	inhibits mRNA synthesis	inhibits RNA polymerase II
rifamycin (rifampin or rifampicin)	inhibits mitochondrial RNA synthesis	inhibits mitochondrial RNA polymerase
camptothecin	inhibits RNA synthesis	probably blocks ribosome assembly
cordycepin	inhibits mRNA function	blocks the addition of polyadenylic acid sequences to mRNA
fluorouracil	inhibits RNA synthesis (and thymidine synthesis)	incorporated into RNA as fluorouridine (as fluorodeoxyuridylic acid, inhibits thymidylate synthetase)
ethidium bromide	inhibits mitochondrial RNA synthesis	binds to double-stranded circular DNA

D. Drugs that affect protein synthesis:

  (a) inhibitors of mitochondrial protein synthesis (70S ribosome) only

Drug	Action
chloramphenicol	prevents binding of aminoacyl-tRNA to ribosomes

  (b) inhibitors of cytoplasmic protein synthesis (80S ribosome) only

Drug	Action
cycloheximide, acetoxy-cycloheximide, streptovitacin A	inhibit chain elongation

Drug	Action
emetine	unknown
diphtheria toxin	inhibits peptide bond synthesis
anisomycin	inhibits peptide bond synthesis

(c) inhibitors of mitochondrial and cytoplasmic systems

Drug	Action
puromycin	causes false chain-termination releasing nascent peptides attached to puromycin, disaggregates polyribosomes
sparsomycin	inhibits peptide bond formation
aurintricarboxylic acid	inhibits initiation of polypeptide chains
pactamycin	inhibits initiation of polypeptide chains
amicetin, gougerotonin blasticidin S	inhibit translocation
ethionine	substitutes for methionine in protein

E. Drugs that affect neural conduction:

Drug	Effect	Mechanism
anesthetics (procaine, novocaine, xylocaine, etc.; halothane, fluothane, etc.), barbiturates	inhibit axonal conduction	probably by decreasing Na^+ permeability
tetrodotoxin	same	blocks Na^+ channels
ouabain	same	blocks Na^+ pump (Na^+, K^+-ATPase)

F. Drugs that affect neurotransmitter metabolism:

(a) Acetylcholine

Drug	Effect	Mechanism
hemicholinium	lowers tissue ACh	blocks choline uptake
botulinus toxin	antagonist	blocks ACh release
d-tubocurarine (active principal of curare), gallamine (Flaxedil)	antagonists	reversibly block ACh receptors
hexamethonium, decamethonium, succinylcholine		
naja naja toxin, α-bungarotoxin	antagonists	bind ACh receptor
atropine, scopolamine	antagonist	blocks muscarinic receptors
nicotine	nicotinic agonist	mimics ACh at nicotinic receptors
oxotremorine	elevates brain ACh	cholinomimetic in CNS
carbachol (carbamylcholine)	agonist	mimics ACh
eserine (physostigmine), neostigmine	agonist	reversibly inhibit AChE
di-isopropylphosphorofluoridate (DFP)	agonist	irreversibly block AChE

(b) Catecholamines

Drug	Effect	Mechanism
α-methyl-p-tyrosine (αMpT)	depletes catecholamines	inhibits tyrosine hydroxylase
Ro 4-4602	depletes catecholamines	inhibits DOPA decarboxylase

Drug	Effect	Mechanism
reserpine	depletes catecholamines	inhibits vesicular storage (see also serotonin)
diethyldithiocarbamate,	depletes NE	inhibits DBH by chelating Cu^{2+}
fusaric acid	depletes NE	inhibits DBH
amphetamine	noradrenergic agonist	probably multiple: stimulates release *and* mimics NE
bretylium, guanethidine	inhibits NE release (PNS only)	unknown
γ-hydroxybutyrate	inhibits dopamine release	unknown
phenoxybenzamine, ergot alkaloids, phentolamine	α-antagonist	blocks α-receptors
dichloroisoproterenol, propanolol	β-antagonist	blocks β-receptors
haloperidol, spiroperidol, phenothiazines (chlorpromazine, fluphenazine)		block dopamime receptors
lithium salts	depress NE	unknown
isoproterenol	β-agonist	
pargyline, tranylcyclopropylamine (tranylcypromine), nialamide		inhibit MAO
pyrogallol		inhibits COMT
cocaine, amitryptyline, imipramine, desmethylimipramine (DMI)	deplete NE	inhibit NE re-uptake
6-hydroxydopamine	destroys catecholamine-containing neurons	unknown; probably taken up into catacholaminergic cells by the selective re-uptake systems

(c) Serotonin

Drug	Effect	Mechanism
p-chlorophenylalanine (pCPA)	depletes 5HT	inhibits tryptophan hydroxylase (and tyrosine hydroxylase)

Drug	Effect	Mechanism
probenicid	elevates 5HT	blocks 5H1AA efflux
reserpine (see also catecholamines)	depletes 5HT	inhibits vesicular storage
amitryptyline	agonist	inhibits re-uptake
methysergide, cinanserin, cyproheptadine	antagonist	block postsynaptic receptor
lysergic acid diethylamide (LSD)	complex effects	may both block and mimic 5HT action (LSD also inhibits the degradation of substance P)
5,6-dihydroxytryptamine	destroys 5HT containing neurones	unknown but probably analogous to 6-hydroxydopamine

(d) Gamma-aminobutyric acid

Drug	Effect	Mechanism
hydroxylamine, amino-oxyacetic acid	increase GABA	inhibit GAD and GABA-T, but GAD less than GABA-T
tetanus toxin	cerebral excitant	inhibits GABA (and gly) release
bicuculline	cerebral excitant	blocks GABA receptors
picrotoxin	cerebral excitant	may block GABA receptors

(e) Glycine

Drug	Effect	Mechanism
tetanus toxin	cerebral excitant	inhibits glycine (and GABA) release
strychnine	cerebral excitant (convulsant at higher doses)	blocks glycine receptor activity

(f) Glutamate

Drug	Effect	Mechanism
glutamic acid diethyl ester	antagonist	blocks glutamate receptor

Drug	Effect	Mechanism
glutamic acid dimethyl ester	agonist	competitively blocks re-uptake

G. Drugs that affect axoplasmic transport:

Drug	Effect	Mechanism
colchicine, vinblastin	block fast and slow axoplasmic transport	bind to tubulin and disrupt neurotubules
	also inhibit cell division	disrupt microtubules formed during mitosis

H. Drugs that affect cyclic nucleotide metabolism:

Drug	Effect	Mechanism
$N^6, O^{2'}$-dibutyryl-cyclic-AMP		mimics $3',5'$-cyclic AMP, but more readily taken up by cells and less readily destroyed by phosphodiesterase
methylxanthines (theophylline, caffeine, aminophylline), papaverine	elevate cyclic AMP	inhibit cyclic AMP and cyclic GMP phosphodiesterases
fluoride	stimulates adenyl cyclase *in vitro* only	unknown

I. Miscellaneous drugs:

Drug	Effect	Mechanism
concanavalin A		binds specifically to α-methyl-D-mannose and α-methyl-D-glucose especially on cell surface

cytochalasin B	disrupts neurofilaments	unknown
flurothyl (Indoklon), pentylenetetrazole (Metrazol)	convulsants	unknown
diphenylhydantoin (Dilantin)	anticonvulsant	unknown but affects excitable membranes

Index

Acetazolamide (Diamox), 5, 180, 254
N-Acetylaspartate, 33, 34, 36, 73
Acetylcholine (ACh), 75, 115–118, 121, 124, 125, 127–130, 142, 159, 161, 162, 179, 182, 184, 187, 257
    assay of, 130
    axoplasmic transport of, 103
    learning and, 217
    phosphoinositides and, 188–190
    receptors, 129, 130, 162, 184
    synthesis, 127, 128
Acetylcholinesterase, 75, 109, 128, 129, 159, 230
    environmental enrichment and, 219
    in neuroblastoma, 17
Acetoxycycloheximide, 205, 255
N-acetylhistidine, 37
N-acetylmannosamine, 92, 149
N-acetylserotonin, 139–141
ACTH (adrenocorticotrophic hormone, corticotrophin), 166–168, 213, 214
Actinomycin D, 54, 55, 181, 206, 255
Action potential, 8, 72–75, 241
Adenine nucleotides, 42–47, 185, 188, 208, 222
Adenine phosphoribosyl transferase, 45, 188
Adenohypophysis, 166–172, 241
Adenosine, 44, 45, 47, 185, 188, 231
Adenosine $3',5'$ cyclic monophosphate *see* cyclic $3',5'$-AMP
Adenosine monophosphate (AMP), 36, 43–47
S-adenosylmethionine (SAM), 38, 83, 127, 131, 133, 136, 137, 139, 141, 254
    synthesis, 38
Adenyl cyclase, 46, 47, 134, 171, 174, 185–188, 260
    in glia, 14
    hormone action on, 171
    neurotransmission and, 174, 185–188
    in pineal, 141
Adrenalin(e) *see* epinephrine
Affective disorders, 219–221
Aging and DNA, 53
Allostery, 64, 242
Alzheimer's disease, 18, 19
α-Amanitin, 57, 206, 255
Amicetin, 256
Amino acids, 28, 31–38, 76, 123, 179, 230, 232
γ-Aminobutyric acid *see* GABA
δ-Aminolevulinic acid, 232
Amino–oxyacetic acid, 143, 180, 259
Aminophylline, 260
Amitryptiline, 137, 140, 220, 258, 259
Ammonia, 36, 179

Amphetamine, 220, 223, 258
Amytal, 254
Anesthetics, 256
Anisomycin, 205, 256
Anoxia, 28, 178, 185, 205
Antimycin A, 254
Aplysia neurons
  acetylcholine receptors, 125
  cyclic AMP in, 187
  DNA content, 52
  proteins of, 61
  protein synthesis, 184, 185
  RNA synthesis, 184
Arachidonic acid, 173
Arachnoid membrane, 2, 3
Arginine, 36, 39
L-aromatic amino acid decarboxylase, 132, 138, 139, 144, 145
Ascorbic acid
  as cofactor for DBH, 132
Aspartate, 33–36, 76, 142, 144, 179, 215, 230
Aspirin (acetylsalicylate), 173
Astroglia (astrocytes), 14, 94, 231, 242
  nuclei of, 51
ATP (adenosine triphosphate), 26–29, 41–46, 76–78, 107, 117, 124, 177–179, 183, 188, 203, 222
  in chromaffin granules, 117
  microassay, 20
  in synaptic vesicles, 118, 128, 133
ATPase (adenosine triphosphatase)
  in synaptic vesicles, 133
Na^+, K^+-ATPase, 65, 76–78
  corticosteroids and, 65
  sodium pump and, 76–78
Atropine, 129, 189, 257
Autoregulation, 24, 242
Aurintricarboxylic acid, 256
Axon, 6–8, 11–14, 59, 71–75, 159, 242
  transport of proteins into, 185
Axon hillock, 6, 8, 11, 63, 72, 73, 242
Axoplasmic transport, 102–109, 120, 134, 144, 145, 164, 182, 260
  mechanism of, 106–108
  of neurotransmitters, 103, 134, 144, 145
  of proteins, 19, 103, 164
  rates of, 104, 105
  of RNA, 106

  tracing fiber tracts, 19
8-Azaguanine, 206, 255
6-Azauridine, 45, 254
Azide, 254
Barbiturates, 210, 212, 256
Bicuculline, 143, 259
Bird song, 237
Black Widow Spider venom, 117
Blasticidin, 256
Blood–brain barrier, 3–5, 209, 231
Blood flow, 23, 24, 191, 192, 208, 211
  effect of attention, 211
  visual deprivation and, 191, 192
Blood supply, 3, 23, 178
Botulinus toxin, 257
Brain composition, 32
Brain slices, 178
Bretylium, 258
2-Bromo LSD, 140
α-Bungarotoxin, 129, 130, 162, 257
  denervation sensitivity, 162
  myasthenia gravis and, 162
Caffeine, 47, 260
Calcium ion (Ca^{2+})
  adenyl cyclase and, 47
  in neuronal conduction, 75
  S–100 and, 61
  synaptic transmission and, 124, 147
Camptothecin, 206, 255
Carbachol (carbamylcholine), 187, 257
Carbamyl phosphate, 36
  carbamyl phosphate synthetase, 39
Carbon monoxide, 254
Carbonic anhydrase, 5, 180, 254
Catecholamines, 123, 130–138, 180–183, 217, 219–221, 223, 224, 257, 258
  anatomical distribution of, 219, 220
  assay of, 137
  axoplasmic transport of, 103
  catabolism of, 134–137
  learning and, 217
  sleep and, 223, 224
  synthesis, 131–133, 180–183
Catechol-O-methyltransferase (COMT), 134–137, 221, 258
Ceramide (cer), 88–90, 92, 93
Cerebrosides, 18, 32, 81, 88, 89, 98, 99, 231
Cerebrospinal fluid (CSF), 3–5, 146, 222
Chloramphenicol, 59, 148, 255

p-Chlorophenylalanine (pCPA), 138, 223, 259
Chlorpromazine, 258
Cholera toxin, 147
Cholesterol, 31, 80, 81, 94, 95, 98
Choline, 82, 83, 86, 127, 128, 192
Choline acetylase (choline-O-acetyltransferase, 75, 109, 127, 128, 159, 164, 182, 221, 230
  induction of, 182
Cholinesterase, 14, 128, 129
  environmental enrichment and, 219
Choroid plexus, 4
Chromaffin granules, 117, 118, 133
Chromatolysis, 62, 63, 164
Chromogranins, 117, 133, 134
Chromosomes, 54
  abnormality in, 233
Cinanserin, 259
Citric acid cycle see tricarboxylic acid cycle
Citrulline, 36, 39
CMP-NANA, 92, 93, 97, 149
Cocaine, 258
Colchicine, 107, 108, 119, 162, 166, 260
Compartmentation, 47–49
Concanavalin A, 260
Contact inhibition, 158
Convulsions, 177, 180, 261
Cordycepin, 255
Corticosteroids, 65, 168
  induction of enzymes, 65
  and myelination, 101
Corticotrophin see ACTH
Corticotrophin releasing-hormone (CRH), 168
Creatine phosphate, 28, 222
Cretinism, 234
Creutzfeldt–Jacob disease, 94
Criteria for neurotransmitter identification, 126
Curare see α-tubocurarine
Cyanide, 254
Cyclic 3′,5′-AMP, 14, 18, 43, 46, 47, 49, 141, 151, 158, 165, 171, 174, 180, 183, 185–188, 231, 260
  compartmentation of, 49, 188
  convulsions and, 180
  in glia, 14, 165
  hormone effects on, 171

in pineal, 141
prostaglandins and, 174
as second messenger, 171, 186
stimulation and, 185–188
synaptic transmission and, 151, 186–188
2′,3′-Cyclic AMP phosphodiesterase, 100
3′,5′-Cyclic AMP phosphodiesterase see phosphodiesterase
Cyclic 3′,5′-GMP, 42, 46, 47, 187, 260
  neurotransmission and, 187
Cycloheximide, 59, 148, 162, 181, 182, 255
  catecholamine synthesis and, 181, 182
  denervation sensitivity and, 162
  learning and memory and, 205
Cyproheptadine, 259
Cystathionine, 33, 34, 37, 38
Cysteine and cystine, 33, 38, 253
Cytidine, 31, 44, 55, 82–84, 209
Cytidine nucleotides, 42–46, 82–84, 88, 89, 92, 94, 97, 127, 149, 189, 208
Cytochalisin B, 119, 261
Cytochrome oxidase, 15, 29, 165, 229
Cytosine arabinoside, 205, 206, 255
Dale's law, 124
Deamination (of nucleotides), 36, 179
Decamethonium, 257
Delta factor, 223
Dendrites, 6–8, 11, 12, 59, 60, 71–73, 163, 164, 242
  environmental enrichment and, 219
  flow of ribosomes in, 60
Dendritic spines, 72, 160, 192, 193, 243
  visual deprivation and, 192, 193
Denervation supersensitivity, 162
Deoxyribonucleic acid see DNA
Depression, 219, 220
Deprivation dwarfism, 169
Dibutyryl cyclic AMP, 260
Dichloroisoproterenol, 134, 258
Diethyldithiocarbamate (DDC), 258
DFP (di-isopropylphosphofluoridate), 254, 257
5,6-Dihydroxytryptamine (DHT), 259
Dilantin (diphenylhydantoin), 180, 261
Dinitrophenol (DNP), 254
Diphtheria toxin, 256
Diurnal rhythm
  of acetylcholine, 192
  in pineal, 140, 141

of protein synthesis, 222
of RNA synthesis, 222
of serotonin, 138, 140, 141, 192
DNA (deoxyribonucleic acid), 52–54, 171, 218, 219, 231
 environmental enrichment and, 218, 219
 malnutrition and, 101
 mitochondrial, 53, 54, 59
 synthesis, 53, 54, 205, 209, 255
DOPA (L-DOPA), 126, 130–138, 146, 181, 182
DOPA decarboxylase, 131, 132, 181, 182, 257
Dopamine (DA), 19, 47, 126, 130–138, 165, 181–183, 219–221, 257, 258
 anatomical distribution of, 219, 220
 cyclic AMP and, 47, 165, 186–188
Dopamine-β-hydroxylase (DBH), 117, 118, 124, 131–134, 181–183, 221, 258
Down's syndrome, 233
Duchenne muscular dystrophy, 162
Electrical stimulation
 of *Aplysia* neurons, 184, 185
 of cortex, 183, 185, 186
 of slices, 178, 183, 184, 185, 188
 of superior cervical ganglion, 184, 185
Electroshock and electroconvulsive shock, (ECS), 178–180, 183–185, 187, 236
 ATP and, 61, 178, 179, 183, 203
 learning and, 203–205
 norepinephrine and, 146, 147, 203
 protein synthesis and, 61, 184, 203, 205, 236
 RNA and, 183, 236
Emetine, 256
Energy utilization, 23–30, 177, 178, 203, 204, 222
Environmental enrichment, 218, 219
Enzymatic recycling, 20, 21
Enzyme induction, 64, 65, 181, 244
Enzyme repression, 181, 247
Epilepsy, 15, 78, 236
Epinephrine, 117, 119, 130–138, 168
Epinine, 131, 133
Eserine (physostigmine), 182, 257
Estrogen, 168
Ethionine, 254, 256
Ethydium bromide, 255

N-ethylmaleimide, 253
Exocytosis, 116, 243
 of synaptic vesicles, 116–118
Experimental allergic encephalomyelitis (EAE), 4, 100
Experimental allergic neuritis, 100
Fabry's disease, 93
Fatty acids, 31, 78, 81, 82, 85, 86
 oxidation, 30
FDNB (dinitrofluorobenzine), 254
Flaxedil, 257
Fluorescence histochemistry, 19, 103, 137
Fluoride, 254, 260
Fluoroacetate, fluorocitrate, 254
Fluorouracil, 255
Fluphenazine, 258
Flurothyl (Indoklon), 261
Follicle stimulating hormone (FSH), 166–170
Follicle stimulating hormone releasing hormone (FSHRH), 168, 169
Freeze-blowing, 43
Fucose, 31, 96, 149, 216
 axoplasmic transport of, 105
Fucosidase, 93
Fucosidosis, 93
Fusaric acid, 258
GABA (γ-aminobutyric acid), 33–37, 123–125, 142, 143, 179, 180, 219, 230, 259
 axoplasmic transport of, 103
 convulsions and, 179, 180
GABA shunt, 29, 30, 37, 142
GABA-transaminase (GABA–T), 142, 143, 259
Galactosemia, 232
α-Galactosidase, 93
β-Galactosidase
 in neurons, 17
Gallamine, 257
Gangliosides, 18, 32, 75, 82, 89–94, 147, 150, 207, 230
 axoplasmic transport of, 105, 106
 excitability and, 91
 learning and, 216
 location of, 91
 in myelin, 98
 synthesis of, 92
Gangliosidosis, 93, 94
Gaucher's disease, 93

INDEX

Genetics, genetic diseases, 65–67
  cerebellar mutants, 158
  factors in development, 229, 231–233, 237
  mosaics, 66
Glia (neuroglia), 14–17, 61, 101, 114, 164–166, 243
  adenyl cyclase in, 14
  potassium and, 14, 15
Glial–neuronal ratio, 15
Glucosamine, 31, 97, 149, 150
Glucose (glu), 26–30
  oxidation, 23–30, 222
  uptake, 5, 25, 123
Glucose–6–phosphate dehydrogenase, 20, 231
Glutamate, 28, 33–35, 48, 49, 73, 76, 124, 141, 142, 179, 215, 230, 259
  compartmentation of, 48, 47
Glutamic acid decarboxylase (GAD), 36, 37, 124, 125, 142, 143, 180, 230, 259
Glutamic acid diethyl ester (GDEE), 142, 259
Glutamic acid dimethyl ester (GDME), 142, 260
Glutamine, 28, 33, 35, 48, 49, 254
  compartmentation of, 48, 49
γ-Glutamyl cycle, 39–41
Glutathione (GSH), 39–41
Glycine, 33, 34, 123, 143, 144, 259
Glycogen, 27–29
Glycolysis, 25–29, 178, 229, 235, 243
  aerobic, 26–28, 229
  anaerobic, 26–28, 178
Glycoprotein, 81, 95–97, 114, 119, 148–150, 158, 170, 216
  axoplasmic transport of, 105, 106, 149, 150
  learning and, 216
  of synaptic vesicles, 119
  of synaptosomes, 119, 148–150
Gougerotonin, 256
Gout, 233
Growth hormone (GH), 166–168
Growth hormone releasing hormone (GHRH), 168, 169
Growth hormone release–inhibiting hormone (GHRIH), 166, 168
Guanethidine, 258
Guanine nucleotides, 42–47, 55, 97
Guanosine 3′,5′–cyclic monophosphate see cyclic 3′,5′–GMP

Habituation, 151, 180, 181
Haloperidol, 258
Hemicholinium, 257
Hexamethonium, 257
Hexosaminidase, 93
Histamine, 144, 145
  cyclic AMP and, 47
Histidine decarboxylase, 144, 145
Histochemistry, 17–19
Histones, 54, 62, 171, 216
  acetylation of, 54
  learning and, 216
  phosphorylation of, 54, 171, 216
  turnover of, 62
Homoanserine, 42
Homocarnosine, 42
Homovanillic acid (HVA), 135, 221
Horseradish peroxidase
  retrograde transport of, 109
  in synaptic vesicles, 119
Huntington's chorea, 143, 219
Hybridization see nucleic acid hybridization
γ-Hydroxybutyrate, 222, 258
6-Hydroxydopamine, 118, 139, 138, 181, 182, 258
5-Hydroxyindoleacetic acid (5HIAA), 139, 140, 259
5-Hydroxyindole-O-methyltransferase, 139–141
Hydroxylamine, 143, 259
p-Hydroxymercuribenzoate, 129, 253
5-Hydroxytryptamine (5HT) see serotonin
5-Hydroxytryptamine N-acetylase, 139–141
5-Hydroxytryptophan (5HTP), 138–140
Hyperoxia, 138, 179, 235
Hypoglycemia, 5, 25, 28
Hypophysiotropic neurons, 166–168
Hypophysis see pituitary
Hypoxanthine–Guanine phosphoribosyl transferase, 45, 46, 232, 233
Hypoxia, 25, 179, 244
Imipramine, 137, 258
Immunological reactions, 4, 100
Imprinting (in chicks), 192, 211, 213
Indoklon, 261
Informosomes, 55, 57
Inosine monophosphate (IMP), 36, 43
Inositol phosphatides see phosphoinositides
Insulin, 5, 28, 236

Iodoacetate, iodoacetamide, 253, 254
Isoproterenol, 258
Ketone bodies, 25, 30
Krabbe's disease, 93
Krebs' cycle *see* tricarboxylic acid cycle
Learning and memory, 197–218, 221
   chemical correlates of, 200, 202, 206–217
   disruption of, 198, 200, 202–206
   neurotransmitters and, 217
   protein synthesis and, 203, 205, 212–215
   RNA synthesis and, 206–212
   transfer of, 58, 217, 218
Lecithin *see* phosphatidylcholine
Lesch–Nyhan syndrome, 46, 232, 233
Leucine, 32, 33, 215
   incorporation into proteins, 149, 212, 213, 215
Lipidoses, 88, 93, 94
Lithium, 200, 258
LSD (lysergic acid diethylamide), 42, 140, 259
Luteinizing hormone (LH), 166–170
Luteinizing hormone releasing hormone (LHRH), 168–170
Lysine, 33, 254
   incorporation into protein, 191, 212, 213, 215, 222
   in regenerating neurons, 63
   during learning, 212, 213
Lysolecithin, 85
Magnesium pemoline, 206
Malnutrition, 101, 235
Mania, 219, 220
   cyclic AMP and, 165
Median eminence (of neurohypophysis), 166, 167
Melanin, 126
Melanocyte stimulating hormone (MSH), 141, 214, 218
Melatonin, 139–141
Membranes
   composition of, 80
   fluid mosaic model, 79, 81
   structure of, 78–81
   unit membrane hypothesis, 78, 79
Memory *see* learning
Metachromatic leucodystrophy, 88, 93, 102
Methionine, 33, 38, 256
Methionine sulfoximine, 179, 254
N–methylhistidine, 144, 145

α-Methyl–p–tryosine (αMpT), 132, 146, 223, 257
Methylxanthines, 47, 260
Methysergide, 259
Metrazol (pentylenetetrazole), 179, 261
Microglia, 14, 15, 245
Microwave fixation (for cyclic nucleotides), 46
Miniature endplate potential (MEPP), 115
Mitochondria, 10, 29, 49, 58, 59, 234
   DNA of, 53, 54, 59
   heterogeneity of, 58, 59
   protein synthesis in, 59
   RNA of, 59
   thryoxin and, 234
Mitomycin C, 255
Mongolism, 233
Monoamine oxidase (MAO), 134–137, 139, 146, 147, 220, 221, 230, 258
   inhibitors, 146, 220, 223
Morphine tolerance and addiction, 64
Multiple sclerosis, 5, 100
Muscular dystrophy, 162, 163
Myasthenia gravis, 162
Myelin, 14, 72, 80, 97–102, 245
   composition, 80, 98–100
   development of, 101, 159
   mutants, 65, 101, 102
   proteins, 61, 62, 99, 100
   purification, 98
Myelination, 101, 159, 231
NAJA NAJA toxin, 257
NANA (N–acetylneuraminic acid) *see* sialic acid
Nauta technique, 19
Neostigmine, 257
Nerve growth factor (NGF), 235, 236
Nerve-muscle interaction, 161–164
Neuraminidase *see* sialidase
Neurin, 119, 120
Neuroblastoma, 17, 186
Neurofibrils, 245
Neurofilaments, 12, 72, 107, 245, 261
Neuroglia *see* glia
Neurohypophysis, 166–172, 245
Neuron, 5–14, 15, 17, 61, 71–75
   degeneration of, 19, 62, 63
   regeneration of, 62, 63, 156–158, 161–163
Neuronal conduction, 73–76
Neuronal death, 53

Neuronal–glial ratio, 15
Neuronal–glial separation, 16, 17
Neuronal–glial transport, 15, 165, 183, 185, 191, 207, 208
Neuronal–glial unit (hypothesis), 15, 164, 165, 207
Neurophysins, 170
Neurosecretion, 163, 164, 166–171
Neurostenin, 119, 120
Neurotrophism (neurotrophy), 158–165, 245
Neurotropism (neurotropy), 156–158, 246
Neurotubules, 12, 72, 73, 107, 108, 246, 260
Nialamide, 258
Nicotine, 129, 257
Nicotine adenine dinucleotide (NAD), 26, 27, 29, 34, 36, 43
Niemann-Pick's disease, 93
Nissl substance, 9, 10, 12, 59, 63, 246
  in chromatolysis, 62, 63
Non-histone proteins, 54, 216
  learning and, 216
  phosphorylation of, 54, 216
Noradrenalin(e) *see* norepinephrine
Norepinephrine (NE), 14, 123, 125, 130–138, 146, 147, 165, 174, 180–183, 217, 219–221, 257, 258
  anatomical distribution of, 219, 220
  cyclic AMP and, 14, 47, 165, 174, 186–188
  learning and, 217
  sleep and, 223
  synthesis, 131–133, 180–183
Normetanephrine, 135
Nucleic acid hybridization, 52, 57, 211, 217, 244
Nucleolus, 9, 51, 63
  in chromatolysis, 63
Nucleosides, 31, 32, 44, 45
Nucleotides, 36, 42–47, 52, 210
Nucleus (cell), 8–11, 51–55, 246
  in chromatolysis, 62, 63
  polyploidy, 52
  tetraploidy, 52
Nutritional requirements, 30–32
Octopamine, 131–133
Oligodendroglia (oligodendrocytes), 14, 246
  nuclei of, 51
Oligomycin, 254
Organophosphates
  myelin and, 101

Ornithine, 36, 39
Orotic acid, 44, 46, 65, 210, 212
  orotic aciduria, 46, 65
Ouabain, 5, 76, 205, 256
Oxotremorine, 257
Oxygen consumption, 23, 24, 28, 222
Oxytocin, 166–171
Pactamycin, 256
Papaverine, 260
PAPS (3'phosphoadenosine–5'phosphosulfate), 88
Paradoxical sleep *see* REM sleep
Pargyline, 146, 258
Parkinson's disease, 125, 137, 219
Pasteur effect, 26
Pentose phosphate pathway, 231
Pentylenetetrazoe (Metrazol), 179, 261
Peptides, 39–42, 166–172, 214, 217, 218
  pituitary, 166–172, 214, 218
  sleep, 222, 223
Perfused brain, 31
Perikaryon, 10–12, 164, 246
Perphenazine, 258
Phenothiazines, 258
Phenoxybenzamine, 134, 181, 258
Phentolamine, 134, 258
Phenylalanine, 31–33
  hydroxylase, 31
Phenylethanolamine–N–methyltransferase (PNMT), 131, 133
Phenylketonuria (PKU), 31, 32, 61, 66, 132, 232
Phosphatidylcholine (lecithin), 82–85, 127
Phosphodiesterase, 189
  for cyclic nucleotides, 46, 47, 185, 186, 260
Phosphoinositides (MPI, DPI, TPI), 75, 80, 82–85, 188–190
  neuronal conduction and, 75
  neurotransmission and, 188–190
Phospholipases, 84, 85, 173
Phospholipids, 75, 78–88, 98, 99, 127, 142
  axoplasmic transport of, 105
  in synaptic vesicles, 119
Phosphomonoesterase, 84, 189
Physostigmine *see* eserine
Pia, 2, 3
Picrotoxin, 143, 259
Pineal, 140, 141
Pituitary, 166–172

Plasmalogens, 32, 86
Poliomyelitis virus, 17
Poly A, 57, 58
  poly C, Poly G, poly U, 58
Polyribosomes (polysomes), 10–12, 56, 57, 60, 205, 214, 215
  ECS and, 184, 205
  learning and, 205, 210
  visual stimulation and, 191
Porphyria, 232
Postsynaptic potential (PSP), 8, 114, 246, 247
  cyclic AMP and, 186
Potassium ion (K^+), 73, 74, 76–78, 177, 178, 180, 182, 184, 210
  glia and, 14, 15
  transport of, 76–78
Precursor pool problem, 191, 209, 215
Probenicid, 259
Progesterone, 168
Prolactin, 166–168
Prolactin releasing hormone (PRH), 168
Prolactin release–inhibiting hormone (PRIH), 166, 168
Propanalol, 134, 258
Prostaglandins, 63, 126, 172–174, 187, 188, 230
  cyclic AMP and, 174, 187, 188
  synthesis, 172, 173
Protein, 61, 62
  axoplasmic transport of, 19, 103, 164, 182
  brain–specific, 61, 62
  catabolism of, 62
  fractionation, 16
  malnutrition and, 101
  membrane, 78–81
  modification by stimulation, 185
  myelin, 61, 62, 99, 100
  synaptic vesicle, 119
  synaptosome, 119, 148, 216, 217
Protein phosphorylation, 54, 171, 185, 187, 203, 207, 216, 217
  during learning, 216, 217
  during sleep, 222
  synaptosome, 187, 203, 216, 217
Protein synthesis, 60, 61, 63, 65, 182, 185, 190–192, 215
  axonal, 185
  inhibitors, 255, 256
  inhibition by 5HT, 217
  learning and, 203, 205, 212–215, 217
  mitochondrial, 60
  nuclear, 60, 148
  regulation of, 62, 63, 181, 182
  stimulation and, 184, 185, 190, 191
  synaptosomal, 60, 105, 148, 182
  visual deprivation and, 190
Proteolipid protein (of myelin), 99, 102
Psychosine, 88
Purine nucleosides and nucleotides, 32, 42–47, 210, 212
  synthesis, 43–46
Purkinje cells, 12, 174, 186–188
  cyclic AMP and, 174, 186
  nuclei of, 51
  ploidy of, 52
  receptors of, 134, 174
Puromycin, 205, 256
  cyclic AMP and, 205
  glycogen and, 205
  learning and, 205, 214
  peptides, 205
  seizures and, 205
Pyramidal cells of hippocampus
  cyclic AMP and, 174
  ploidy of, 52
  receptors of, 134, 174
Pyridoxal phosphate (vitamin B_6), 34–37, 131, 132, 138–140, 142–145
Pyrimidine nucleosides and nucleotides, 31, 32, 35, 42–46, 210, 212
  synthesis, 43–46, 65
Pyrogallol, 136, 258
Raphé nuclei, 141, 220, 223, 224
Reeler mutant, 158
REM sleep, 221–224
  blood flow and, 24
  dark maintenance and, 192
  norepinephrine turnover during, 147
  oxygen consumption and, 24
Reserpine, 103, 139, 181, 182, 217, 223, 258, 259
Respiratory quotient (RQ), 25
Retinal cell specificity, 156, 157
Retrograde transport, 109, 164
Ribonucleic acid see RNA
Ribonucleoprotein particle (RNP), 55, 57
Ribosomes, 10–13, 54–60, 72, 114, 115, 148
  ECS and, 184

learning and, 210
visual stimulation and, 191
Rifamycin, 255
RNA (ribonucleic acid), 18, 54–60, 64, 65, 148, 183, 184, 231
  ACTH and, 214
  axoplasmic transport of, 106
  base composition, 16, 191, 207, 208, 210, 211
  environmental enrichment and, 219
  histochemistry, 18
  learning and, 58, 206–212, 217
  malnutrition and, 101
  uridine incorporation into
    chromatolysis and, 63
    diurnal rhythm of, 222
    environmental enrichment and, 219
    learning and, 209, 210
    stimulation and, 183, 184, 190
    testosterone and, 234
  RNA synthesis, 54–59, 163, 183, 184, 206, 208–212
    inhibitors of, 255
    learning and, 206–212
    stimulation and, 183, 184, 190, 191
  hnRNA (heterogeneous nuclear RNA), 54–58
  mRNA (messenger RNA), 54–59, 64, 65, 171
  rRNA (ribosomal RNA), 54–59, 106
  tRNA (transfer RNA), 54–56
Ro 4-4602, 257
S-100 protein, 17, 61, 165, 212, 230
Salicylate, 173
Schizophrenia, 219–221
Schwann cell, 14, 72, 247
Scopolamine, 257
Scotophobin, 217, 218
Seizures, 178–180, 203, 205, 236
Serine (ser), 33, 34, 254
Serotonin (5-hydroxytryptamine, 5HT), 32, 124, 126, 136, 138–141, 147, 220, 223, 224, 258, 259
  anatomical distribution of, 138, 220
  cyclic AMP and, 47, 187
  inhibition of protein synthesis, 217
  learning and, 217
  sleep and, 223, 224
Sialic acid, 75, 88–94, 96, 106, 147
  synthesis, 92
Sialidase (neuraminidase), 93, 94, 140

Sleep, 221–224
Sodium ion (Na^+), 73–78, 177, 178
  permeability of, 73–78, 187, 256
  transport of, 73–78, 142
Sodium pump, 76–78
Sparsomycin, 256
Sphingomyelin, 80, 86, 88, 89
Sphingosine, 86–89
Spiroperidol, 258
Stenin, 119, 120
Steroid hormones, 65, 95, 168, 171, 234
Streptovitacin A, 205, 255
Stress, 212–214
Strychnine, 144, 206, 259
Substance P, 41, 42, 140, 144
Succinic Dehydrogenase, 15, 27, 29, 165, 229
Succinylcholine, 257
Sulfatides, 32, 37, 81, 88, 89, 98, 99, 231
Superior cervical ganglion, 140, 181–186
Supraoptic nucleus (of hypothalamus), 170
Sympathectomy, 137, 138, 236
Synapse, 8, 13, 14, 113–115, 248
Synaptic junction (see also synapse), 219
  isolation of, 123, 150
Synaptic modification, 150, 203, 204, 206, 207
Synaptic vesicles, 13, 114–124, 248
  depletion of, 117
  recycling of, 119, 120
Synaptosomes, 105, 121–123, 185, 219, 248
  glycoproteins of, 119, 148–150
  protein synthesis in, 60, 105, 148, 182
Synephrine, 131
Taurine, 33, 37, 38
Tay–Sachs disease, 66, 91, 93
Testosterone, 234
Tetanus toxin, 147, 259
Tetrodotoxin, 76, 256
Theophylline, 47, 185, 186, 260
Thymidine, 44, 255
Thyroid hormone (Thyroxin), 168, 169, 234
  and myelin synthesis, 101
Thyroid–stimulating hormone (TSH) (thyrotropin), 158, 166–170
Transneuronal transport, 108, 109, 151, 164
Tranylcypromine, 258
Tricarboxylic acid cycle (citric acid cycle, Krebs' cycle), 25, 27, 29, 30, 34, 35, 36

Tricyclic antidepressants, 137, 140, 220, 258, 259
Trophic effects, 156–164
Tryptophan, 32, 33, 126, 138–140, 147
Tryptophan hydroxylase, 138–140, 258
d-Tubocurarine, 130, 257
Tubulin, 61, 108, 120, 248
Tumors, 17, 163, 186
Tyramine, 131, 132, 134
Tyrosine (tyr), 31, 33, 131, 146, 181, 192
Tyrosine hydroxylase (TH), 131, 132, 180–183, 257
Unit membrane hypothesis (Davson–Danielli), 78–81
Urea, 37–39
Urea cycle, 37–39
Uric acid, 232–233

Uridine, 31, 44, 48, 65, 183, 184, 209
Uridine nucleotides, 42–46, 88, 89, 92, 97, 149, 184, 209, 210, 212
  learning and, 209, 210
  stimulation and, 184
Vasopressin (lysine vasopressin), 166–171, 187, 206, 214
Vesiculin, 128
Vinblastin, 107, 108, 119, 120, 162, 260
Visual system
  axoplasmic transport in, 103–106
  deprivation, 190–193
  development of, 156, 157, 159–161, 165
  organization of, 160–161
  stimulation of, 190–193
Wallerian degeneration, 62, 165
Wolfgram proteins, 99, 100

DATE DUE

DE 20 '77		
FE		
OC 18		
5-15-95		
DEC 1 2 1997		

HIGHSMITH 45-220

612.822 D92   89969

DUNN

FUNCTIONAL CHEMISTRY OF THE BRAIN

College Misericordia Library
Dallas, Pennsylvania 18612